EVALUATION CONCEPTS & METHODS:
Shaping Policy for the Health Administrator

Health Systems Management
Series editor, **Samuel Levey, Ph.D.,** University of Iowa

EVALUATION CONCEPTS & METHODS:
Shaping Policy for the Health Administrator

Paul C. Nutt
Associate Professor,
Graduate Program in Hospital & Health
Services Administration,
Ohio State University,
Columbus, Ohio

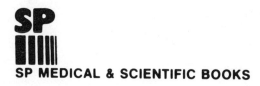

SP MEDICAL & SCIENTIFIC BOOKS

New York

SPECTRUM PUBLICATIONS, INC.
175–20 Wexford Terrace, Jamaica, N.Y. 11432

Library of Congress Cataloging in Publication Data

Nutt, Paul C
  Evaluation concepts & methods.

  Includes index.
  1. Evaluation research (Social action programs)
2. Health services administration—Evaluation.
I. Title. [DNLM: 1. Evaluation studies. 2. Health
services—Organization and administration. 3. Hospital
administration. W84.1 N978e]
H62.N87   361′.007′2   79-27349
ISBN 0-89335-094-X

For Nancy, Suzi, Lynn, and Charles

Contents

Preface

I constructed four miniature houses of worship—a Mohammedan mosque, a Hindu temple, a Jewish synagogue, a Christian cathedral—and placed them in a row. I then marked 15 ants with red paint and turned them loose. They made several trips to and fro, glancing in at the places of worship, but not entering.

I then turned loose 15 more painted blue; they acted just as the red ones had done. I now gilded 15 and turned them loose. No change in the result; the 45 traveled back and forth in a hurry persistently and continuously visiting each fane, but never entering. This satisfied me that these ants were without religious prejudices—just what I wished; for under no other conditions would my next and greater experiment be valuable. I now placed a small square of white paper within the door of each fane; and upon the mosque paper I put a pinch of putty, upon the temple paper a dab of tar, upon the synagogue paper a trifle of turpentine, and upon the cathedral paper a small cube of sugar.

First I liberated the red ants. They examined and rejected the putty, the tar and the turpentine, and then took to the sugar with zeal and apparent sincere conviction. I next liberated the blue ants, and they did exactly as the red ones had done. The gilded ants followed. The preceding results were precisely repeated. This seemed to prove that ants destitute of religious prejudice will always prefer Christianity to any other creed.

However, to make sure, I removed the ants and put putty in the cathedral and sugar in the mosque. I now liberated the ants in a body, and they rushed tumultuously to the cathedral. I was very much touched and gratified, and went back in the room to write down the event; but when I came back the ants had all apostatized and had gone over to the Mohammedan communion.

I saw that I had been too hasty in my conclusions, and naturally felt rebuked and humbled. With diminished confidence I went on with the test to the finish. I placed the sugar first in one house of worship then in another, till I had tried them all.

With this result: whatever Church I put the sugar in, that was the one the ants straightway joined. This was true beyond a shadow of doubt, that in religious matters the ant is the opposite of man, for man cares for but one thing; to find the only true Church; whereas the ants hunts for the one with the sugar in it.[1]

---

[1]Reprinted with permission from Mark Twain, "On Experimental Design" in Scott W.K. and L.L. Cummings, *Readings in Organizational Behavior and Human Performance*, Irwin: Homewood, Ill., p. 2, (1973).

Drawing sensible conclusions from an evaluation can be tricky. The best planned evaluation can be totally misunderstood. The misunderstanding can be without guile or deliberate. Examples of each can be found in most organizations.

In some instances, evaluation is used to posture. Sponsors set up a sophisticated-sounding experiment, but do so in a way that limits the ability of the evaluation to draw definitive conclusions. Paint the ants carefully and move the sugar cube about creatively. In other instances, the sponsor of an evaluation effort may mix the sugar cubes with the "intervention program" and conlcude that the intervention tastes good. In this case, the evaluation findings provide little in the way of policy guidance.

This book is designed to help the interested reader separate sugar cubes and interventions and cope with divisive sponsors. First, a methodological foundation is built to point out what constitutes a good evaluation. This discussion stresses the conceptual and methodological aspects of evaluation. The planning of data acquisition, its analysis, and its interpretation are treated as largely inseparable aspects of an evaluation project. Tests are provided that can be used to judge quality of the evaluation findings. Guides are described to aid the reader in assessing the prospects of a successful evaluation effort. Several illustrations are used to show how evaluations can go wrong—really wrong. Such politically sensitive studies as Coleman's assessment of the potential for bussing to influence school performance and Head Start, as well as managers who attempt to evaluate their own intervention program, are considered. Both evaluations which threaten administrators and evaluations which lack controversy are described.

Part I of the book provides basic analytical and conceptual evaluation skills. Chapter 1 describes evaluation concepts, including methods of evaluation, types of evaluation, uses of evaluation, and some barriers to various types of evaluations. Chapter 2 introduces the reader to basic concepts and describes options in the collection of evaluation information. Examples are used to show how evaluation methods can be used to plan and structure an evaluation effort. Chapters 3 and 4 describe several evaluation methods in detail. The discussion couples analytic skills with interpretation and application insights. The analysis approaches were selected to illustrate concepts, *not* efficient data analysis. Chapter 5 describes nonexperimental methods like time series, matched groups, and naturally occuring groups. Chapters 3, 4, and 5 stress two interrelated topics: the planning of data collection activities and the interpretation of this information. Chapter 6 contrasts evaluation findings, derived from these methods, in terms of their interpretability and generalizability.

Part II deals with behavioral issues. Chapter 7 discusses how measures can be devised for causes and effects. Ways to identify evaluation objectives, criteria, and measures, and the distinction between reliabilty in measurement and validity in results are discussed. Chapters 8, 9, and 10 discuss behavioral factors that can dictate the success of an evaluation. The evaluation process and various dialogues that occur between the evaluator and the sponsor are sketched in Chapter 8. Chapter 9 provides a model which can be used to diagnose the prospects of a successful project and to predict problems. The relationship between decision making and evaluation is discussed in Chapter 10. This chapter describes several forensic and analytical decision strategies, illustrates how the adoption of a particular strategy is strongly influenced by the manager's decision style, and provides guides in selecting a decision strategy that considers the nature of the decision task.

Paul C. Nutt, Ph.D.
The Ohio State University
Columbus, Ohio

Acknowledgments

This book presents an integration of ideas, techniques, and concepts gleaned from many people. It attempts to build on a foundation provided by Edward Suchman's conceptual treatment of evaluation, by Donald Campbell and Julian Stanley's quasi-experimental designs, and by the conceptually based treatment of analysis offered by G.E.P. Box and his collegues. The behavioral concepts applied to evaluation were drawn from a wide variety of sources. In particular, David Gustafson, George Huber, and Andre Delbecq should be acknowledged. My colleagues and students at The Ohio State University offered many helpful ideas and provided many useful comments. Joanne Jones should be recognized for her conscientous assistance in preparing this manuscript. Joanne shepherded the book through all its many revisions. Finally, my family merits special recognition for putting up with me during the book's lengthy gestation.

Foreword

In reviewing this book I am struck by several aspects that make it desirable reading for the student of program evaluation. The book touches on a broad range of evaluation topics including evaluation design, model building, analysis, and implementation of results (decision-making based on results of the evaluation). Evaluation is all these and possibly more. It is important to understand evaluation as a whole and Dr. Nutt has attempted to present that perspective. Some evaluation books address individual components of an evaluation, but few address the components together in a coherent whole.

The individual components also have much to recommend them. Dr. Nutt attempts to address analysis in a way that presents both the conceptual structure as well as the mathematical/statistical logic. There is no question in my mind that any person involved in evaluation needs both of these perspectives.

Dr. Nutt also presents an intriguing approach to evaluation design. He reinterpretes the Campbell and Stanley prospective and suggests a cyclical design aimed at the organization unable to identify external control groups.

Methods to identify objectives, to derive measures from objectives, and to interpret the resulting measures are presented in a new and refreshing way, with many examples. Measures are linked to evaluation model building, effectively drawing on literature from both the philosophy of science and operations research.

Entirely new topics of managerial diagnosis and evaluation implementation are presented. Dr. Nutt links evaluation-problem finding to model building and decision making to implementation, drawing on several new ideas in behavioral sciences.

So for those of us who believe that evaluation should be relevant to promoting organizational change, this book offers several reasons to recommend it—and that is not surprising considering the author's background.

Dr. Nutt comes to the health care field with considerable. experience in conducting, observing, and sponsoring evaluations. He worked in aerospace and commercial industries before pursuing his doctorate at the University of Wisconsin. He played a major role in the design and operation of Wisconsin's Regional Medical Program and has served as a consultant for many health care organizations. This experience provided many opportunities to observe as well as conduct evaluations in health care. After earning his Ph.D. at the University of Wisconsin, Paul has published actively in the evaluation arena and acted as an advisor to the governmental and private sectors on a wide variety of evaluation issues. This book is the culmination of that experience and effort.

David H. Gustafson, Ph.D.
University of Wisconsin
Madison, Wisconsin

EVALUATION CONCEPTS & METHODS:
Shaping Policy for the Health Administrator

PART I

EVALUATION METHODS

Quantification at any stage depends on qualification. What is qualified at one stage must be quantified at another; but at any stage some qualitative judgements are made.

Russell Ackoff

CHAPTER 1

Evaluation Strategies

May I in my brief bolt across the scene not be misunderstood in what
I mean.

Robert Frost, *The Fear Of Man*

EVALUATION INTENT AND APPROACHES

The following report was submitted by a work study engineer after
visiting the symphony orchestra at the Royal Hall in London:

(1) For considerable periods, the four Oboe players had nothing to do. The
number of Oboe players should be reduced and the work spread more evenly
over the whole concert, thus eliminating the peaks of activity.

(2) All twelve violinists were playing identical notes, which seems to be an
unnecessary duplication of effort. The staff in this section should be cut, and
if greater volume is required, it could be obtained through electronic
amplification.

(3) There is too much repetition of some musical passages. Scores should be
pruned because no useful purpose is served by the horns repeating passages
already played by the strings. If all the redundant passages were pruned, the
playing time of the concert could be reduced from two hours to twenty
minutes. There would be no need for an intermission and the players would
not need to be paid for the redundancies.

(4) Obsolescences of equipment is another matter that could bear further
investigation. It was reported in the program that the leading violinist's
instrument was already two hundred years old. If normal depreciation
schedules had been applied, the value of this instrument should have been
reduced to zero and it is probable the purchase of more modern equipment
could be considered...[1]

Evaluation is often misunderstood. It represents a field of study that must
sharpen its definition of both purpose and methods. Confusion over means
and ends has led to evaluation projects which produce carefully solicited
testimonials, outright misrepresentations, or careful analysis that yields
meaningless information, like the work study engineer's report.

According to Suchman, evaluation provides a judgment of worth or an appraisal of value.[2] Increasingly the administrators of human service organizations must direct their attention toward the cost–effectiveness of existing and proposed services, internal operations, and managerial actions. Evaluation can be used to establish the merits of these programs, measuring the extent they meet the needs of their clientele vis-à-vis their cost. In many public and quasipublic organizations, funds to support new initiatives may soon depend on internal reallocations. Evaluation can provide essential information in this reallocation process.

Periodicals, data files, and statistical records; surveys, simulation, and mathematical models; and experiments represent a small sample of methods that have been used to carry out an evaluation. This diversity in method has stemmed from the need to study a wide assortment of phenomena and from the preferences, skills, and outright bias of evaluators. But diverse methods lead to evaluation findings that lack comparability. As Suchman points out, "different results obtained by different methods based on different criteria [produce] confusion that is difficult to resolve..."[3]

As a consequence, evaluation is often seen as a methodological jungle where the perceptive mind of the administrator must save the day. Evaluation is perceived to be more of an art than a science. Administrators tend to be unaware of methods that can be used to carry out an evaluation, let alone which method is appropriate for the evaluation task at hand. In Part I, this book seeks to overcome some of these method–related problems. First, several methods of evaluation are presented, followed by a discussion of their application to problems in human service organizations, with emphasis on the health care industry. Guides that aid in the selection of an evaluation method are provided. In Part II, behavioral issues in evaluation are considered. A schema of evaluation is provided to illustrate steps in an evaluation process and the transactions that must occur between the sponsor of an evaluation and the evaluator to establish measures and interpret the evaluation findings. The process of managerial diagnosis is outlined to depict how the sponsor shapes the evaluation process. Finally, the relationship between evaluation and decision making is discussed. Decision making is pictured as a judgmental process that sifts and weighs evaluation information.

THE STATUS OF EVALUATION

In the past twenty years organizations have attempted to remedy increasingly complex problems. Today programs attempt to curb health expenditures via planning,[4] to deal with educational deprivation by stimulating pre-schoolers from low–income families, to control safety hazards in places of work, to provide environmental protection, to reduce the time lag between medical discoveries and their application, to name just a few. The success of these programs depends on several factors; some only partially amenable to control by the implementing agency. For instance, the success of a Head Start program depends on the participation of the preschooler's parents as well as the program's design and long–term commitments of federal resources. Regional medical programs had to rely on medical schools to provide consultation services and continuing education in their attempt to reduce the lag between medical discoveries and their application.

Program goals are often stated in terms of total problem eradication, like the proclamation by the Nixon administration to wipe out cancer in our lifetime. Broad goals create programs correspondingly broad in scope, and may create unrealistic expectations. These complex, multifaceted programs often find they must engage in a painful appraisal to select a mission which seems achievable and, at the same time, merits the required funds. The period of racing expectations is followed by an assessment which isolates what is feasible, given resources and other constraints. This leads to the delivery of services that have modest but realistic objectives. When administrators announce revised objectives, stating that the problems cannot be ameliorated but merely contained, critics are quick to condemn the program.

The growth and subsequent disenchantment with action programs has become common in many organizations, following trends set nationally. This disenchantment has stimulated considerable interest in program evaluation. Suchman points out that the type of demonstration found to be acceptable depends on the level of trust between the program's sponsor and those that support and/or use the program's services.[5] As skepticism grows, so does the need for unassailable proof of program effectiveness, which leads to costly evaluation projects.

USES OF EVALUATION

To describe the initiatives of organizations, their programs will be termed "interventions." Intervention has a fairly broad meaning encompassing managerial actions, organizational services, an organization's internal procedures, and the actions of third parties. Attempts by an administrator to change worker productivity through a set of discrete activities such as incentives, would be called an intervention. Similarly, the services that an organization offers to its clientele, the operations and procedures within the organization which support these services (such as a management information system), and the actions of outsiders (such as the initiation of hospital price–controls by government) are also interventions. *Program evaluation* is defined as an assessment process aimed at specifying the merit of an intervention program.

A principal use of program evaluation is to measure the extent to which objectives of intervention programs have been achieved. Some additional uses of evaluation are listed below:

1. Identifying ways to make a service program more effective through a modification of current operations or by comparing different modes of operation in various organizations.[6]
2. Acquiring information to describe the outcomes of a planned intervention.[7]
3. Characterizing the results that stemmed from an unplanned or unintentional intervention.
4. Comparing the merits of delivery mechanisms, with varying levels of resources, that could be used by an intervention program.[8]
5. Demonstrating the needs for a service program or how the program can alleviate social problems.[9]
6. Measuring service program's accomplishment against the total needs of its target group.[10]
7. Establishing priorities among programs with the same, or similar, missions to isolate the mechanisms that seem best in delivering a particular service.[11]
8. Creating a ranking of an organization's programs as a means to phase out some of these programs.
9. Establishing a means to periodically measure the attainment of objectives as a management control mechanism.
10. Determining whether a service program can be transferred to new settings and/or applied to new target groups.[12]
11. Checking for unintended side effects (negative and positive extranalities) that may stem from an intervention.
12. Providing public accountability for the use of resources in publicly subsidized programs.[13]
13. Developing, in administrators, skills in examining assumptions used to establish interventions and to interpret results; and in staff, developing skills in devising relevant and measurable objectives and data collection devices.
14. Developing information which describes effective delivery mechanisms, given setting and target groups, to aid in the planning of service programs in the future.
15. Providing ways to tie program administrator's rewards to program achievement.
16. Measuring the long–range effects of an intervention.

TYPES OF INTERVENTION PROGRAMS

Figure 1.1 identifies three basic types of intervention programs. Indigenous conditions combine with causes to create opportunities for *primary* intervention programs. Causes combine with effects offering *secondary* intervention opportunities. Effects combine with consequences identifying *tertiary* intervention programs. Evaluation can be focused on interventions at any point in the causal sequence.

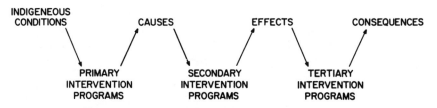

Figure I.I TYPES OF INTERVENTION PROGRAMS

Adapted from Suchman, E.A., *Evaluation Research,* Russell Sage Foundation, New York, p. 173, (1967).

An intervention program can be carried out with primary, secondary, or tertiary intervention objectives. The earlier the intervention, the greater the benefits. Primary intervention programs have more value because they eliminate causal factors. Secondary interventions can only minimize undesirable effects, and tertiary interventions deal with the residual effects. When the point of intervention is inappropriately selected, opportunities may be lost. For example, home safety programs and child abuse programs may be a more effective intervention than expanding the number of burn centers. Similarly, enforced housing codes may reduce the incidence of ghetto children ingesting plaster coated with lead paint, which may reduce the need for poison control centers or the treatment of lead poisoning (Table 1–1).

The relationship between these links is often unknown or ambiguous. For example, diabetes can't be prevented, but it can be cheaply and reliably controlled. In contrast, the prepayment mechanisms of neighborhood health centers are supposed to induce low–income people to use health services and thereby prevent health problems from occurring. The indigenous factors which cause a population to seek health care are not clear and may not be related to prepayment. If so, a secondary intervention program, with a direct provision of needed services to the target group, may be a more effective intervention program.

In some instances, primary intervention programs are infeasible. For example, cancer has been linked to smoking; but programs designed to change smoking behavior have been ineffective. Genetic studies of prospective parents provide a basis for eliminating birth defects, but counseling, which attempts to dramatize the potential for birth defects, may be viewed by its target group as discriminatory and thus be ignored.

Intervention programs are dictated by the state of the art, the size of a target group, the importance of the anticipated effect, and the likelihood of achieving these effects. The state of the art can be used to identify viable links between

Table 1-1: Examples of Intervention Programs

Health Care Treatment Programs	Primary Intervention Programs	Secondary Intervention Programs	Tertiary Intervention Programs
Cancer	change smoking behavior	surgery, radio-therapy, chemotherapy	rehabilitation
Lead Poisoning	housing codes	hospital poison control center (for lead plant ingestion)	treat after effects of lead poisoning
Burns	home safety & child abuse programs	stabilization & acute burn care	restorative & rehabilitative care
Birth Defects	sex education and counseling	identification of defects and their prognosis	sheltered workshops

Health Management Programs	Primary Intervention Programs	Secondary Intervention Programs	Tertiary Intervention Programs
Performance	study employee motivation	explore appraisal program effectiveness	investigate turnover discharge & rates
Structure	investigate lags in response to requests for information	study the reporting relationships in organization	examine the organization structure
Planning	study the need for health service in hospital catchment area	investigate ways to enlarge medical staff with primary admitting privileges	study reasons to HSA rejection of hospital expansion program

indigenous conditions and causes. The Salk Vaccine, which eliminated the causes of polio, is an example of an effective primary intervention. In other cases, the state of the art is largely unknown, making primary interventions controversial. There appears to be a link between air pollution and cancer, but authorities have yet to discover effective air pollution programs.

   The size of the target group helps to determine the focus of an intervention program. Programs can be ranked according to the target group's size. For instance, screening programs to identify people with hypertension and renal disease have vastly different target groups. In a population of five million, half a million hypertensives can be found, and probably no more than one hundred will have end–stage renal disease.

The effects of programs can also be used to determine where a program should intervene. The survival rate in burn centers can be compared to prospects for preventing child abuse, in order to judge which type of program has the greatest potential benefits. (Pathetically, parents who inflict burns on their children by holding them in boiling water as a form of punishment contribute many pediatric burn cases.) Serious burns often leave the victim with little to hope for in terms of quality of life: limited mobility of limbs, extensive disfigurement, and few prospects for employment. Suicide is common. This provides a real motivation to seek ways to eliminate the causes of burns. Thus, effects themselves offer important ways to discriminate between programs.

Like health care delivery, the interventions of managers can be primary, secondary, or tertiary in nature; and one type of intervention may be more appropriate than another. For instance, when performance of employees of a particular department is perceived to be low, management can search for the causes of low performance with a primary intervention program which investigates employee motivation and ability. Employee satisfaction instruments, interviews, and the like might be used to assess employee job satisfaction. Performance requirements of the job can be used to determine whether employees' dissatisfaction stems from being over or under–qualified for their jobs. A secondary intervention program might concentrate on the organization's employee appraisal program. The effectiveness of the appraisal program in diagnosing and dealing with poor performers can be explored. A tertiary evaluation might investigate turnover and discharge rates.

Programs are more likely to be effective when they intervene early in the causal sequence. For example, managers often respond to lags in their requests for information by investigating the need for changes in organization's structure. It might be better to assess the indigenous conditions which slow information requests, rather than assessing reporting relationships (a secondary intervention), or examining the organization's structure (a tertiary intervention). Similarly, an evaluator may be asked to determine the reasons behind the rejection of hospital expansion programs rather than studying the need for health services implicitly assumed in the expansion, or investigating ways to enlarge the medical staff. A study of needs might clearly justify more health services. Also, more hospital admissions lead to a higher occupancy rate, which might justify the expansion. In summary, the evaluator must consider the need for the program, look for missed opportunities to intervene, and then assess the merits of the intervention.

THE EVALUATION OF INTERVENTION PROGRAMS

Intervention programs typically provide services to some client group or help to change a management practice. These programs can vary across several dimensions, depending on the kind of objectives sought, the type of organization that provides the service, the mechanisms used to deliver the service or carry out a program, the newness of the activity, its budget, revenues available to support the program, and still other factors. For instance, a service program may have comparatively narrow objectives, like making chest x-rays available in an Indian reservation. Alternatively, the program could seek a reduction of Indians' age-specific mortality rates. The objectives of the intervention program dramatically alter the nature of an evaluation effort.

The means to achieve an intervention program's objectives include staff, funding arrangements, administrative structure, and other physical features such as the location of the service. For example, an outreach service program could be initiated in a medically underserved area, and supported by the revenues derived from the delivery of the program's services. The outreach program could be administered locally, at a satellite center, or rely on the administrative structure of the sponsoring hospital. A variety of services could be provided ranging from health information to hands-on care. Altering the means used to deliver a given bundle of services leads to dramatically different types of service programs.

Funding for the outreach program could be sought from Medicare payments, government programs, or by prepayment mechanisms based on cooptation. After its initiation, administrators are interested in the program's performance, given its objectives and the resources that have been expended.

The Evolution of Intervention Programs

Tripodi *et al.* identified three stages of program development: initiation, contact, and implementation.[14] Evaluation can and should take place at each level. *Initiation* refers to the development of a plan to carry out the program. Thus the planning process itself could be evaluated vis-à-vis its objectives. *Contact* refers to locating and initiating services. Activities might include renting space and hiring physicians for an outreach clinic, and overcoming obstacles in the delivery of services, such as coping with resentment in the medical community which historically provided services in the area to be served by the outreach clinic. Evaluation findings may isolate information that suggests how to modify the program plan to overcome obstacles to its success. *Implementation* refers to providing services; often called the operational phase of a program. Evaluation considers the extent the service program meets its objectives and the resources expended in this process.

The Nature and Impact of Evaluation Objectives

Evaluation depends on objectives in the same way that research relies on a formal statement of a hypothesis. It is essential to know what is being evaluated. An evaluation project demands a clear specification of objectives before an intervention program can be assessed. The objectives must specify several components which include the target group to be served, the nature of the service to be rendered or activities to be carried out, expected performance levels, and contraints such as time and budget. For example, an outreach service program located in a ghetto, might have an objective of providing physical examinations to a certain portion of the target group annually, within budgetary provisions. Evaluation can be inhibited or even stymied if objectives for programs are not formulated with this level of specificity. Much of the conflict between program administrators and evaluators stems from the evaluators' attempt to define and understand program objectives. Unclear objectives lead the evaluator and sponsor into unproductive discussions often aimed at defending the program or its lack of objectives.

Program objectives are often inferred during an evaluation, not preselected by the sponsor. Suchman points out that administrators may change the objectives to match what they believe has been achieved by the program.[15] For example, when HEW issued a contract to evaluate the achievement of minority children in public schools, their objectives were quite fluid. Rossi and Williams indicate that HEW policy makers called the study "preliminary," asking for a pilot study to relate the performance of minority children to public school resources.[16] Thus, HEW commissioned a study of the status of the public school system. But new schools, educational parks, parallel systems, and the like were discussed by policy makers as though the study would aid them in selecting among these options. When the findings failed to confirm that resource-intensive public schools could improve the performance of minority youngsters, critics like Cain and Watts blasted the report for failing to develop a "theory of education" from which policy questions could be viewed.[17] The objectives of the evaluation effort are often distorted to bolster the claims of its critics. Unless objectives are carefully specified at the outset, they may tend to shift as evaluation findings turn up. Shifting objectives often shrouds evaluation findings with controversy, limiting their value in policy making. Thus, a careful specification of objectives is a critical task in any evaluation effort.

Methods of Evaluation

A statistical format is required to evaluate most interventions. In other fields of study, different approaches are used. For example, the natural sciences stress the measurement process. Telescopes and cyclotrons are examples. In behavioral psychology, the intervention must be carefully controlled. For example, a patient is exposed to a carefully constructed operant conditioning program designed to elicit a particular chain of responses. If the patient behaves in the way specified, the program works. No other interpretation of the data is plausible and the evaluator counts percent successes. To illustrate, operant conditioning is used to train autistic children to develop certain desirable social behaviors like dressing and eating. Once the child performs these functions without assistance, the program is a success. Similarly, desensitization is used to aid people to diet and to quit smoking. As before, the desired behavior is measured directly without the use of statistical methods.

The effects of managerial interventions are rarely this conspicuous. Statistical procedures are required for several reasons. First, the evaluation methodology must be sufficiently sensitive to isolate the effects of the program in a noisy environment. The magnitude of the noise can obscure the effects of the program. Secondly, the objectives of most interventions are both complex and multiple, lacking clear cut norms. As a result, single measures can be misleading, and multiple measures are often difficult to combine or interpret. Finally, service programs and other types of interventions are carried out in a dynamic milieu. Many factors can have dramatic effects upon results. These factors must be carefully controlled in the evaluation methodology.

Methods useful in assessing intervention programs that are discussed in this book fall into three general categories: post hoc observation, quasi–experimental designs, and experimental designs.[18]

Post hoc observation is often used to generate evaluation information. For example, a case study essentially measures an effect as it occurs. As a result, this approach lacks the power to tie changes in one or more measures of effectiveness to the intervention. The power to relate interventions and results can be enhanced when a baseline exists to compare against the results. For example, a careful study of unit costs in a hospital's outpatient department, along with some idea of the type of people reached using this approach, could be used as a baseline to evaluate the results of a satellite clinic to be operated by the hospital. Baselines improve evaluation information.

Quasi–experimental designs can dramatically improve the precision of evaluation findings. Typical examples of quasi–designs are time–series data and matched and/or naturally occurring groups. The time–series approach serially tracks success indicators before a program is implemented, and for a period of time after it has been implemented. Several samples of important indicators, collected before an intervention, are compared to several samples after the intervention. Time–series approaches attempt to model important patterns in the data. Changes in key indicators can be appreciated when trends can be examined. For instance, to evaluate an outreach program it is helpful to consider how the utilization rates, unit costs, and other hospital indicators have been changing over several time periods prior to the initiation of a satellite clinic. After the clinic (intervention) has been established, several factors may have caused initial utilization rates to fall below expectations. For example, knowledge of the program's existence often spreads slowly. Also, endorsement by important figures in the area may be necessary before utilization rates climb to representative levels. Thus several discrete measurements are needed to detect the impact of intervention programs after its initiation.

Another type of quasi–design is called the matched group. A matched group is used when the recipients of the services in a satellite clinic cannot be randomly placed in two groups: those receiving and not receiving the clinic's services. A comparison group is sought whose characteristics are very similar to the target group of the clinic. The comparison group does not have access to services like the outreach program, but in all other ways must be similar to the target group. The comparison groups are often equated in terms of income, ethnicity, and the like. Utilization rates, cost, and health status indicators for those receiving the services at the outreach clinic are collected and compared to these same measures observed for people with a similar profile of income and ethnic composition in another part of the city. The comparison is made using the baseline of a similar group.

The most powerful methods of evaluation are called *experimental designs.* Experimental designs require a random assignment of recipients of a particular service to two categories: those who receive the service and those who do not. The precision of information in these designs is usually superior to the information in quasi–designs. However, there may be barriers to implementing this type of evaluation method. For instance, certain groups perceive that the use of control groups will deny them benefits. Administrators attempt to avoid this type of controversy. As a result, evaluation sponsors often mandate that *all* people receive the benefits of the program even before the benefits are verified. Nonetheless, experimental methods can be widely used in a wide variety of settings.

Types of Evaluation

Suchman describes five types of evaluation: effort, performance, adequacy of performance, efficiency, and process.[19] *Effort* reflects the level of activity within an intervention program. For example, during the initiation phase an evaluation project may seek to determine the capacity for effort. Assessing the availability of resources to carry out a program can often provide useful information. Unless carefully qualified, effort–based evaluations can be misleading. For example, accreditation commissions measure the presence of resources, so accreditation must be based on the capacity to perform, not the performance itself.

A *performance* evaluation attempts to assess the output or result of an intervention program. A check is made to see if changes mandated by the program's objectives occurred. For example, to evaluate a satellite outpatient center, a variety of performance measures can be used: the number of cases treated in a satellite center, the type of referrals, mortality or morbidity measures, rehabilitation successes, and the like, depending on the program's objectives. The number of cases treated can be an appropriate performance measure when program objectives stress contact. A referral program in a neighborhood health center could adopt such an objective, but a clinic could not. A performance evaluation isolates the accomplishments of an intervention program, which are often compared to the program's objective.

A *performance adequacy* evaluation determines the extent that performance meets a need. For instance, an outreach program may reach thousands of people, but only a small proportion of the target group to which it was directed. Adequacy has goal ingredients. It represents a desirable, but not necessarily attainable, state of affairs. For instance, a performance adequacy evaluation might determine the extent that the swine flu innoculation program eliminated mortality due to flu, recognizing that zero mortality probably exceeds our technological capabilities. In short, a performance adequacy evaluation judges a program by using a denominator of need. It also embodies a notion of progress increments. A neighborhood health center moves from an initial 10 percent penetration of their target group to higher percentages in succeeding years. Thus an evaluation may carefully track the number of premiums paid to signal when corrective action is needed. This suggests recursive evaluation, like that carried out when administrators monitor financial reports. Performance adequacy is judged by the extent that a goal such as 100 percent involvement of the target group in a neighborhood health center is reached.

Efficiency is concerned with the evaluation of both costs and results. It represents a ratio of output and input in which outputs are measured in performance terms and inputs in resource terms. One of the key ingredients in service programs is the cost of providing a service. Intervention programs, while needed, may be too expensive. An efficiency evaluation relates program results to unit costs.

Program strategy evaluation seeks to discover why an intervention program works.[20] A strategy evaluation compares various ways to deliver service programs to see which is best. The means used to deliver a service represents the strategies to be compared. Each strategy must be carefully and fully defined. For example, the Head Start program used several strategies, including organized play, two–month summer programs with part–time teachers, and full–year programs with specified classroom experiences and full–time teachers.[21] Clearly these strategies were quite different. Program benefits are likely to depend on the specific intervention processes used by the strategy that is applied. A strategy evaluation can also explore the impact of the population served and the environment in which the program is to function. Evaluation is applied in order to learn whether the program can work for another population or in another environment. In this instance, a strategy evaluation is used to weight the importance of factors that dictate the generalizability of evaluation information: the characteristics of the Head Start children and particular environments may limit or enhance the benefits of the program when applied on a large scale.

Uses of Evaluation Information

Evaluation can be used to accumulate ritualistic, operational, and behavioral information. *Ritualistic* evaluation information provides indices which have little diagnostic value.[22] For example, departments of health routinely collect mortality data for particular kinds of cancer patients, but seldom classify the data and refer it back to treatment centers for their utilization review or quality assessment activities. Nurses in a surgical intensive–care unit are often required to record, every two hours, blood intake levels, urine output, temperature, blood pressure, spirometry readings, and a host of other factors which describe a patient's condition when physicians use only arrhythmias to signal the needs for an intervention.[23] Apparently, requiring nurses to record data gives physicians a way to insure that patients were "looked in on" every two hours.

Operational evaluation information stresses cost–benefit or cost–effectiveness indices to determine the merit of services and intervention programs. Administrators monitor programs and other activities comparing outputs to inputs or outputs to objectives. Operational evaluation information helps administrators select and refine missions for their intervention programs. For example, outpatient services in a clinic can be pruned, enlarged, or modified, based on the findings of operational evaluations.

Behavioral evaluation information is used to project an organization's ability to respond to new conditions. Contingency plans require evaluation to determine strategy in the plan that seems best. For example, a hospital with an expansion objective may have several options on the drawing boards, such as satellite clinics, new beds, or new services. A behavioral evaluation projects the impact of each option on the hospital's occupancy, revenues, and community reactions; judging the likelihood of approval by regulation bodies, hospital trustees, and others. Behavioral evaluations can be difficult to carry out.

Evaluation information is a critical component of effective decision making in organizations. Unfortunately, evaluation often threatens those being evaluated, which encourages the ritualistic accumulation of data. Volumes of data are difficult to interpret, protecting program administrators from a probing assessment of their activities. Ritualistic data are often collected when a more definitive form of data collection can and should be carried out. Ritualistic evaluations are as pervasive as behavioral evaluations are infrequent. Shifting evaluation resources from ritualistic to operational applications will dramatically improve information for decision making. Operational evaluation provides critical information which aids administrators in improving programs and making related decisions. Behavioral evaluations can aid administrators in formulating their "visions" into achievable programs, and should be used more frequently.

Data Sources

Data for evaluation can be obtained from archives or collected prospectively. *Retrospective* data are drawn from an organization's records or its management information system. Retrospective data are often cheap, readily available, and seldom subject to manipulation. Manipulation can be controlled because retrospective data are collected for multiple purposes (or as a ritualistic exercise), so the chances for tampering, altering the data to fit expectations, are minimal. However, evaluation projects often find that available data are riddled with errors, inaccessible, and lack important categories. For instance, to discover factors that influence nursing home costs, using retrospective data, an information system must be found that contains the annual cost reports from each nursing home with the homes categorized by factors such as the home's size, its occupancy rate, its proportion of skilled nursing personnel to total personnel, and the like. Errors in the data, such as 1,000 percent occupancies or cost–per–patient–day greater than an acute care hospital's per diem costs, make these data impossible to use. The evaluation cannot assume that entries of 1,000 percent occupancy were intended to be 100 percent and erroneously entered. Without a basis to correct the data, obviously erroneous information must be discarded. In other cases, important data categories may not be recorded. For instance, the staffing practices of the home must be recorded to detect whether homes control cost by limiting services to their patients. If these data are missing from the nursing home cost report, the evaluation project cannot determine whether costs are low because the home is well run or because the nurse–patient ratios are restricted.

Retrospective data can also make evaluation findings difficult to interpret.

Causality is frequently hard to demonstrate when using historical data. For instance, an evaluation using Medicaid cost reports may find that nursing home daily costs were low when occupancy exceeded 85 percent, when homes are larger than 100 beds, *and* when the home had few Medicare patients. These findings suggest that the size of nursing homes should be increased and that incentives should be offered to increase occupancy. However, large homes with high occupancy may avoid Medicaid patients because the Medicaid Program reimburses them at less than their actual costs. This provides homes with few (or no) Medicaid patients, and therefore additional revenues which could have been used to improve their management, which may lead to low cost in these homes. With historical data, the policy maker is faced with several plausible explanations of the findings, and has no basis to select among these explanations.

Prospective data collection follows an explicit data collection procedure. Prospective data are tailored to answer specific evaluation questions, which forces the evaluator to carefully define each evaluation question. For instance, a maternal and child health agency can use prospective data to assess the benefits of a program to improve the health of newborns through a food service for expectant mothers. A "Hollister Maternal Newborn Record System" could be used to record information in clinics and health centers that do and do not offer the nutrition program. The effects of the nutritional program can be determined by measuring a newborn's birth weight, APGAR score,[24] complications, and abnormalities. Comparisons are made for groups of mothers who participated and did not participate in a program that had comparable age and race profiles, numbers of prenatal visits, previous problem children, and the like.

The disadvantages of prospective data stem from the delays in developing and carrying out data collection and the problems that tend to arise as the data are accumulated. Data collection can be quite reactive. Participants are sensitized because their actions are being monitored, which may entice them to behave in atypical ways. Further, it is often difficult to get administrators to endorse prospective data collection when data are available in archives. The choice between prospective and retrospective data should rest on the quality of existing data as compared to the increased precision of data that could be generated prospectively.

EVALUATION STRATEGIES

In this chapter an evaluation project was described as including six factors: the intervention's focus and stage, evaluation methods, data source, types of evaluation, and uses of evaluation information. Figure 1-2 lists evaluation strategies which can be derived from all combinations of these six factors. An evaluation project's strategy can be identified by a particular combination of factors, as shown in Figure 1.2. For instance, an evaluation project could be initiated by the chief executive officer (CEO) to determine why occupancy is down in a hospital, applying a case study approach and retrospective data which relate historical events with changes in occupancy (performance) for ritualistic purposes (the CEO is not sure how the information will be used). An evaluation strategy which focuses on a service program during its initiation stage, may use prospective data, collected using a quasi–experimental approach, to characterize the performance of an intervention program to detect the program's merit (operational purposes). In all there are (4 × 3 × 3 × 2 × 5 × 3) or 1,080 distinct evaluation strategies shown in Figure 1.2. Some of these strategies will be infeasible for particular classes of evaluation projects. For instance, case studies with retrospective data *cannot* be carried out when information systems fail to collect data during the initiation of a service.

The evaluation strategies in Figure 1.2 provide several ways to visualize an evaluation project. Evaluations often have obscure origins and may develop

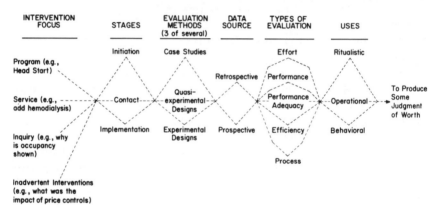

Figure 1.2 EVALUATION STRATEGIES

inappropriate constraints. The evaluator should review each evaluation project to test the appropriateness of its initial, and often implicit, strategy. Selecting a counter strategy can help to detect whether changes in procedure are warranted. For instance, prospective data may be more suitable when the sponsor intends to base wide–ranging changes on the evaluation information. In other instances, the use of evaluation data can be questioned. To illustrate, the Early Periodic Screening Testing and Treatment (EPSDT) program was devised to detect correctable health conditions in people. A recent review of the program suggested that policy makers should carry out evaluations to find out ways to increase enrollment in the program.[25] However, an evaluation that demonstrates the benefits of the EPSDT program (substituting a performance adequacy for effort evaluation) may suggest defensible ways to expand the EPSDT program's services and budget (a behavioral application).

Evaluation information must also meet the test of decision–making utility. For instance, evaluation of the initiation stage of a program must be completed before the initiation has been carried out, in order to offer aid in improving the initiation process. (This of course assumes a one–of–a–kind program.) In the ensuing chapters, skills will be built up to help select evaluation methods, select between retrospective and prospective data generation, and specify the types of evaluation that seem appropriate.

THE FLOW OF TOPICS

Apser points out that administrators who hope to carry out an effective evaluation must learn the requirements for a meaningful evaluation project.[26] This book presents a scheme to formulate and carry out an effective evaluation of an intervention program. Experiments are described in the early chapters to begin the discussion of evaluation methods with the ideal method of generating evaluation information. Subsequent material permits the reader to compare other mechanisms of generating evaluation information with the more precise evaluation methodologies. This flow of topics is aimed at helping the reader to gradually amass skills in assessing the precision of evaluation findings. For instance, correlational studies have less explanatory power than an evaluation which carefully isolates the intervention program, and then measures its effects. Reports, journal articles, and the claims of consultants can be tested against the standards described in the early Chapters. Part I concludes by comparing the methods of evaluation in terms of their ability to interpret and generalize their findings.

Part II presents behavioral issues. First, measurement is described. The process of deriving proxy measures from criteria and criteria from program objectives is presented and some behavioral problems in measurement process are described. Next, behavioral models are provided which help the evaluator anticipate contentious debates that often arise during an evaluation and provide strategies to help the evaluator cope. The last Chapter illustrates the interrelationship of evaluation and decision making.

In short, the reader is exposed to methods, then purposes, and finally rationale. This sequence in the material seeks to build an awareness of pragmatic considerations, after a repertoire of skills has been developed. Pragmatism is stressed vis-à-vis opportunities to enlighten our understanding of a program and why it works.

NOTES

1. The origin of this bit is obscure. This piece was adapted from the *British Bulletin,* printed in 1952.
2. Suchman, E.A. *Evaluative Research: Principles and Practice in Public Service Organizations.* Washington, D.C.: Russell Sage Foundation, 1967, p. 11.
3. *Ibid.,* p. 27.
4. PL 93–641, for example, requires that Health Systems Agencies (multicounty planning federations) devise health service plans that specify where services, by type, should be located when little is known about the origin of a population's health needs, let alone how profiles of health services can be used to cope with peoples' needs.
5. Suchman, p. 2.
6. Wholey, J.S., J. Scanlon, H. Duffy, J. Fukumoto, and L. Vogt, *Federal Evaluation Policy: Analyzing the Effects of Public Programs.* Washington, D.C.; The Urban Institute, 1970, p. 23.
7. Roos, N.P., "Evaluation, Quasi–Experimentation and Public Policy," in *Quasi Experimental Methods.* Evanston, Ill.: Northwestern Univ. Press, 1973, p. 285.
8. Wholey, et al. p. 25.
9. Tripodi, T., P. Fellin, and I. Epstein, *Social Program Evaluation: Guidelines for Health, Education, and Welfare Administration.* Itasca, Ill.: Peacock, 1971, p. 4.
10. Suchman, p. 141.
11. Wholey, et al., p. 26.
12. Suchman, p. 141.
13. Tripodi, et al., p. 6.
14. *Ibid.,* p. 51.
15. Suchman, p. 144.
16. Rossi, P.H. and W. Williams, (eds.) *Evaluating Social Programs: Theory, Practice And Politics.* New York: Seminar Press, 1972.
17. Cain, G. and H.W. Watts, "Problems in Making Policy Inferences From the Coleman Report," in P. Rossi and W. Williams (eds.) *Evaluating Social Programs.* New York: Seminar Press, 1972.
18. Operations Research, Decision Analysis, Baysian methods, and many other techniques can also be used for evaluation. Statistical techniques are stressed because they provide the most generally useful set of methods. For a somewhat different view, see Guttentag, M., "On Qualified Sachel," *Evaluation,* Vol. 4, 1977; pp. 7–8. Guttentag contends that "sachel" (Yiddish for a well–informed judgment) rests on whether evaluation information is useful in a decision process. She also contends that Baysian methods are a superior evaluation approach. There is no disagreement over the need for evaluation to aid decision making. However, method selection is a substantive issue and few, including Guttentag, have offered concrete guides.
19. Suchman, p. 61

20. Wholey, et al., p. 26.
21. Williams, W. and J.W. Evans, "The Politics of Evaluation: The Case of Head Start," in P. Rossi (eds.), and W. Williams *Evaluating Social Programs*. New York: Seminar Press, 1972.
22. Suchman, p. 142.
23. Nutt, P.C., "The Accuracy and Acceptance of Decision Analysis Methods," Working Paper Series 78–75. The Ohio State University, College of Administrative Science, Columbus, Ohio, 1978.
24. The APGAR score is a subjective measure assigned by the attending physician, based on the newborn's heart rate, respiration, muscle tone, reflexes, skin color, and other factors.
25. Currier, R., "EPSDT: An Experience in Preventive Health," *Urban Health*, Vol. 7, No. 3, April 1978, pp. 18–34.
26. Appler, R., "In Defense of the Experimental Paradigm as a Tool for Evaluation Research," *Evaluation*, Vol. 4, 1977, pp. 14–18.

CHAPTER 2

Generating Evaluation Information

"It is demonstrable," said he [Pangloss, the professor], "that all is necessary for the best end. Observe that the nose has been formed to bear spectacles, legs were visibly designed for stockings, stones were designed to construct castles, pigs were made so we could have pork year around..."

Voltaire, *Candide*

EVALUATION AND CAUSATION

Evaluation is the study of causation. This approach to etiology is dissimilar from that advocated by systems and field theorists, who see causation as a mosaic of interrelated components. Evaluation rests on the belief that observable effects can be related or attributed to a set of causes. The relationship between an independent or "causal" agent(s) and an "effect" variable is weighed to detect its significance. Tsatsos calls evaluation *teleological,* arguing that "...to lay a sound foundation for the management of any social activity we [should] base our study on the *law of final causes.*"[1]

According to Suchman, evaluation seeks to relate "y," some desirable set of goals, with some intervention program "x."[2] The program x is intentionally devised to change y. The relationship between x and y is tested, attempting to hold other possible causes constant. For instance, evaluation was used to determine how Head Start (the intervention) improved youngsters' achievement on standard tests in public school, given the youngsters' age, grade in school, and the like.[3] Head Start would have been termed a success if the school performance of the Head Start children was superior to other youngsters with similar characteristics.

Interventions occur within what Thompson called a naturalistic or open system, making it difficult to trace or to isolate causal agents.[4] The intervention is one of many plausible explanations of the effects that are observed. Suchman defines several aspects of an open system, contending that an intervention is influenced by "initial condition" and by "intervening events," and leads to "consequences" that may not be anticipated.[5]

Figure 2.1 describes evaluation in an open system and identifies several major sources of confounding variables and biasing events. *Initial conditions* are factors that are present before the intervention begins that may influence its effectiveness. For instance, an evaluation of the cost–effectiveness of a shared service arrangement among hospitals in a city may have different levels of acceptance of the shared service notion within each hospital's medical staff and board. Similarly, the participating hospital's costs may be above or below the national norms for comparable hospitals.

Intervening events occur as the evaluation is being carried out. Some hospitals may undergo a reorganization or change in the membership of their board of trustees, which may alter their expectations and level of cooperation. The new management team may exert considerable changes in hospital efficiency, creating an intervening variable for the evaluation to consider.

Consequences flow from the effects of an intervention and may not be fully measurable or observable. Serendipitous outcomes, unanticipated benefits or problems may not show up immediately, and thus evade measurement. For instance, a shared service program may reduce costs but become a coordinational nightmare for the participating hospitals. If the shared service organization operates at a profit, an antiprofit stigma may turn up which alters the attitude of hospital contributors, leading to declining contributions. The

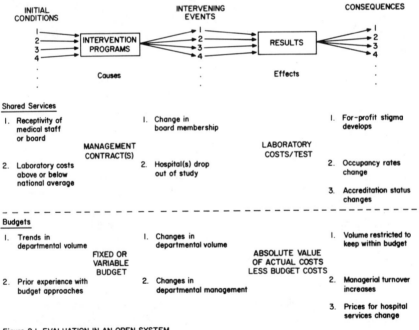

Figure 2.1 EVALUATION IN AN OPEN SYSTEM

Adapted from: Suchman E.A., *Evaluation Research,* Russell Sage Foundation, Wash. D.C., 1967.

medical staff may dislike the control procedures used to constrain costs and refer patients to local hospitals that do not participate in the shared service consortium.

Multiple causation makes it essential to identify events that may influence the benefits of an intervention. Preconditions and intervening events must be identified when they occur, to attempt to account for their effects. Consequences indicate that the measurement of effects was incomplete. Longitudinal studies may be necessary to fully comprehend the downstream effect of an intervention.

Suchman points out that some administrators may not believe that it is necessary to demonstrate that observed effects were caused by the intervention.[6] According to this view, so long as the desirable effects continue, it doesn't matter what caused them. This may lead to expensive interventions, because one of several mechanisms in the intervention program may have produced the desirable results. Even worse, programs may be instituted only to find that the relationship was spurious: the apparent link between cause and effect proved to be fleeting.

DISTINCTIONS BETWEEN EVALUATION AND RESEARCH

Evaluation is used to explore the relationship between an intervention program and the benefits and costs that occur following its application. Its purpose is to determine which effects can be attributed to the intervention program and to specify the value of these effects. The evaluator examines the objectives of the program, deduces the results suggested or specified by the program's objective, and develops a data collection scheme that isolates the results that stemmed from the intervention. Evaluation seeks to determine whether an intervention program can be relied on to produce the desired result and if this result can be cost justified. For example, an evaluation of a mass inoculation program can be carried out to verify that improvements in the health of people can be related to the vaccine, and whether these improvements can be justified in terms of the program's cost.

Research, in contrast, seeks to explore why an intervention program has certain results. The researcher is more apt to study a few well–defined variables, attempting to generalize the findings. For example, the researcher may study how people respond to various incentives to participate in mass–inoculation programs. The cause (various types of incentives)—effect (response rates) relationship is studied over a wide range of circumstances so the findings will generalize to a wide variety of settings. The need for information, as identified by the state of the art in the subject under study, stimulates research. A hypothesis, which provides a formal statement of a cause–and–effect relationship, is drawn to generate new knowledge.

The objectives of an intervention program determine what evaluation projects will study. The evaluator derives measures of performance from objectives, whereas the needs for new knowledge dictate measures used by the researcher. As a result the researcher and the evaluator develop distinct cause–and–effect relationships. Once the cause–and–effect relationship has been established, evaluation and research studies proceed following the same dicta. The researcher and evaluator have somewhat different purposes when they study an intervention program, but apply *the same methods* and adhere to the *same standards*.

ACTORS IN AN EVALUATION

The term *intervention* refers to a deliberate act initiated for implicit or explicit reasons by organizations. Table 2–1 lists some intervention programs undertaken by adminstrators in the human services industry. Some interven-

Table 2-1:   Some Intervention Programs

Intervention	Program Administrator	Evaluation Sponsor
mass innoculations (e.g., swine flu)	State department of Public Health	HEW - National Institutes of Health
Satellite clinics	local hospital	Health systems agency
Neighborhood health centers	OEO - CAP Agency	Funding agent in HEW
Hospital initiated cost control program	Hospital that initiated the program	Hospital (contracting with consultant)
Hospital labor control program	State hospital association's management engineering group	hospital's administration
Expanding Radiotherapy Services	Physician group	Hospital that rents the space to the physician group
Establishing a Burn Center	Hospital's medical staff	Accreditation team
An Appraisal System for Hospital Administrators	Hospital's CEO	Hospital's board of trustees
Priority scheme for United Way project review	United Way staff	United Way board of directors

tions are imposed. Inoculation programs (e.g., swine flu) were administered locally by health departments, but federal agencies retained evaluation prerogatives. Other intervention programs flow from the deliberate acts of management in an organization. For instance, a management appraisal program may be initiated, managed, and evaluated by the hospital's chief executive officer (CEO). Alternatively, the board of trustees may initiate an evaluation of the appraisal program. Thus an intervention program may be initiated, managed, and evaluated by the same person or by three different parties.

THE REQUISITES OF EVALUATION

The essential components of an evaluation project are described in Figure 2.2. A stratified sample is drawn from a target population and divided into

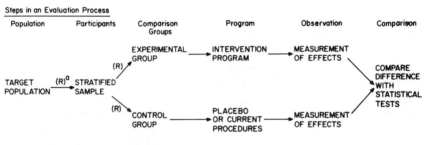

Steps in an Evaluation Process

| Population | Participants | Comparison Groups | Program | Observation | Comparison |

TARGET POPULATION → (R)[a] STRATIFIED SAMPLE

(R) → EXPERIMENTAL GROUP —— INTERVENTION PROGRAM —— MEASUREMENT OF EFFECTS

(R) → CONTROL GROUP —— PLACEBO OR CURRENT PROCEDURES —— MEASUREMENT OF EFFECTS

COMPARE DIFFERENCE WITH STATISTICAL TESTS

Principal Ingredients in an Evaluation Project

1. Constructing equivalent comparison groups
2. Administering the intervention, placebo, or current processes to the comparison groups
3. Defining and measuring effects

[a](R) signifies that participants were selected by a random process

Figure 2.2 ESSENTIALS OF EVALUATION

comparison groups. One comparison group, called the experimental group, is exposed to the intervention. The other comparison group, termed the control group, is exposed to a placebo or the current program. The comparison groups are exposed to some process of measurement to document the effects of the intervention. A comparison of these effects is made using tests of statistical significance.

There are three essential activities in evaluation: constructing equivalent comparison groups; exposing these groups to some type of intervention; and the definition, measurement, and comparison of effects that can be attributed to the intervention.

The Measurement of Effects

Evaluation weighs the factors or conditions that limit or enhance the success of an intervention. A careful definition of what marks success is required. All interventions tend to produce certain types of results, but the evaluation must identify those results the intervention has been designed to create.

The five types of evaluation described in Chapter 1 offer some guidance in the selection of measures. For instance, Suchman points out that professionals, like physicians, tend to define effort and performance in terms of professional standards.[7] The goals and practices of administrators often dictate using measures such as adequacy and efficiency. Process measures stem from academics and others concerned about ways to improve the intervention program.

Measures can be defined which represent the interests of the program's clients, advocates, or administrators, the public, or professionals who carry out the intervention. These groups tend to frame unique evaluation questions and thus advocate different measures. For instance, the advocates of a suicide prevention program may stress the number of calls as a measure of success, while professionals may attempt to measure the number of suicides averted, and administrators may use contact–cost indices. In large part, the objectives and thus the measure of success for an intervention are dictated by those in positions of power in the organization sponsoring the evaluation project.

The process of measurement follows the dicta of clinical investigations, often using blind or double–blind observational arrangements and placebos. Placebos are used to control for the symbolic power of many formal activities to alter the views, behavior, and performance of people. Blind measurement insures that the evaluation participants do not know whether they will be exposed to the intervention program or to a placebo. In a double–blind evaluation, neither the participant nor the observer (or even the investigator in certain types of studies) knows whether a participant has been exposed to the intervention, a placebo, or the current practices of the organization.

Methods to extract measures from objectives and ways to test the validity and reliability of measures are discussed in Chapter 7. Chapter 8 details how measures fit into the overall process of evaluation and how restrictive assumptions, which dictate certain types of indices, can be relaxed.

Statistical tests are used to compare the effects that stem from each comparison group. Chapters 3 and 4 detail the calculation procedures needed to assign both operational and statistical significance to these comparisons.

Carrying Out the Intervention Program

Intervention programs must specify the protocol to be used by the intervention, documenting procedures, staff qualifications, and the environment in which the program is to operate. Title III of ESEA, the Elementary and Secondary Education Act of 1965, provided funds for innovative public school programs. Bardach describes a program in which administrators encouraged teachers to become "catalytic role models," stimulating children to become self-motivated and responsible for their own learning and education.[8] An evaluation found that only 16 percent of the available class time was devoted to this approach. Perhaps the teachers did not understand how to become catalytic role models.

The protocol of the intervention is carefully defined so the program can be carried out in the same way at different points in time and in different settings. For instance, the Head Start evaluation findings were difficult to interpret because the achievement scores for youngsters who attended full-year programs were mixed with scores for those in the six-week programs. Each Head Start site also varied in terms of teacher qualifications and learning programs that were attempted.

Evaluation is one type of a search for causes. As pointed out in Chapter 1, several causal factors must be accounted for, requiring a test of the association between each factor and the performance measure selected. Evaluation becomes cumbersome, and even impossible, if the intervention program is carried out in a different way at different sites or evolves during the collection of evaluation data.

Suchman contends that the description of the intervention program must detail *what* the program will change and *why* such a change may stem from the intervention.[9] In the Head Start program, the "why" stemmed from the belief that a "public preschool" would stimulate low-income children and interest them in school, thereby improving their school performance. As we have seen, the "what" for Head Start was carelessly defined.

Comparison Groups

Comparison groups are drawn from the target population of the intervention program (see Figure 2.2). For instance, the target group of the Head Start program was specified by the eligibility requirements in the enabling legislation. The evaluation was carried out to generalize its findings to all youngsters with these characteristics (e.g., age, income of parents, ethnic identity). Statisticians call the target group the "population" or the "universe." Usually economy dictates that the evaluator must draw a sample which represents a subset of the population. This sample must be drawn in such a way that the evaluator can make valid assertions about the performance of this program when applied on a large scale.

The best sample is a random one. To create a random sample, a list of youngsters in the first grade is made and matched to a list of random numbers. When the youngster's place on the list corresponds to the digit 1 (in a set of digits from 0 to 9), he or she is asked to participate, creating a 10 percent random sample of first graders for the study. (The "R" adjacent to the population in Figure 2-2 indicates that participants were selected by a random process.)

Randomization insures that the participants in an evaluation will tend to match the target group, eliminating various types of selection biases. As Suchman points out, evaluation studies often select participants who are easy to work with, or willing to participate in a study, or sympathetic to the aims of the evaluation.[10] "Cooperative volunteers" will provide few insights into the behavior, preferences, or performance of the larger population because the population may be apathetic or even antagonistic toward the program.

To construct a stratified random sample, participants are selected at random, proportional to the size of each strata used to identify the target group. Using the Head Start example, each stratum is defined by levels of parents' income, as well as by age and race of the preschoolers. The evaluator matches the proportions in each stratum with those found (or thought to exist) in the target group. For instance, 20 percent of the population of preschoolers may be black, fall between the ages of four and five, and have parents whose income is above $5,000 annually. The evaluator draws a sample of this population so that the strata of race–age–income equals 20 percent.

The *sample size* or number of participants often creates problems for the evaluator. Formal rules for the selection of a sample size requires a historical measure of the variability of performance for the target group. This information is seldom available. For instance, raw scores on standard achievement tests for children must be available by grade, age, and year to measure the variability in these scores for each stratum. Without this information, the sample size is based on the number of strata to be considered and the anticipated size of the intervention's effect. Many population subgroupings or strata and an intervention that is expected to have a small but potentially important effect leads to large samples and vice versa. Sample size is frequently dictated by practical necessity, considering the cost of data acquisition and the availability of participants.

The evaluator draws from the pool of participants to set up the comparison groups that are equivalent. In well–controlled situations, participants can be assigned to comparison groups by a random process such as a coin flip. Comparison groups are formed, making the recipients of services in each group as much alike as possible. The intervention program is applied in half of these groups, called "experimental groups." The remaining groups are called "control groups." The control groups are not exposed to the program and may or may not receive a placebo. Control groups establish a baseline for the evaluation project indicating the attitude, behavior, or performance of people *not* exposed to the intervention. For instance, comparing disability or sick days for those who received and did not receive a swine flu vaccination may be misleading. People who neglected or refused to take the vaccine may differ from the people who were vaccinated, perhaps in terms of their susceptibility to disease. If so, people's "susceptibility" would be mixed or *confounded* with the effects of the vaccine. To control for factors like susceptibility, people are assigned to treatment and nontreatment comparison groups by a random process.

Comparison groups are constructed by controlling their membership. For example, a multihospital system could evaluate the performance of its management appraisal program by randomly selecting several hospitals in the system to try out the new appraisal program. Management performance in the remaining hospitals (the control group) provides a baseline to use in judging the effects of the new appraisal program. Similarly, to judge the effects of a new service, patients would be randomly assigned to the new service (experimental group) and the old service (control group) categories.

People often respond in unique ways to identical stimuli. Randomization insures that capricious responses to the program are equally likely in each comparison group. For example, suggestibility, resistance to change, natural immunity, and a host of other factors may dictate how people will react to intervention programs. Like people, organizations often exhibit unique responses to an intervention. For instance, administrators cannot pilot–test a new intervention program in one department of an organization and obtain a good indication of the program's value. Randomly selecting departments to receive the intervention program controls for differences among departments.

In some instances, random assignment is impractical or impossible, and other methods must be adopted. For example, some administrators of human service programs have restricted or eliminated the use of control groups. They fear that people who find they were in a control group will perceive they have been denied benefits, even if these benefits have yet to be demonstrated. For example, the target populations of intervention programs like Head Start and Job Corps, and the negative income tax experiments, expressed such views.[11] The beneficiaries of such programs often believe that control groups deny them the opportunity to receive benefits or to participate. In certain settings these criticisms have become so intense that evaluation sponsors are reluctant to employ control groups in any evaluation project.

In other instances, structural limitations prohibit the use of randomization. For instance, it is not feasible to assign people to health maintenance organizations, clinics, or private practitioners when they have particular ailments, in order to compare these modes of health care delivery. The evaluator has no control over the flow of participants. Hyman, *et al.*, point out that case–work agencies and similar organizations implicitly recruit their clients, which leads to clients with a predisposition to the agency and its programs.[12] These favorable attitudes may color their response to any change made by the agency. Everything is viewed positively, even when control and experimental groups are used. Suchman notes that the services of such an agency may be impossible to assess using a control group.[13] Program clients are self–selected, and there is no way to make those who rejected the service participate in an evaluation.

When randomization is prohibited, matched or naturally occurring groups or time series data are used to provide the comparison groups. The control group can be constructed in several other ways, including observing the preintervention state of the experimental group and measuring performance in a matched group or naturally occurring group whose members are unaware of the evaluation. For example, neighborhood health centers (NHC) in different cities form naturally occurring groups. Each center operates independently. Classifying these centers by their attributes (such as payment mechanisms, community involvement, or physician reimbursement methods) provides an excellent way to determine how these attributes influence NHC performance. Unfortunately, evaluators may find that important attributes, such as NHC payment mechanisms, do not vary in the naturally occurring groups. Using matched groups to assess the effect of a satellite clinic on a community, health indicators for those using the clinic could be compared to similar people in a community that lacks a clinic's services. The matched group must be carefully selected or bias will result. Time series analysis tracks important indicators before and after an intervention to see if the trends are favorable. The before–and–after data sets become the comparison groups. These approaches are called quasi–experimental designs. They have several useful applications and each has important limitations. These methods are discussed in detail in Chapter 5. In the discussion that follows, randomization is assumed. On occasion, a matched or naturally occurring group is used to illustrate data collection in constrained situations.

Several approaches to the planning of evaluation experiments will be illustrated. Two examples are used: the evaluation of various budgeting methods applied in several hospital departments, and the impact of shared services on hospital costs.

THE BUDGET ILLUSTRATION

There are several ways departments in an organization can budget, including fixed, variable, and semivariable approaches.[14] A brief description of these budgeting approaches is provided below:

Fixed Budgets: Expenditures for the department in past budget periods are estimated. The budget is based on previous years' experiences, with adjustments for inflation.

Variable Budgets: Unit costs in past years are estimated and volume is forecast for the budget period. The budget is determined by the unit costs multiplied by the volume anticipated in the budget period.

Semivariable Budgets: The budget is based on adjusted historical costs that have a fixed *and* a variable component.

The *objectives* of a budget may be either planning for or control of departmental activities within the organization. Assuming a control objective, several *criteria* could be used such as the appropriateness of rewards, attainability, controllability, and participation (see Table 2–2). For the purpose of this illustration, appropriateness of reward will be used as the criterion. Reward appropriateness can be measured by the variation of the budget from the actual costs. As both positive and negative deviations are equally undesirable, the absolute value of the difference will be used as a measure of budgeting effectiveness. This is shown graphically in Figure 2.3. When volume is low, and a fixed budget is used, rewards are given even though there is a budget overrun that cannot be justified. Rewards are given for cost control when the department failed to exercise cost control. When volume is high, a fixed budget suggests a cost overrun, and penalties may be assigned inappropriately.

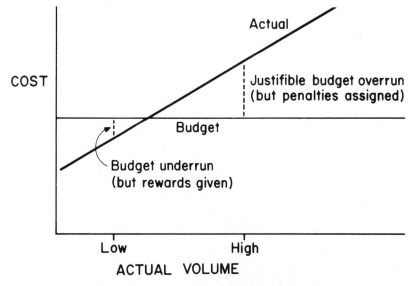

Figure 2.3 REWARDS & PENALTIES STEMMING FROM A FIXED BUDGET

THE SHARED SERVICE EXAMPLE

Shared services programs seek to reduce the cost of hospital operations by creating a consortium which attempts to secure some of the economies of scale offered by a large organization. Shared service activities often include laundry, joint purchasing, and the laboratory. Evaluation could be used to determine the impact of a shared services program on hospital costs. A related question concerns the *type* of shared service arrangement (intervention) that is the most cost-effective. There are several options that a hospital could adopt, including management contracts with multihospital systems (both profit and nonprofit), local consortia, state and local hospital associations, and still others.

Shared service evaluation questions can be proposed from several prospectives. Multihospital systems offering shared service contracts should be vitally concerned with the impact of these contracts on hospitals that purchase their services. Obviously, a favorable cost picture can aid the multihospital systems in marketing their management contract services. The hospital exploring the merits of sharing seeks to answer the same question from a slightly different vantage point: which shared service approach provides the most benefits to a subscribing hospital? The objectives for both perspectives concern efficiency and effectiveness. Some potential program options and indicators of program success are shown in Table 2-3. Specific measures for laboratory shared

Table 2-2.

BUDGETING EXAMPLE

Causes or Intervention Program Options

    (1) Fixed Cost Budgets
    (2) Variable Cost Budgets
    (3) Semi-Variable Cost Budgets

Effects or Indicators of Program Success
    (1) Participation
    (2) Reward Logic (accuracy of control activities)
    (3) Controllability
    (4) Attainability

Table 2-3.

SHARED SERVICES EXAMPLE

Causes or Intervention Program Options
    (1) Profit Hospital Chain Management Contract
    (2) Non-Profit Multi-Hospital System Management Contract
    (3) Hospital Association Management Contract
    (4) Local Consortia Management Contract

Effects or Indicators of Value of A Shared Service Program
    (1) Costs (Total, Variable or Fixed Component, Etc.)
    (2) Revenues
    (3) Operating Statistics (Occupancy, Costs Per Patient Day, Etc.)
    (4) Price Level (Charges) for Services Shared
    (5) Quality (Infection Rates)
    (6) Services (Number Elective & Complex Surgical Procedures)
    (7) Acceptance - (The views of physicians, the hospital's management, the community, the Board of Trustees, etc.)

service include the cost per test in a laboratory and test errors, determined by repeating a sample of tests each day.

COMPARING TWO INTERVENTION PROGRAMS

The Before–and–After Study

Often administrators implicitly require before–and–after studies. In such an evaluation, indicators are collected from data archives to represent past performance. These same performance indicators are collected again after the program had been installed. The after indicators are compared to the before indicators to determine the effect of the intervention program.

The before–and–after observations may not be representative. For example, the benefits of a management contract observed in one hospital may not occur in hospitals that have more beds or fewer services. To verify these benefits, they must be observed in a variety of hospitals with different characteristics. Consider an evaluation project to determine the effect of a management contract on hospital laboratory costs. Laboratory costs vary due to absenteeism of key personnel, equipment breakdowns, and unusually low volumes of activity. These factors will induce variability in costs before and after a shared service contract has been implemented. The variability in hospital laboratory costs may be large enough to mask differences in average costs determined before and after the program was installed. If so, the evaluation findings become inconclusive. The participation of many hospitals over an extended time period is required to keep unusual occurrences from artificially inflating the variability in costs.

A before–and–after evaluation for shared service programs is shown in Table 2-4. The data in the first column (no sharing) represent the average laboratory costs in several hospitals prior to the adoption of a management contract. The second column represents the same indicators collected after the hospital's laboratory has been operated by contract. The evaluator determines whether costs have declined enough to justify the cost of the contract.[15]

Administrators often call for before–and–after evaluations, because they appear to be a quick and inexpensive way to carry out an evaluation project. But the quantity of data needed to make accurate measurement of performance indicators is often badly underestimated. Extensive data acquisition dramatically hikes the costs of an evaluation project. Administrators also tend to assume that data in archives are more accurate and accessible than practice dictates. Merely reformatting data can dramatically increase costs when large amounts of data must be processed. Also, transformations may introduce errors and misinterpretations. Finally, measures are dictated by what is

Table 2-4:   Before and After Studies With and Without Pairing

Shared Service Example

C1 = laboratory cost in hospital 1 (The Effectiveness Measure)

Hospitals in Study	No Sharing	Management Contract	Differences In Cost (d)
Hospital #1	C4	C1	d_1 = C1 - C4
Hospital #2	C5	C2	d_2
Hospital #3	C6	C3	d_3
Hospital #4	C7	C4	d_4
-	-	-	-
-	-	-	-
-	-	-	-

Budget Example

Actual Cost - Budgeted Cost = V (The Effectiveness Measure)

Departments in Study	Fixed Budget	Variable Budget	Differences In Performance (d)
Department #1	V1	V2	d_1 = V1 - V2
Department #2	V2	V1	d_2 = V2 - V1
Department #3	V1	V2	d_3 = V1 - V2
Department #4	V2	V1	d_4 = V2 - V1
-	-	-	-
-	-	-	-
-	-	-	-

recorded in data files, when other measures may be far more meaningful. Before–and–after evaluations have several important limitations, and other modes of data acquisition should be explored before they are adopted.

The Data Pairing Concept

To evaluate a shared service program using a pairing approach, the costs of each participating hospital would be paired with cost data from the Hospital Administrative Service (HAS) program of the American Hospital Associations for similar hospitals. The pairing strategy controls for differences among the hospitals. The management contract data (Table 2–4) would contain laboratory costs in hospitals with shared services. The no–sharing column would list hospital laboratory cost data found in HAS reports for hospitals matched to hospitals participating in the shared service program, using size or some other characteristic. Data from similar hospitals permit an analysis of the difference in cost across the hospitals (see Table 2–4).

Other types of data collection approaches could also be used. For instance, the cost performance of hospitals that adopted *and discontinued* a comparable shared–service arrangement for laboratory operation could be compared. The available data would be paired by the year that the contract was added or dropped. Hospitals in the no–sharing column (Table 2–4) would have dropped a shared service program. They would be paired with a comparable hospital maintaining the arrangement. If the cost decreases in the hospitals that use a shared service concept are similar to the cost increases experienced by those abandoning shared service, a compelling demonstration of the shared service concept can be made. The evaluator attempts to find creative ways to *pair* the evaluation data to wash out particular kinds of biases.

The budgeting example illustrates a different approach to paired data. Asking each participating hospital department to budget first with fixed approaches and then with the variable approach may induce learning which may improve the variable budget's performance. A learning effect will be mixed (confounded) with the effects of the variable budget. Some departments in a hospital may learn how to get around the control elements built into particular kinds of budgets. For example, departments with high volume potential may be able to manipulate variable budgets by meaningless increases in their activity, whereas departments with very stable volumes may take advantage of fixed budgets by restricting their activities. The pairing approach controls both volume and learning by distributing their effects to each comparison group.

A coin flip is used to decide which budget approach would be carried out first in each department. After the budget was completed, the department would be asked to budget with the second approach. The data arrangement is shown in Table 2–4. The numbers associated with each effectiveness measure indicates the order in which the departments carried out the budgeting process (determined by a coin flip). As a result, the effects of learning are equally represented in both sets of performance measures. Pairing the data *blocks* out the effects of learning. Without pairing, learning effects would be *confounded* with the marginal improvement (or decrease) in performance associated with a variable budget.

COMPARING MORE THAN TWO INTERVENTION PROGRAMS

A hospital association may be interested in comparing the cost effectiveness of several types of shared service programs. Laboratory costs could be collected in hospitals that participate in a local consortium, purchase the services from a multihospital corporation, and provide their own services.

Equivalent Populations

In Table 2–5, the data for the shared service example represent laboratory costs averaged over the past year. The entry in each column represents the cost experience of a particular hospital with a particular type of shared service arrangement. To make the results comparable, the hospitals in each sample (column) were required to be similar in terms of their size, ownership, complexity, and other factors that are likely to influence laboratory efficiency. The hospitals that fall into the categories "no shared services," "shared services–local consortium," and "management contract with a multihospital system," are carefully matched.

The validity of the conclusions that can be drawn is dependent upon the precision of this matching. The matching process may lead to selecting hospitals with deceptively similar characteristics. For example, hospitals with a similar bed size may differ markedly in terms of volume and type of activity in their laboratories. A thousand–bed military hospital is not comparable to a thousand–bed teaching and research institution. The missions of these hospitals require that they serve distinct patients with unique health problems, leading to different profiles of laboratory tests which can cause dramatic differences in hospital laboratory efficiency. In this case, bed size created a misleading match of hospitals.

To make populations in the budget example equivalent, the order that departments apply each budget approach is randomized.

Accounting for Block Variables

An index, based on the type or number of services, is often used to sort hospitals into comparison groups (Table 2–6). This permits the evaluator

Table 2-5: Comparing Several Program Options

Shared Service Example

	OPTIONS	
No Sharing	Management Contract	Consortia
Hosp. #1 Costs	Hosp. #11 Costs	Hosp. #70 Costs
Hosp. #2 Costs	Hosp. #21 Costs	Hosp. #90 Costs
Hosp. #3 Costs	Hosp. #50 Costs	Hosp. #32 Costs
Hosp. #4 Costs	-	Hosp. #45 Costs
-	-	Hosp. #65 Costs
-	-	-

Budget Example

	OPTIONS		
Participants	Fixed	Variable	Semi variable
Dept. #1	$(1)^a$	$(2)^a$	$(3)^a$
Dept. #2	(3)	(1)	(2)
Dept. #3	(2)	(3)	(1)
Dept. #4	(1)	(2)	(3)
Dept. #5	(3)	(1)	(2)
Dept. #6	(2)	(3)	(1)

[a]Order in which budget was prepared

to control hospital complexity, measured by number of services. The controlled factor, complexity, is called a "block" variable. Accounting for block effect dramatically improves the quality of evaluation data. But block effects increase data demands. The sensitivity of paired data is less than the sensitivity of the same data examined independently. To put it another way, when one stratum is added in an evaluation, the amount of data must be doubled to maintain a given level of sensitivity. When accounting for block

Table 2-6: Blocking For Unwanted Effects

Shared Example

Type of Hospital	No Sharing	Management Contract
Hospital 1	Hosp. 1 Costs	Hosp. 10 Costs
Hospital 2	Hosp. 2 Costs	Hosp. 20 Costs
Hospital 3	Hosp. 3 Costs	Hosp. 30 Costs
Hospital 4	Hosp. 4 Costs	Hosp. 40 Costs
Hospital 5	Hosp. 5 Costs	Hosp. 50 Costs

1 & 10 : Hospitals with "few" services (Category 1)
2 & 20 : Hospitals with "some" services (Category 2)
3 & 30 : Hospitals with "typical" services (Category 3)
4 & 40 : Hospitals with "many" services (Category 4)
5 & 50 : Hospitals with a "full complement" of services (Category 5)

Budget Example

Participating Departments	Fixed Budget	Variable Budget	Semi variable Budget
Department 1	(1)[a]	(2)[a]	(3)[a]
Department 2	(3)	(1)	(2)
Department 3	(2)	(3)	(1)
Department 4	(1)	(2)	(3)
Department 5	(3)	(1)	(2)
Department 6	(2)	(3)	(1)

[a]Order budgeting was carried out

effects with a fixed sample size, sensitivity is lost directly proportional to the number of blocks considered. For example, to control for hospital size, three categories might be selected, 75 to 150 beds, 400 to 600 beds, and 1,000 beds and above. The sample size is tripled to control for the size variable.

Factors not considered by the block effect will cause the hospital laboratory to perform somewhat differently. This makes it necessary to measure the performance of several hospitals within each cell, defined by the type of sharing program and level of the block variable, to characterize laboratory costs for that cell. This concept is called replication.

The budget example (Table 2–6) illustrates an evaluation that compares the performance of fixed, variable, and semivariable budgets. Each entry represents a particular department's performance, using a particular budgeting approach. As in Table 2–5, the order in which departments carry out the

Table 2-7:   Factorial Evaluation Studies

Budget Example

Contrast	Budget (Policy)	Volatility (block)	Observation
1 (Dept. A)	Variable	Low	Deviation of
2 (Dept. B)	Fixed	Low	actual from budget
3 (Dept. C)	Variable	High	
4 (Dept. D)	Fixed	High	
5 (Dept. E)	Variable	Low	

Coding :   Type of Budget Used (policy variable)

   -Variable
   -Fixed

Volatility (block variable)

   -Small volume changes: ±10%
   -Large volume changes: ±25%

Sharing Example

Contrast	Shared Service (policy)	Beds (Block)	Observation
Hosp. 1	None	100	Measures unit
Hosp. 2	Sharing	125	costs, such as $/pound in the
Hosp. 3	None	700	laundry of each
Hosp. 4	Sharing	695	hospital
Hosp. 5 [a]	None	125	

Coding: Policy variables defined as

   -sharing
   -no sharing

Block variable defined by hospital size ranges

   -500 to 700 beds
   -100 to 150 beds

[a] Contrast E provides a replication of Contrast 1 and hospital 5 is a replication for hospital 1.

budgeting process is randomized, as shown by the numbers in parentheses in Table 2-6. The quality of the evaluation data can be improved by accounting for the block factor. In this example, each department becomes a block. Each department's performance over several distinct time periods, when budgeting with each of the three approaches, is measured. This type of evaluation can determine which budgeting approach works best, independent of the block effect (departmental performance). Administrators may also be interested in the block effect: average departmental performance. Thus, some block effects can be translated into meaningful information for managerial control purposes.

MORE COMPLEX EVALUATION STUDIES

It is often useful to weigh the interactions among the causal factors. For instance, a variable budgeting approach may favor departments that have large changes in volume from month to month. This often leads to an interaction between departmental performance and budget approach, or a "budget–department" interaction. Laboratory costs, with a particular shared service strategy, might be affected differently in small hospitals compared to large hospitals. This causes an interaction between size and the shared service arrangement: some arrangements are superior for large or small hospitals.

To explore the interaction effects between block variables and intervention programs, a somewhat different data arrangement is used. Table 2-7 provides an example of this data–generating device, which is called a "factorial design."

As shown in Table 2-7, four distinct contrasts are used to provide a prospective study of all combinations of the causal variables: volatility (the block variable) and budgeting approach (the policy variable). A replication is obtained by measuring the performance of several departments with high (or low) volatility that use a particular budget approach. For contrast (Table 2-7) the performance of a "low volatility" department which applied the variable budget approach (department A) is measured. Contrast two records performance for department B, which had low volatility and used a fixed budget. The other contrasts are interpreted in the same way.

Several replications are required for each contrast. A replication can be provided by having department E, which has only modest swings in activity, like department A, also prepare a variable budget. Replications can also be created by having each department use both budget approaches. For example, department A (low volatility) could rebudget with the fixed approach to create another observation for contrast 2; department B (high volatility) could use the variable budget approach, creating another observation for contrast 1; and so on.

In the shared service example, historical data for laboratory performance in hospitals are sought. The data are sorted into particular bed size categories, according to their shared service arrangement. Hospitals are matched according to size (the block variable) and whether or not they have a shared service (the policy variable). Laboratory costs for all hospitals with shared services, in the 100 to 150 bed size range, are included in comparison group one. All hospitals with (or without) shared service arrangements that fall into a particular size become replications.

SUMMARY

This chapter described several modes of collecting evaluation data. Principles in defining and collecting data for an evaluation were illustrated. The collection, analysis, and interpretation of data from evaluation experiments are largely inseparable concepts, making these illustrations somewhat artificial. They do, however, serve to demonstrate the power of prospective data collection and the need to control extraneous factors that can influence the evaluation data. In Chapters 3 and 4, additional examples will be used to illustrate how evaluation data are collected, analyzed, and interpreted.

A short glossary of evaluation terms follows:

GLOSSARY

Bias: Contamination or errors in the measures used to assess an intervention program causes bias. For instance, questionnaires may suggest desired answers or the respondent may be influenced by overhearing others as the questionnaire is filled out.

Block Variables: Factors that will influence results if not controlled, but often not subject to direct control by the sponsor.

Blocking: Blocking screens an unwanted effect from the evaluation data. For instance, blocking can be used to control for learning effects in data depicting performance. When a factor is blocked, it is equally distributed between the programs being compared or subtracted out to remove its influence.

Confounding: Confounding occurs when some block effect is mixed with a program effect. For example, to compare hospitals with and without a management contract, hospital size may be mixed or confounded with the effect of the shared service program.

Contrast: A specific observation which defines population to be sampled; for instance, the performance of departments with low volatility using a fixed budget.

Control Group: A baseline is established to measure the views, behavior, or performance of a population to provide a basis of comparison. Control groups are essential when a clear and unambiguous history of relevant performance measures has not been retained in an organization's data banks.

Degrees of Freedom: The total observations in a given stratum, minus the one which is used to compute the mean of the stratum.

Experimental Group: Comparison groups that are exposed to an intervention program.

Interaction: The *joint* effect of several variables. For example, hospital departments with high volatility that perform better using a variable budget.

Placebo: People often contend that inert substances improve a variety of physical ailments. To control for suggestibility, an inert substance; or placebo, is often administered to a control group.

Policy Variables: Intervention program options and other variables that can be manipulated by the sponsor.

Prospective Evaluation Data: Data that are collected following a prescribed evaluation plan.

Proxy Measures: The objectives of intervention programs are often broad and general. Specific measures can consider only elements of the program's objectives. A good proxy is a measure that captures the intent of these objectives. For example, when evaluating a neighborhood health center the number of previously undetected health problems per contact is a better proxy than the number of visits.

Randomization: Randomizing eliminates many kinds of order effects in the evaluation data. For example, the sequence in which evaluation data are collected is randomized to eliminate practice effects, maturation, and the like.

Replication: Repeated observations for particular combinations of the policy and block variable. For example, the number of hospitals falling into a particular size range and using a given sharing arrangement.

Sample Size: The total number of observations taken in an evaluation study.

Sensitivity: The precision of estimates of important parameters, such as means and variances, improve as the amount of data available for analysis increases. For a fixed sample size, sensitivity declines proportional to the number of strata considered.

Treatments: Treatments refer to intervention program options that are being compared in the evaluation project. Treatments may also include the absence of a program or the use of a placebo.

Validity: An intervention program is thought to be valid when it can be shown that it invariably creates a particular result after repeated evaluation studies.

NOTES

1. Tsatsos, H.E.C.D., "Methodology and Teleology," *Management Science,* Vol. 24, No. 7, March 1978, pp. 709–711.
2. Suchman, E.A., *Evaluative Research: Principles and Practice In Public Service and Social Action Programs.* Washington, D.C.; Russell Sage Foundation, 1967, p. 78.
3. Williams, W. and J. Evans, "The Politics of Evaluation: The Case of Head Start," in P. Rossi and W. Williams (eds.) *Evaluating Social Programs.* New York: Seminar Press, 1972.
4. Thompson, J.D., *Organizations In Action,* New York: McGraw–Hill, 1967.
5. Suchman, p. 84.
6. *Ibid.,* p. 87.
7. *Ibid.,* p. 109.
8. Bardach, E., *The Implementation Game,* Cambridge, Mass.; MIT Press, 1977, p. 2.
9. Suchman, p. 106.
10. *Ibid.,* p. 104.
11. Rossi, P. and W. Williams (eds.) *Evaluating Social Programs,* New York: Seminar Press, 1972.
12. Hyman., C. Wright, and T. Hopkins, *Applications of Methods of Evaluation: Four Studies of the Encampment for Citizenship,* Berkeley: University of California Press, 1962, pp. 23–24.
13. Suchman, p. 104.
14. These budgeting strategies were selected to illustrate evaluation methods and may not represent the most sophisticated budgeting approaches available.
15. This illustration assumes that inflationary trends in the case data have been removed.

CHAPTER 3

The Scheduling, Analysis and Interpretation of Evaluation Studies

In the investigation of hidden causes, stronger reasons are obtained from sure experiments and demonstrable arguments than from the probable conjectures and the opinion of philosophical speculations.

William Gilbert (1600)

A REVIEW OF STATISTICS FOR EVALUATION

Populations and the Samples

Ideally, an evaluation compares several *populations*. Populations are ideal because they contain the entire target group for a particular type of intervention program. For instance, to determine the influence of contract management on laboratory costs, two populations would be compared: all laboratories managed by hospitals and all those managed by a specific type of contract.

Typically, data which describe a population cannot be obtained at a reasonable cost. The evaluator must draw a *sample* of the populations to be compared. For instance, laboratory costs can be estimated by sampling costs in hospitals with and without contract laboratory management. Each sample is used to represent the population of hospitals with local or contract management. The number of observations in this smaller group is referred to as the *sample size*. Thus, each comparison group, in an evaluation project, can be described by its population or, more often, by a sample drawn from its population.

Characteristics of Populations and Samples

Both the population and its sample are described by two parameters: its mean and variance. The *mean* is the arithmetic average of the sample:

$$\bar{x} = E(x) = \sum_i x_i/n \qquad (\mu = \text{true mean})$$

where: x_i = the ith observation in a sample
n = sample size
$E(x)$ = the expected value of the observations

The mean is the most common or the expected value of x. The sample mean is denoted by $\bar{x}$. μ represents the true mean, the mean of the population. The second parameter of interest is the *variance,* the range or dispersion of values in a population or sample. The variance is the sum of squared deviations between the mean and each observation used to compute the mean. The arithmetic calculation of the variance is shown below:

$$s^2 = V(x) = \sum_i [(x_i - \bar{x})^2/(n - 1)] \qquad (\sigma = \text{true variance})$$

The variance of the sample is denoted by s^2 and the variance of the population by σ^2. Variances are often converted to a "standard deviation" to compare variation in costs with average costs, using the same scale units, as shown below:

$$s = SD(s) = \sqrt{V(x)} \qquad (\sigma = \text{true standard deviation})$$

The evaluator typically relies upon a sample drawn from a population to calculate the mean and variance. The variance of the population is represented by the sample variance; and the mean of the population, represented by the sample mean. The calculation's format for the variance of a sample is given by:

$$\sigma^2 = s^2 = \sum_i (x_i - \bar{x})^2/\text{degrees of freedom} = [\sum x_i^2 - n\bar{x}^2]/(n - 1)$$

(One degree of freedom is lost because the variance computation requires a prior estimate of the mean.) the notation σ^2 is often used to designate an estimate of the variance.

Distributions

The distribution of values in a *population* take on a specific shape. Many populations have *a normal* distribution (see Figure 3–1). The standard deviation measures the spread of the population, at the inflection point of the normal curve. The standard deviation identifies a range that encloses one–third of the population.

THE NORMAL DISTRIBUTION

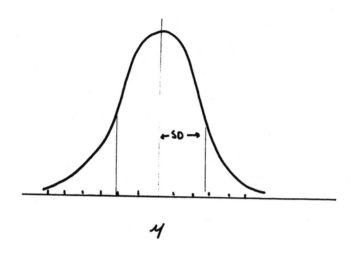

THE FREQUENCY DISTRIBUTION

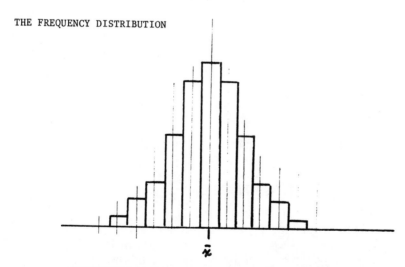

FIGURE 3.1 POPULATION DISTRIBUTION

The distribution of *samples* is usually drawn as a frequency diagram. Several ranges, like those shown in Figure 3.1, are defined, and the number of times that samples fall into each range are counted. A bar diagram is used to describe how often data fall in each range.

The sample distribution drawn from a normal distribution is called the "t" distribution. The "t" distribution is formed by drawing samples from a population, described by a normal distribution. Note that the "t" distribution in Figure 3.2 is always broader than the normal distribution. This can

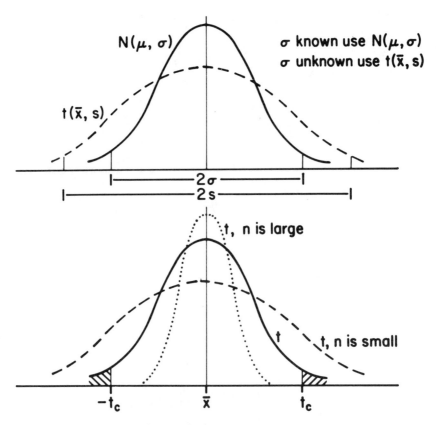

Figure 3.2 t DISTRIBUTIONS

be verified by inspecting the computational formula for the variance. Because n, the sample size, is always much smaller than the size of the population, the estimated variance (s^2) is always larger than the true variance σ^2. As n increases, the estimate of the variance s^2 gets smaller as it approaches the variance of the population σ^2. The variance parameter (properly scaled) measures the spread of the distribution, so the "t" distribution will be broader than the corresponding normal distribution. As n approaches the size of the population, the "t" distribution shrinks, as shown in Figure 3–2.

A sample is called unbiased if the "t" distribution and the corresponding normal distributions are centered at the same point. If not, the sample mean will shift to the left or right of the population mean. (The sample distribution, shown in Figure 3.2, has an unbiased estimate of the population mean.)

Significance Tests

To determine the merits of a management contract, the costs from a sample of hospitals with a management contract and the costs from sample hospitals providing their own management services could be compared. The analysis begins by stating a "null hypothesis." The difference between laboratory costs, with and without a contract, is assumed to be zero. Stated somewhat differently, the evaluator begins by viewing the costs as roughly the same and tries to prove or disprove this view.

Statistical tests are applied to determine whether the evaluator should "accept" or "fail to accept" (reject) the null hypothesis. Failing to accept the null hypothesis suggests that there were differences in laboratory costs. The intervention program with the lowest cost would be adopted.

The index used to make this determination is called a "t" statistic. The calculation for the t value is shown below:

$$t = \frac{\text{estimated mean of the data} - \text{true mean}}{\text{standard deviation of the data}}$$

or

$$t = \frac{\overline{x} - \text{expected value}}{s/(n)^{1/2}}$$

The null hypothesis makes the expected value of a difference in costs zero. The calculation's form of the t statistic is given by:

$$t = \frac{(\overline{x} - 0)}{s/(n)^{1/2}}$$

The t statistic is made up of the mean of the sample, less the mean of the population, divided by a standard deviation of the samples, corrected by the size of the sample. Thus, the t statistic is a composite measure of the central tendency (mean) and spread (variance) in a sample drawn from a population.

To find that a difference exists, the t value must be "large" compared to a table value, denoted t_c in Figure 3–2. These values are found in Table A–1 in the Appendix. For example, when n = 20 and a level of significance (α) of .05 is used, t_c = 2.09. α represents the percentage of total area that falls into the cross hatched portions of the t distributions, beyond the critical values t_c (Figure 3–2). The critical value from the table is written as

$$t_c = t_{n-1,\ \alpha} = t_{19,\ .05} = 2.09$$

If the t statistic ($t = (\bar{x} - \mu)/s/\sqrt{n}$) is larger than t_c, the null hypothesis is discredited. This comparison requires that

$$t \geqslant t_c$$

The t statistic can be made large in two ways. First, the differences in costs may be substantial, suggesting that one of the management approaches is superior. But to detect these differences the variation in these costs must be small. To enhance the chance that differences between intervention programs are detected, the variance in the data must be reduced. The magnitude of the standard deviation can be reduced if the sample size is increased. Standard deviation is measured by $\Sigma_i(x_i - \bar{x})^2/(n - 1)$. As the sample size, n, goes up, the standard deviation will get smaller. The t statistic is measured by $t = \bar{x}(n)^{-.5}/s$. The t value will increase with a decrease in the standard deviation. A higher t value increases the chance the evaluator can find the difference between two populations, ($t \geqslant t_c$), if a difference exists.

Notice that the t distribution is broader than the normal distribution (Figure 3.2). As the sample increases, the t distribution gets closer and closer to the normal distribution. When the evaluator has information for each element in the population, a normal distribution is used. Significant tests are based upon critical values drawn from the normal distribution. However, in most evaluation studies the true variance is unknown, so the sample variance and a t distribution must be used to carry out significance tests.

Confidence Intervals and Their Relationship to Significance Tests

A confidence interval is constructed so it will enclose a specified percentage of the samples drawn from a population. The level of confidence is denoted as α. $1 - \alpha$ is the probability that a particular sample will fall in this range which is expressed as a percent. The confidence interval (CI) defined by

$$CI = \text{Mean} \pm (t_{n-1,\ \alpha/2}) \quad \text{standard deviation}$$

$$= \bar{x} \pm t_{n-1,\ \alpha/2}\ s/\sqrt{n} = 1 - \alpha$$

The CI defines a set of values that will fall in this range $1 - \alpha$ percent of the time.

$$-t_{n-1, \alpha/2} \, s/\sqrt{n} \leqslant \bar{x} \leqslant t_{n-1, \alpha\backslash 2} \, s/\sqrt{n}$$

For example, a 95 percent confidence interval ($\alpha = .05$) describes the range in laboratory costs that will occur 95 percent of the time in hospitals that manage their own labs. Only a small percentage of laboratory costs (5 percent) are expected to fall outside the range defined by the confidence interval. When costs for laboratories run by management contract fall outside the range, the evaluator concludes that this difference in cost is not due to chance (normal variations in the practices of a laboratory), but rather can be attributed to the management contract.

A close examination of formulae for confidence intervals and the t statistic points out the similarity between a confidence interval and a significance test. Each determines whether the costs associated with alternatives (management contract and hospital operation) came from the same or from different populations. If the confidence intervals of hospital costs overlap, or if the t statistic fails to exceed a critical value, the evaluator concludes that the costs are the same. If not, the management contract may be a useful way to reduce laboratory costs.

Errors in Statistics

Statistical analysis admits to two types of errors. They are illustrated by the areas where the two t distributions overlap in Figure 3.3. A *type I* error is made when the evaluator concludes that an intervention program caused a difference, when in reality no difference exists. A 5 percent chance of making this kind of error is tolerated in the example shown in Figure 3.3. In medicine this is called a "false positive": concluding that someone is sick when in fact he/she is fine. For example, the two populations in Figure 3.3 can be used to represent norms for well and sick individuals, measured by a certain diagnostic test like blood pressure. t_c represents the critical value for the blood pressure indicator. When this level of blood pressure is exceeded, an intervention, like a medication, is prescribed. According to this curve, 5 percent of the time the physician is willing to make a type I error, concluding that the high blood pressure is high enough to prescribe a medication when a patient is not sick. Again type I error is synonymous with a false positive.

A *type II* error makes the reverse mistake. The type II error is synonymous with a "false negative," concluding someone is well when in fact he/she is sick. 10 percent of the values between t_1 and t_c in Figure 3.3 are subject to a type II error.

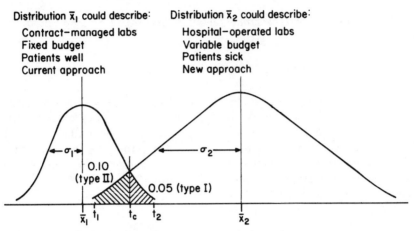

Figure 3.3   ERRORS IN STATISTICS

Values between t_c and t_2 represent a type I error and occur 5 percent of the time in Figure 3.3.

Type I and type II errors are inversely related. When few type II errors can be tolerated, the number of type I errors will increase. For example, physicians attempt to minimize type II errors (false negatives), which causes more type I errors (false positives) to occur. Reducing the risk of concluding that someone is well, when in fact he is sick, will increase the number of false positives. concluding that well people are sick. People are placed in the right hand distribution when in fact they are in the left hand distribution. Table 3–1 summarizes the circumstances leading to false negatives and false positives and true negatives and true positives.

Decision rules are needed to select the probabilities for the type I or type II error. These probabilities must be consistent with the consequences associated with each error. For example, if the management contract requires a minimum commitment of five years, as opposed to one year, the tolerance for a false positive (or Type I error) diminishes. In essence, with a five–year contract an increased demand is placed upon the quality of evaluation information. Relatively *more* certainty, or lower error rates, are sought. The permissible error rate can be reduced by moving the value of t_c to the right in Figure 3.3. This forces the decision maker to adopt a smaller level of confidence (α). In the example shown in Figure 3–3, the level of confidence, (α), equals .05. This means that 95 percent of the time the values would fall to the left of t_c. To reduce the chance of a false positive the confidence level is decreased, perhaps to .01. The significance test becomes more conservative, which is reflected by the longer contract. When only one year's commitment is required, a .05 level of

Table 3-1: Conclusions From Statistical Tests

TRUE CONDITION

		Present	Absent
	Present	true positive	false positive
TEST CONCLUSION			
	Absent	false negative	true negative

significance may be adequate. A five-year contract, however, may demand an .01 level of significance.

Adopting a more stringent test by increasing the level of significance always increases the chance of making a type II error (false negative). In contrast to medical practice, evaluation applied by a manager attempts to avoid finding differences when differences do not exist. Managers have an aversion to erroneously concluding that an intervention will have favorable impact on cost. Before implementing an intervention program, managers hope to be quite certain of the intervention's benefits when applied on a regular basis to their clientele. When the costs of analysis are low, compared to the losses from ineffective interventions, this is rational strategy.

Summary

Statistical methods aid the evaluator in describing and understanding samples drawn from a population. There are two salient parameters in any sample, the population's mean and variance. Evaluation compares parameters of samples drawn from populations which represent a current approach and a new approach. For example, consider an evaluation that compared the average costs of laboratories managed locally by hospitals or by a contract. Considerable variability in these costs is likely because hospitals differ. If the distributions of laboratory costs drawn from these two populations tend to overlap, the evaluator concludes that the costs came from the same population. Costs in a laboratory were not reduced as a result of a management contract. Conceptually, this can be illustrated by a confidence interval for the sample of laboratory cost for hospitals *with* and *without* the contract management service for this laboratory. If these confidence intervals overlap, costs were not reduced by the management contract.

Statistics recognize two types of errors. When a false positive or type I error is made, the evaluator concludes that costs were reduced by the management contract, when in fact they were not. A false negative or type II error occurs when the evaluator concludes that costs were not reduced through sharing, when in reality costs declined. Most evaluation studies seek to minimize false positives, in contrast to medicine, which seeks to minimize the false negatives. In medicine, the consequences of making an incorrect judgment can be measured in terms of human life. In management, economic concerns dictate a balance between Type I and Type II error, and reflect the cost of carrying out more evaluation studies on the one hand, and the cost of implementing ineffective programs on the other.

In the discussion that follows, a .05 level significance is used. It is assumed that this level of significance balances the consequences of Type I and II errors. Managers who believe that the consequences of making a wrong decision are extreme would adopt a more conservative test, using a lower significance level.

EVALUATION USING PAIRED DATA

Evaluation data can be paired to screen out unwanted effects. Factors like maturation, learning, and the like can distort evaluation findings. By pairing, these effects are eliminated or blocked.

Take, for example, the introduction of a nurse–practitioner program within a hospital outpatient clinic. To assess the merits of this intervention program, the outpatient clinic's management can determine the extent to which the program's objectives were met. The evaluator examines the program's objectives and defines criteria based on the objectives. The criteria are used to define performance measures. For example, physicians seldom take the time needed to explain the rationale behind their instructions. The nurse–practitioner can be used to interpret instructions to patients. Nurse–practitioner advocates believe that an interpretation will increase the proportion of patients who comply with medical instructions.

Compliance can be used as a proxy to measure the nurse–practitioner program's effectiveness. As patients leave the clinic, they could be asked to recall the instructions they were given, to measure compliance. The percentage of the instructions that were accurately recalled by the patients could be used as a surrogate measure of the success of the nurse–practitioner program. Proxy measures do not measure all facets of an intervention objective. Rather, a good proxy measure captures salient elements of the intervention process to provide an indication of its merit.

Data Collection

To test the value of the nurse practitioner, patients with certain types of presenting conditions would be assigned to one of two queues. In the first queue, a physician identifies an appropriate treatment and instructs the patients. In the second queue, a nurse-practitioner interprets the physician's instructions to the patient after a treatment has been selected by the physician. Patients are asked to recall their instructions by answering questions pertaining to their problem. For instance, flu victims could be asked what to do if symptoms persist in order to self–treat this illness, and to list activity precautions, using a multiple choice questionnaire.

Several extraneous factors can influence the results of such an evaluation. People with life–threatening conditions, chronic conditions (where patients have had a considerable opportunity to learn the ramifications of their ailment, proper treatments, and the need for compliance), and mild or self–limiting problems are likely to have unique rates of compliance. Further, a person's ability to assimilate instruction is influenced by his/her age, educational level, and many other factors. Factors like the time of day may dictate the type of people who come to the clinic. People with unique characteristics may use the clinic at particular times during the day or particular days during the week. Working professionals, for example, who can quickly assimilate the instructions, may tend to visit an outpatient clinic early in the morning. The evaluator attempts to *block* out the influence of these factors to control for their effects.[1]

An example is shown in Table 3–2. Patients with life–threatening and chronic conditions were excluded to control for factors stemming from patient condition. Data were collected on Monday mornings, to control for the "day of the week" effect. On the first Monday, patients who came between 7 and 9 A.M. were assigned a physician. Patients who arrived between 10 A.M. and 12 noon saw a nurse–practitioner after the physician. The next Monday, patients arriving early saw both a physician and a nurse–practitioner; those coming later saw a physician. This procedure blocked for the time of day that patients visited the clinic. The evaluation data are paired by time blocks.

The numbers in parentheses in the example (Table 3–2) indicate the order in which the data were taken in each week. In practice, order is determined by

Table 3-2: Paired Data

Week Number Observation Was Taken	Intervention I Physician Instructs Patients	Intervention II Physician Instructs & Nurse Practitioner Interprets	Difference (d_i)
1	73.2(1)[a]	74.0(2)	.8
2	68.2(2)	68.8(1)	.6
3	70.9(2)	71.2(1)	.3
4	74.3(1)	74.2(2)	-.1
5	70.7(1)	71.8(2)	1.1
6	66.6(2)	66.4(1)	-.2
7	69.5(1)	69.8(2)	.3
8	70.8(2)	71.3(1)	.5
9	68.8(2)	69.3(1)	.5
10	73.3(1)	73.6(2)	.3

$$\Sigma_i \, d_i = 4.1$$

Code (1)   patients who arrive between 7 Am. & 9 Am.
(2)   patients arriving from 10 Am. to Noon

[a] Data measure the percent compliance of all patients exposed to a particular intervention in a given week

something as simple as the flip of a coin. If people who come to the clinic between 7 and 9 in the morning were better able to assimilate instructions, this procedure insures that susceptibility would be equally represented in each comparison group. Using the symbol + for the increased ability to assimilate instructions, randomization distributes susceptability across the interventions as shown in Table 3-3.

Patients were questioned prior to their departure from the clinic. The numbers 73.2 and 74.0 in Table 3-2 indicate the observed compliance rates for patients exposed to physicians and nurse-practitioners (respectively).

A second objective of the nurse-practitioner program might be to improve patients' perceptions of services in the outpatient clinic. A questionnaire could be administered to patients before they leave the clinic to elicit their views. Checks on rating scales, with numbers that range from no satisfaction to 100 percent satisfaction, could be used to quantify patient perceptions. The

Table 3-3

Week	Intervention I	Intervention II
1	+	
2		+
3		+
4	+	
5	+	
6		+
7	+	
8		+
9		+
10	+	

numbers shown in Table 3–2 could represent the average percent satisfaction expressed by patients. In this case, the block would be each patient. A random process, like a coin flip, can be used to select the treatment process. In Table 3–2, the first patient was initially exposed to the physician. On his next clinic visit this patient was seen by the physician, with the nurse–practitioner there to explain the instructions. The second patient was seen by the physician–nurse–practitioner tandem on his first visit, and the physician on his second visit (for a similar problem). This procedure measures perceptions of the nurse–practitioner program, blocking individual differences.

Many other examples could be envisioned in which evaluation data are collected to mask for unwanted effects. The key to quality evaluation information stems from devising clever blocking arrangements.

Analysis Procedure

Evaluation data are shown in Table 3–2. A paired t test is used to isolate differences in the data, controlling for block factors. In the example, time–of–day effects were controlled. The changes in compliance rates caused by the intervention programs were measured so the effects of the block factor could be removed in the analysis.

Statistical tests with paired data are performed using a t statistic. For the data in Table 3–2, the t statistic is formed by subtracting the expected value of the difference in compliance for the nurse practitioner instructions from compliance resulting from the physician's instructions. The observed value of this difference is divided by the variability of the difference. The null hypothesis demands that the expected value of this difference must be zero. The t test permits the evaluator to determine if the observed difference is large, compared to the variation in compliance rates.

First, the mean difference is computed.

$$\bar{d} = \Sigma_i d_i / n = 4.1/10 = .41$$

The standard deviation is computed.

$$s^2 = (\Sigma_i d_i^2 - n\bar{d}^2) / (n - 1) = (3.03 - 1.68) /9 = .15$$

$$s = \sqrt{.15} = .39$$

The t statistic is computed.

$$t = \frac{\text{observed difference} - \text{true difference}}{\text{variability in the observed difference}}$$

$$
\begin{aligned}
t &= (\bar{d} - 0) / s/ \sqrt{n} = \\
&= (.41 - 0) / .39/ \sqrt{10} = \\
&= .41/.12 \\
&= 3.42
\end{aligned}
$$

This value is compared to the critical value t_c (see Table A–1 in the Appendix). The critical value is given by

$$t_c = t_{n-1}, \alpha = t_{9, .05} = 2.262$$

The t statistic exceeds the critical value t_c (3.42 > 2.262), so the evaluator concludes that the nurse–practitioner increased the rate of compliance. (In evaluation a one–tailed test is typically used because, for example, the costs associated with an intervention are expected to be lower than costs stemming from a current practice.)

The confidence interval leads to the same conclusion. The confidence interval is computed by the relationship:

$$\text{Probability } (t_c \leqslant t) = 1 - \alpha$$

Setting $\alpha = .05$ for the data in Table 3–2 yields $t_c = 2.262$. The confidence interval is given by

$$\text{Probability } (2.262 \leqslant \bar{d}\sqrt{n}/s)$$

Expanding, the relationship becomes

Probability $(.14 \leqslant \bar{d} \leqslant .68) = .95$

Ninety–five percent of the time the difference will fall between .14 and .68. Because the confidence interval does not include zero, the difference is termed statistically significant.

Interpretation

The results of the analysis were statistically significant. The nurse–practitioner instructions created more compliance (or more satisfaction) compared to the physician instructions. In each case, the administrator must be concerned with the operational, as well as the statistical, significance of these differences. The average physician's compliance rate was 70.63 percent, and the average nurse–practitioner compliance rate was was 71.04 percent, a difference of less than 1 percent. The cost of the nurse–practitioner program is compared to its performance factors. The administration must ask, "Does a 1 percent increase in patient compliance or a 1 percent increase in patient satisfaction justify the salary and related expenses of a nurse–practitioner?" In the latter case, the answer is probably no. In the former, the consequences of a 1 percent drop in compliance in terms of the health and welfare of the patient must be determined and balanced against the costs of the intervention program. The example illustrates that both the statistical and the *operational* significance of evaluation findings must be considered, and that a statistically significant difference may not yield an important difference.

Data in this example were collected to eliminate several sources of bias, providing a good test of the nurse–practitioner program's benefits. Nevertheless, a judgment must be made by the administrator which balances the increase in compliance (or other benefits) against the costs of the program. This judgment rests upon a stronger foundation because paired data eliminated several sources of bias in the evaluation data.

RANDOMIZATION WITH TWO POPULATIONS

Structural limitations can prohibit the collection of paired data. For example, paired data for a shared service evaluation would require cost information from an equal number of comparable hospitals which dropped and added a particular type of shared service arrangement in a particular year. Hospitals dropping a shared service arrangement are unlikely to make data available for an evaluation. Further, hospitals which add and delete a shared service arrangement in a particular year are unlikely to have similar characteristics.

The same type of problems apply to the nurse–practitioner program evaluation. For instance, to block for individual differences, it was proposed to have patients exposed to one intervention and then the other. Insuring that patients are exposed to a particular form of instruction when they next visit the clinic may prove to be a formidable task. The second visit may be for a completely different problem. The nature of the problem easily could influence satisfaction. Instructions that deal with a serious illness may cause apprehensions that mask any satisfaction a nurse–practitioner could generate.

Data Collection

When data pairing is not feasible, the evaluator attempts to describe samples of two populations. In this example, people's satisfaction after being exposed to the nurse practitioner and to the physician are compared. Randomization is used to insure that the samples of people are similar. For the example shown on Table 3–4, the evaluator randomly assigned patients (except those with chronic or life–threatening problems) to either the nurse–practitioner or the physician as they entered the clinic. As they left the clinic, the patients filled out a questionnaire. The responses to several similar questions were averaged to provide an aggregate satisfaction index for each patient. The numbers shown represent an average of the satisfaction index for all patients assigned to the physician or nurse–practitioner on a particular day. (The numbers in parentheses in Table 3–4 provide a code to recall the week that the data were collected.) A sample question and the response scale are shown in Figure 3.4.

Sample question: "Were the explanations that were provided about your health problems while at the clinic courteous?"

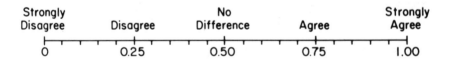

Figure 3.4 SAMPLE SURVEY QUESTION & RESPONSE SCALE

By randomly assigning the patient to a particular treatment process, *each* sample of people should have an equal proportion of the factors that may

Table 3-4.   Independent Data Example

(sample question)   –   "the explanations about my health problem provided while at the clinic were courteous?"

Strongly Disagree	Disagree	No Difference	Agree	Strongly Agree
0	.25	.50	.75	1.00

Intervention I Physician		Intervention II Nurse Practitioner		
62.7	(1)	64.9	(1)	← (sequence data recorded)
61.8	(2)	62.1	(2)	
63.3	(3)	60.7	(3)	
65.2	(4)	63.8	(4)	
60.8	(5)	62.9	(5)	
		69.7	(6)	

$$Ex_1 = 313.8 \qquad Ex_2 = 384.1$$
$$\bar{x}_1 = 62.76 \qquad \bar{x}_2 = 64.02$$
$$n_1 = 5 \qquad n_2 = 6$$

influence perceptions such as income, age, suggestibility, and the like. The variability in the evaluation data may be inflated by each of these factors. (Pairing the data eliminates the influence of such factors by subtraction.)

Analysis Procedure

Evaluation data are shown in Table 3-4. An independent t test is used to compare the average responses, categorized by those exposed to physician or to nurse–practitioner instructions. To carry out this test, the variances from each data set must be pooled. (The example provides an unequal number of samples of patients exposed to the instruction processes, in order to illustrate these calculations.) The variances from each process must be weighted by the differences in sample size. Thus, the pooled variance represents a weighted average of the variance in satisfaction scores taken from patients exposed to the instructions by the physician and the instructions of the nurse practitioner.

The analysis is based on a t statistic, which is given by

$$t = \frac{\text{observed differences} - \text{true difference}}{\text{Pooled variability of observed differences}}$$

$$= \frac{(\bar{x}_1 - \bar{x}_2) - (\mu_1 - \mu_2)}{\sqrt{V(x) \text{ pooled}}}$$

The null hypothesis contends that the satisfaction of people exposed to the nurse–practitioner instructions and physician instructions will be the same. Thus, μ_1 minus μ_2 is zero. The t statistic is formed by subtracting the mean of the data in column one from the mean in column two, divided by the variance of the pooled data.

$$t = \frac{(\bar{x}_1 - \bar{x}_2)}{\sqrt{V(x)}}$$

The pooled variance is a weighted average of the variance for each group, given by

$$s^2_{pool} = \frac{(n_1 - 1)s_1^2 + (n_2 - 1)s_2^2}{(n_1 - 1) + (n_2 - 1)}$$

Carrying out computations

$$s_1^2 = (\Sigma_i x_i^2 - n_1 \bar{x}^2) / (n_1 - 1)$$
$$= 2.75$$
$$s_2^2 = (\Sigma_i x_i^2 - n_2 \bar{x}^2) / (n_2 - 1)$$
$$= 9.81$$
$$s^2_{pool} = 6.67$$

Assuming the covariance is zero, the variance can be pooled

$$V(x) = s_1^2 + s_2^2 = s^2_{pool} \left(\frac{1}{n_1} + \frac{1}{n_2} \right)$$

Finally, the denominator in the t statistic

$$\sqrt{V(x)} = s_{pool} \sqrt{\left(\frac{1}{n_1} + \frac{1}{n_2}\right)}$$

$$= 6.67 \sqrt{\left(\frac{1}{5} + \frac{1}{6}\right)}$$

$$= 1.6$$

The t statistic

$$t = \frac{(64.02 - 62.76) - 0}{1.6}$$

$$= .75$$

This statistic is compared to the critical value, t_c

$$t_c = t_{n-2,\alpha} = t_{a,.05} = 2.262$$

t equals .75 which is less than t_c, at 2.262. The difference in satisfaction is not significant; the null hypothesis is accepted. As before, the confidence interval can be used which will arrive at the same conclusion as the significance test.

Interpretation

No difference in patient satisfaction was found when comparing nurse–practitioner and physician instruction. This is not surprising for two reasons. First, sample size was quite small. Second, and more important, the method of collecting the data had a built–in defect. The evaluator randomly assigned each person, as he/she came through the door, to the nurse–practitioner or the physician for instructions. The variability in people's responses could have masked the effects of the nurse–practitioner program. Stratifying people into various categories helps to eliminate this variability. For example, people could be identified as welfare, self–pay, and third–party–insured. Classifying people by their pay status may control for certain factors like suggestibility or the ability to understand instructions. This procedure reduces the variability in the data, making it easier to find a difference when one exists. For instance, the nurse–practitioner program may be particularly meaningful for low–income people who have difficulty in understanding instructions. If so, the nurse–practitioner program could be directed toward those who can benefit from that program's services. Cost can be reduced because the nurse–practitioners are not needed for all population groups. The program could be directed at population groups where its benefits are demonstrable.

COMPARING PAIRED AND NONPAIRED EVALUATION DATA

The validity and sensitivity of evaluation data trade off. Pairing increases validity. Validity is enhanced because the analysis blocks or screens out the effects of one or more factors, to focus on increases (or decreases) in performance due to the intervention.[1] But pairing observations cuts the available data in half, which reduces the sensitivity of the estimates for the mean and variance.

To illustrate these points, one set of data will be analyzed using both the paired and the independent t test. The purpose of the analysis is to demonstrate the loss of validity that occurs when paired data are analyzed independently. Assume that the data in Table 3–5 represents percent

Table 3-5. Comparing a Paired & Independent Analysis

Observation	Variable Budget Performance (x_1)	Fixed Budget Performance (x_2)	Difference in Performance (d)
1	4	18	14
2	37	37	0
3	35	38	3
4	43	36	- 7
5	34	47	13
6	36	48	12
7	48	57	9
8	33	28	- 5
9	33	42	9
	$Ex_{1i} = 303$	$Ex_{2i} = 351$	$E_i d_i = 48$
	$\bar{x}_1 = 33.67$	$\bar{x}_2 = 39.00$	$\bar{d} = 5.33$

Adapted from Box, G.E.P., et al., *Statistics for Experimentors,* Wiley, New York, p. 179, (1978).

deviation from an actual budget, following the example in the previous chapter. The order in which the departments carried out the budgeting approaches was determined by a coin flip, so the observations could be paired. This procedure blocked for the effects of learning.

The paired t is computed by

$$t = \frac{(\bar{d} - 0)}{s/\sqrt{n}}$$

The variance is given by

$$s^2 = (\Sigma_i d_i^2 - n\bar{d}^2) / (n - 1)$$

$$= 62.25$$

The t statistic is

$$t = \frac{5.33 - 0}{7.89/3}$$

$$= 2.03$$

The table value $t_c = t_{n-1, \; \alpha} = t_{8, \; .05} = 2.31$. A comparison of t and t_c suggests that the difference is significant at the 10 percent level, but not at the 5 percent level. Such a difference would be labeled suspicious but not conclusive.

The independent t is computed by

$$t = \frac{(\bar{x}_1 - x_2) - 0}{s_{pool}/\sqrt{n}}$$

The variance is given by

$$s^2_{pool} = \frac{1192 + 1054}{9 + 9 - 2} = 140.37$$

The t statistic is

$$t = \frac{5.33 - 0}{11.8(1/9 + 1/9)^{.5}} = .96$$

The table value $t_c = t_{n-2, \; \alpha} = t_{16, \; .05} = 2.12$. (Note that the increased sensitivity of the independent t made the critical value smaller.) Because t is much less than t_c, the evaluator finds that the difference is insignificant (unimportant).

In this example the paired data found that the difference between the budgeting approaches merited further study. But when each column of data was analyzed independently, with the variances pooled, no difference was observed. These dramatically different findings can be attributed to the variability among departments which masked the apparent superiority of the variable budgets when the independent t test was used. When paired data can be collected, they are nearly always preferable.

SEVERAL PROGRAM OPTIONS

Up to this point, data collection and analysis procedures have been limited to the comparison of two alternatives, such as comparing costs with and without a shared service program, or patient satisfaction following physician instructions compared to physician instructions elaborated and explained by a nurse–practitioner. The methods described in this section permit the evaluator to compare more than two intervention programs or program options at the same time.

Comparing Several Programs

Continuing with the example in the previous section, several alternatives to physician instructions are compared. The nurse–practitioner program was found to create an increase in patient compliance, but the magnitude of this increase did not seem to justify the costs of the program. This conclusion often stimulates advocates to suggest that a more intensive nurse–practitioner program would produce a justifiable benefit. Nurse–practitioners, trained in a formal educational program, may be able to deal with patients more effectively. Physicians may counter with a proposal of their own, urging the use of a physician–assistant to elaborate their instructions. Such an evaluation considers four instruction programs to determine which has the greatest compliance (or satisfaction). Analysis is carried out to aid the administrator in choosing among various intervention program options.

Data Collection

To collect the needed data, patients as they enter the clinic would be randomly assigned to one of four treatment queues. In one of these queues, patients would receive instructions from the physician. In the others, the instructions would be elaborated by a nurse–practitioner, with and without

Table 3-6: A Comparison of Several Populations

Intervention Program Options

	A	B	C	D
	x_{11}	x_{12}	x_{13}	x_{14}
	x_{21}	x_{22}	x_{23}	x_{24}
	x_{31}	x_{32}	x_{33}	x_{34}
	x_{41}	x_{42}	x_{43}	x_{44}
		x_{52}	x_{53}	x_{54}
		x_{62}	x_{63}	x_{64}
				x_{74}
				x_{84}
Group Averages	$\dfrac{\Sigma x_{1j}}{n_1}$	$\dfrac{\Sigma x_{2j}}{n_2}$	$\dfrac{\Sigma x_{3j}}{n_3}$	$\dfrac{\Sigma x_{4j}}{n_4}$

Grand Mean $\quad \displaystyle\sum_{ij} \frac{x_{ij}}{n}$

Sample Size $\quad n = n_1 + n_2 + n_3 + n_4$

Compliance, x_{ij}, is the average rate of compliance for patients on the ith day exposed to the jth intervention program

training, and a physician–assistant. As before, compliance would be measured by a questionnaire.

The data collection format is shown in Table 3-6. Compliance, X_{ij}, is determined by averaging the compliance rate for patients on day i exposed to intervention program j. The sample size is n and the number of samples in each strata are n_i.

Analysis Procedure

Table 3–7 provides some data which will be used to illustrate the

Table 3–7.   Example Comparing Several Program Options

A	B	C	D	The Interventions are:
62	63	68	56	
60	67	66	62	A = Physician
63	71	71	60	B = Nurse Practitioner
59	64	67	61	C = Nurse Practitioner with formal training
	65	68	63	
	66	68	64	D = Physician's Assistant with formal training
			63	
			59	
Group 61	66	68	61	
Grand Mean 64				

calculation procedures. First, the analysis determines the *variance within*. In this example the variance within is caused by the inherent variability of people's responses. For a difference *between* these options to show up, the variances between the data must be greater than the variances within the data.

The sum of squares for the data in column A (Table 3–7) is calculated as shown below:[2]

$$ss_A = [(62 - 61)^2 + (60 - 61)^2 + (63 - 61)^2 + (59 - 61)^2]$$
$$= 10$$

Sum of squares is one of those fortunate names that indicates the required arithmetic operations. The mean is subtracted from each observation, the difference squared, and each component is added. The subscript A indicates the source of the sum of squares; in this instance the physician's instructions. The remaining sums of squares are calculated in the same manner. These calculations yield

$$ss_B = 40$$
$$ss_C = 14$$
$$ss_D = 48$$

The sum of squares within is given by

$$ss_W = ss_A + ss_B + ss_C + ss_D = 112$$

The sample variance for each program option is the sum of squares divided by its degrees of freedom.

$$
\begin{aligned}
s_A^2 &= ss_A/(n_1 - 1) = 10/3 = 3.3 \\
s_B^2 &= ss_B/(n_2 - 1) = 40/5 = 8.0 \\
s_C^2 &= ss_C/(n_3 - 1) = 14/5 = 2.8 \\
s_D^2 &= ss_D/(n_4 - 1) = 48/7 = 6.9
\end{aligned}
$$

The intrinsic or within–group variation found in the data is given by

$$s_w^2 = \frac{10 + 40 + 14 - 48}{3 + 5 + 5 + 7} = \frac{112}{20} = 5.6$$

The computation for the within–group variation is similar to weighted average of the variation within each column of data. In general, the expression is

$$s_w^2 = \frac{v_1 s_1^2 + v_2 s_2^2 + \ldots + v_n s_n^2}{v_1 + v_2 + \ldots + v_n}$$

where $v_j = n_{j-1}$, the degrees of freedom in sample j

The degrees of freedom in a sample can be understood conceptually. To calculate a variance, another calculation must be carried out. The mean must be determined which uses up one degree of freedom in the data. Again the name implies the operation. The degree of freedom in column A is 3. Put another way, given the mean and three of the four pieces of data in column A, the last piece of information can be deduced. The degrees of freedom for each column of data in Table 3–6 are equal to the number of entries less one. v_i is equal to $n_i - 1$ (v is often used to designate degrees of freedom).

To calculate the *variation between* groups, the data are arrayed as shown below. The group means are listed in the first row. Under that, the grand average is shown. Again, the sum of squares represents the squared deviations of the group means from the grand average.

	A	B	C	D
x_j	61	66	68	61
$\bar{x}$	64	64	64	64
n_j	4	6	6	8
$(\bar{x}_j - \bar{\bar{x}})$	−3	2	4	−3
$(\bar{x}_j - \bar{\bar{x}})^2$	9	4	16	9

where $\bar{x}_j$ = group means

n_j = sample size for strata j

The computation for the sum of squares between, or ss_B, is

$$ss_b = \Sigma_j n_j (\bar{x}_j - \bar{\bar{x}})^2 =$$

$$= \Sigma_j n_j \, ss_j$$

$$= 4(9) + 6(4) + 6(16) + 8(9) = 228$$

The variance between groups is the sum of squares over the degrees of freedom.

$$s_b^2 = \frac{SS_B}{n-1} = \frac{228}{3} = 76.0$$

One degree of freedom was used up to calculate the grand mean; therefore 3 degrees of freedom are left. The sum of squares is divided by the degrees of freedom to give an estimate of the variance.

The data are interpreted using an analysis of variance or ANOVA table. The ANOVA table has five components: source, the source's sum of squares, degrees of freedom, mean square (or variance), and the F ratio. In the ANOVA table, the sum of squares within represents the variation within each column of data. The variance within is the sum of squares divided by its degrees of freedom. Thus, the mean square for the variance within in the ANOVA table is the weighted average of the individual variance components. (It is conceptually similar to the pooled variance used in the independent t test.) The F ratio is constructed by dividing the between-group variance by the within-group variance. If variation within the data is small as compared to the variation between the different intervention programs, the evaluator concludes that the difference between intervention programs may be important. The ANOVA table for the data in Table 3-7 follows:

Source	Sum of Squares	Degrees of Freedom	Mean Square	F Ratio
Between groups	$ss_B = 228$	3	$s_B^2 = 228/3 = 76.0$	$76/5.6 = 13.6$
Within groups	$ss_w = 112$	20	$s_w^2 = 112/20 = 5.6$	
Mean	$n\bar{\bar{x}}^2 = 98,304$	1		
Total	$\Sigma_i\,\Sigma_j\,x_{ij}^2 = 98,644$	24		

To interpret the F ratio in the ANOVA table, a critical value F_c is sought from a table of F values (see Table A-2 in the Appendix). In general, the critical value is given by

$$F_{n_B-1,\ n_w-1;\ \alpha}$$

The degrees of freedom between groups ($n_B - 1$) is 3, and the within–group degrees of freedom is 20 ($n_w - 1$). The critical value at the .05 level

$$F_c = F_{3,\ 20;\ .05} = 3.1$$

The difference between groups was found to be significant, meriting a careful interpretation.

The degrees of freedom in an ANOVA table may be determined in one of several ways. Note that the degrees of freedom for the groups is three. The grand mean is required for this computation, which uses up 1 degree of freedom, resulting in 3 degrees of freedom between groups. Given the total number of pieces of data (24 in the example), the within-group degrees of freedom can be obtained by subtraction ($20 = 24 - (1 + 3)$). To compute the within-group degrees of freedom in another way, recall that 1 degree of freedom is lost for each column of data used to calculate the variance within. Thus, 3+5+5+7, or 20 degrees of freedom, are left.

The total sum of squares in the ANOVA table must equal the sum of squares for the mean plus the sum of squares for the variance within and the variance between comparison groups. In the same way, the total degrees of freedom must equal the degrees of freedom used up in the calculation of the mean, the degrees of freedom assigned to the comparison groups and to the within variation, often called the residual. The total degrees of freedom in the ANOVA table is equal to the sum of the degrees of freedom for each of the source components. The same applies to each mean square, which provides an estimate of the variance associated with each factor in the ANOVA table.

Assumptions

Several assumptions are required in the analysis of variance. Violation of these assumptions may invalidate the ANOVA's conclusions. First, the observations must be independent. To illustrate, if a person is filling out a questionnaire to indicate his/her perceptions and overhears another patient complaining about or praising his/her encounter, this could bias the first individual's views. The evaluator must insure that such an interference did not occur during data collection. A second assumption requires that the strata or cell variances must be equal. The variability within the compliance rates for each of the four intervention approaches should be about the same. (This assumption was somewhat violated in the example. Small sample sizes often cause such problems.) Thirdly, the residual or within–group variation is required to have certain properties. Residuals must be independent, must have a zero mean, and must follow a normal distribution. (The residual variance indicates measurement precision in an evaluation study. Large variances may be unbiased but still may mask important effects.) Finally, the model or cause–and–effect relationship assumed in the evaluation study must be correct. Model correctness is an important assumption that is often ignored or left implicit. For instance, the model dictated by the data in Table 3–7 is

$$y \text{ (observations)} = \text{grand mean } (\bar{\bar{x}}) + \text{group deviations from grand mean } (x_j - \bar{\bar{x}}) + \text{errors } (\epsilon)$$

If this relationship is invalid, the associated statistical analysis can also be invalid.

Conceptual Analysis Procedure

To illustrate the calculations necessary for an ANOVA table conceptually, the data can be decomposed, as shown in Table 3–8. Using the relationships postulated by the evaluation model, several blocks of numbers are constructed to illustrate each of the calculations needed by the analysis of variance.[3]

On the far left in Table 3–7, the observations (average daily patient compliance rates) are shown. Next a data block for the grand mean is shown,

Table 3-8. Decomposition of the Data

Observations x_{ij} (T)				Grand Mean $\bar{\bar{x}}$ (M)				Group Averages x_j (A)				$x_{ij}-\bar{\bar{x}}$ Grand Average (D)				$\bar{x}_j-\bar{\bar{x}}$ Group Deviation (G)				$x_{ij}-\bar{\bar{x}}-x_t+\bar{\bar{x}}$ Residual (R)			
62	63	68	56	64	64	64	64	61	66	68	61	-2	-1	4	-8	-3	2	4	-3	-1	-3	0	-5
60	67	66	62	64	64	64	64	61	66	68	61	-4	3	2	-2	-3	2	4	-3	-1	1	-2	1
63	71	71	60	64	64	64	64	61	66	68	61	-1	7	7	-4	-3	2	4	-3	2	5	3	-1
59	64	67	61	64	64	64	64	61	66	68	61	-5	0	3	-3	-3	2	4	-3	-2	-2	-1	0
	65	68	63		64	64	64		66	68	61		1	4	-1		2	4	-3		-1	0	2
	66	68	64		64	64	64		66	68	61		2	4	0		2	4	-3		0	0	3
			63				64				61				-1				-3				2
			59				64				61				-5				-3				-2

Vector	T	M	A	D	G	R
ss	98,644	98,304	98,532	304	228	112
df	24	1	4	23	3	20

followed by a data block for the group averages. The fourth data block lists the deviations from the grand average. The grand mean is subtracted from each observation. For example, take the upper–left–hand entry in observation matrix 62, and subtract the grand mean (64) from the number, yielding an entry of (–2). The rest of the numbers in the data block were determined in the same manner.

The group deviations were determined by subtracting the grand mean from the group averages. The group average in the first column is 61, and the grand mean 64; thus each of the entries in the first column will be −3. The group averages in the second column is 66 − 64, or +2. The other entries are calculated in the same way.

The residual, as the name implies, is the unexplained variation of the data which remains after the variation associated .with the postulated cause and effect relationship has been accounted for. Essentially the cause and effect relationship (or model) says that the means of the four columns of data can be used to predict any entry in those four columns. The residual is the error in this prediction. To create the residual block of data, the predicted value (group average) is subtracted from its associated observation. In the upper–left–hand entry in this block of data, it is derived by subtracting 62, the observation, from 61, the group average, yielding 1. The rest of the data are calculated in a similar manner.

Beneath these blocks of data in Table 3–8, capital letters are used to designate the ss vectors. The sum of squares computations are shown below the vectors, and below that the degrees of freedom for each block. The sum of squares for each block of data is obtained by squaring and adding in each number in each data block. The sum of squares for the grand mean is calculated in the same way. 64 is squared and multiplied by 24; hence, $n\bar{x}^2$ is the formula for this computation. Sum of squares associated with each data block can be determined by squaring and adding each number in that block of data.

The degrees of freedom can also be determined by a visual inspection of the data. The observations have 24 independent pieces of data. Every observation is different (independent) from every other. The grand mean contains just one piece of information; thus it has one degree of freedom. The group averages have four unique pieces of information: the four group means. The deviations from the grand average, designated by the vector D, have 23 independent pieces of data. This may not be obvious. Recall that the deviation data block entries were derived by subtracting the observations from the grand mean. Thus, with the grand mean, and 23 of the entries in the data block, the last observation can be deduced. As a result, there are 23 degrees of freedom, or 23 independent pieces of data. The group deviations have 3 degrees of freedom. Again, this may not be obvious. Recall that the group deviations were derived by subtracting the group averages from the grand mean. Thus, with three of the group averages and the grand mean, the remaining group averages can be deduced, yielding 3 degrees of freedom. Finally, the degrees of freedom for the residual can be determined by examining each column of data in the residual data block. The residuals in any column must add up to zero. A degree of freedom is lost in each column. For example, with three pieces of information in the first column we can deduce the fourth. There are 3 degrees of freedom in column one, 5 each in columns two and three, 7 in column four; a total of twenty.

Geometric ANOVA

Figure 3.5 presents a geometric interpretation for the ANOVA.[4] A three-dimensional pyramid is pictured using vectors. In this pyramid the total

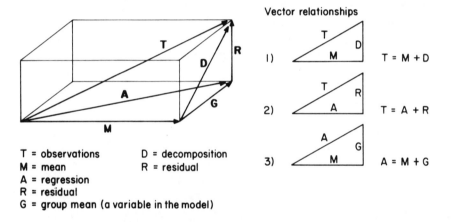

T = observations   D = decomposition
M = mean   R = residual
A = regression
R = residual
G = group mean (a variable in the model)

Recall that the decomposition of the sum of square requires that

$$t^2 = m^2 + d^2 \qquad d^2 = g^2 + r^2$$
$$t^2 = a^2 + r^2 \qquad d^2 = m^2 + g^2$$

Figure 3.5 VISUAL ANOVA

Adapted from: Box, G.E.P., et al., *Statistics for Experimentors,* Wiley: New York, 1978.

sum of squares (T) is equal to the sum of squares associated with the mean (M) plus the decomposition sum of squares (D). Also, the total sum of squares (T) is equal to the regression sum of squares (A), plus the residual sum of squares (R). The regression is a term often used to represent the cause and effect relationship (model) of interest, in this case the four groups' averages. The regression A is made up of two components, the grand mean M and the group effect G. By knowing how to calculate the decomposition vector several other calculations can be avoided. The relationship dictated by the data in Table 3–8 was:

observation = grand mean + group deviations + error

Figure 3.5 illustrates that the same relationship is obtained by following the rules of vector addition:

T = M + G + R.

A geometric explanation of the sum of squares follows the Pythagorean theorem. The square of the long side of each right triangle is equal to the square of the remaining sides, as shown in Figure 3.5.

Both the decomposition of the data and the geometric representation of the sum of squares can be decomposed because the effects are geometrically at right angles. A statistical property called orthogonality results. This allows the ANOVA table to separate the effects of each factor in the model to weigh their importance individually. Other forms of analysis, such as multiple regression, cannot separate out individual effects in the model.

Interpretation

The ANOVA found significant differences in the rates of compliance that stemmed from the four intervention programs. Further analysis is needed to determine which of the four intervention programs to adopt, if any.

A confidence interval must be constructed for each of the four intervention programs.[5] The calculations are shown in Table 3–9. If confidence intervals overlap, these methods of patient instruction provide the same results: patient compliance rates are similar. The 95 percent confidence intervals for the intervention programs are shown in Figure 3.6. They suggest that programs A and D produce lower compliance rates than B and C. Further, the nurse–practitioners with or without formal training (interventions B and C) are superior to either the physician (intervention A) or physician and physician–

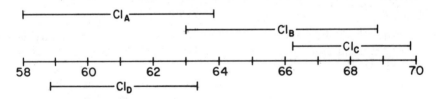

Figure 3.6   CONFIDENCE INTERVALS FOR THE INTERVENTION PROGRAM

assistant (intervention D). The confidence intervals for intervention programs B and C overlap, so the administrator would need additional information to select one of these options. Nurse–practitioners without training might be adopted, should they demand less salary.

Table 3-9.   Selecting an Intervention Program

Recall that:

$$CI = \text{mean} \pm t_{\alpha,n-1}\ s/\sqrt{n}$$

$s_A^2 = 3.3$ $A = 61$

$s_B^2 = 8$ $B = 66$

$s_C^2 = 2.8$ $C = 68$

$s_D^2 = 6.9$ $D = 61$

$$CIA = \bar{A} \pm 1\ t_3, \ _{.05}s_A/\sqrt{n}$$

$$= 61 \pm (3.18)\ \sqrt{3.3/4}$$

or

CIA = 58 to 64

CIB = 63 to 69

CIC = 67.25 to 69.75

CID = 60.6 to 63.4

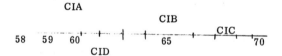

Multifactor Studies with Blocking

When comparing several populations, random assignment to experimental and control groups is used to insure that people with similar characteristics find their way into each comparison group. For instance, certain patients may have more susceptibility to instructions than others. A random assignment of patients controls for susceptibility by attempting to represent the likely range of responses in each comparison group.

Randomization is essential for valid comparisons but tends to inflate the estimate of the residual, called the "variance within" in the last section. The variance in compliance rates for each of the intervention programs will be elevated because the entire range of susceptibility is represented in each comparison group. Large residuals or error variances may conceal important differences in intervention programs which merit further study.

The F and t tests have similar limitations. To increase the chance of finding differences, the error variance must be as small as possible. The error variance is minimal when it captures *only* measurement error. Random assignment will tend to inflate the error variance by including responses caused by a variety of factors which influence people's ability to assimilate information. It is desirable to control for these factors by extracting their effects from the analysis. A technique called a Random Block can be used to collect the evaluation data so the effects of one or more block factors can be extracted in the analysis.

Data Collection

Data for a Random Block are collected as shown in Table 3–10. There are five blocks in this example, defined by levels of income. The compliance rates are classified by income level and by the method used to give patient's instructions. The strata can be defined by the patient's mode of payment: self, third party, Medicare, Medicaid. Patient's pay status is used as a proxy measure of a patient's ability to understand instructions, to block for this effect. Patients are randomly assigned to one of the four queues to receive instructions, hence the name Random Block. The evaluation data are classified into a series of categories as they are collected.

Another block of interest might be patient problems. Patients with serious problems may behave differently from those with minor difficulties. Compliance rates may differ for patients seeking care for routine health problems as compared to chronic or life–threatening problems. Type of problem, as defined by categories in the problem–oriented medical record, could serve as the block. Patients with a particular problem would be randomly assigned to treatment processes A, B, C, or D (Table 3–10). Still other blocks could be considered, including day of the week, sex, age of the patient, and patient condition. In each case, a stratum of patients is randomly assigned to the intervention options.

Many variables may influence the results in an evaluation. To account for several block variables, the data are keyed to strata defined for that variable. For instance, in addition to the patient's mode of payment, patient problem may be recorded. Self–pay, third–party pay, or Medicare and Medicaid

Table 3-10: Comparing Several Populations With Blocking

		METHODS (j)				
		A	B	C	D	(x^i)
	1	x_{11}	x_{21}	x_{31}	x_{41}	$\bar{x}_1$
	2	x_{12}	x_{22}	x_{32}	x_{42}	$\bar{x}_2$
Mode of Payment (i)	3	x_{13}	x_{23}	x_{33}	x_{43}	$\bar{x}_3$
	4	x_{14}	x_{24}	x_{34}	x_{44}	$\bar{x}_4$
	5	x_{15}	x_{25}	x_{35}	x_{45}	$\bar{x}_5$
	$\bar{x}_j$	$\bar{x}_A$	$\bar{x}_B$	$\bar{x}_C$	$\bar{x}_D$	$\bar{\bar{x}}$

x_{ij} is the average complaince observed for people using the ith mode of payment that were exposed to the jth intervention (method)

$\bar{\bar{x}}$ (grand mean) $= \underset{ij}{\Sigma\Sigma}\ x_{ij}/n$

n (sample size) is the cell size times 20

$\bar{x}_A$ is the mean of column A, etc.

patients would also be classified by routine, urgent, chronic, serious, and life–threatening problem categories. To visualize such a data collection scheme, imagine a third dimension running into the page of Table 3–10 in which the data are further segregated. Patients with a particular combination of characteristics would be randomly assigned to one of the four treatment processes. Each observation, at the intersection of a payment mode, patient problem, and method, would represent the average compliance rate for a random sample of patients.

As the number of blocks increase, the data demands go up proportionately.[6] As shown in Table 3–9, controlling for the mode of payment increased the data demands by a factor of five. Five times the data is required for comparable sensitivity. This again illustrates the trade–off between sensitivity and validity. The principles are exactly the same as those described for paired data. When a limited number of block variables can be used to collect data, the variables thought to have the most pervasive effect on the intervention program are selected.

Causal Relationship

Every data collection has an implicit cause and effect relationship or model which the evaluator must make explicit. In the nurse–practitioner evaluation the model states that compliance can be predicted, for a population of patients, by knowing methods of instruction and the patient's mode of payment. This predictive relationship is given by

Observation = prediction + error

And, using the notation in this chapter, by

$$\text{(observation) } x_{ij} = \bar{\bar{x}} + (\bar{x}_i - \bar{\bar{x}}) + (\bar{x}_j - \bar{\bar{x}}) + \epsilon$$

The model has a grand mean, a method effect, a block effect, plus an error term. $\bar{x}_j - \bar{\bar{x}}$ measures the deviations due to method, and $\bar{x}_i - \bar{\bar{x}}$ measures the deviations due to the block factor. The model contends that method variables and block variables, along with the grand mean, can explain the variance in the data. The model predicts an outcome at level i for the block variables and level j for the treatment variable. For example, $\hat{x}_{1A}$ (intervention A for modes of payment 1) can be predicted from $\bar{x}_A$ and $\bar{x}_1$. The prediction equation has the form

$$\hat{x}_{ij} = \bar{\bar{x}} + (\bar{x}_i - \bar{\bar{x}})$$

The error is given by

error = predicted value − observed value

By rearranging terms, the residual (error variance) is computed by

$$\epsilon = \hat{x}_{ij} - x_{ij} = x_{ij} + \bar{\bar{x}} - \bar{x}_i - \bar{x}_j$$

Analysis Procedure

Table 3–11 provides some data to illustrate the steps in the analysis. The data indicate the percent compliance of patients exposed to the four methods, classified by five modes of payment. The analysis follows directly from an understanding of the components of the model, or predictive relationship. Compliance is believed to be influenced by the method used to instruct patients, categorized by the patients' modes of payment.

Table 3–11: Comparison of Several Populations With Blocking[a]

		METHOD				
		A	B	C	D	$\bar{x}_{i\cdot}$
Block	1	89	88	97	94	92
	2	84	77	92	79	83
	3	81	87	87	85	85
	4	87	92	89	84	88
	5	79	81	80	88	82
	$\bar{x}_{\cdot i}$	84	85	89	86	86 = $\bar{\bar{x}}$

x_i average compliance rate when intervention j is used for patients with mode of payment i.

[a]The data in this example were drawn from Box, G.E.P., et al., Statistics for Experimentors, New York: Wiley, 1978.

Three computations are required to construct analysis of variance table: the variance due to method, block, and error.[7] To determine the importance of these factors, the variance explained by the method and the block variables are compared to the unexplained variance or the residual variance. The analysis of variance table lists the results of this analysis.

The data at each intersection of a row and a column in Table 3–11 are the average of several peoples' compliance rates. For instance, an 89 percent compliance rate is shown at the intersection of column A and row 1. Eighty-nine percent is the average compliance rate observed when patients were exposed to Method A (a physician) for payment category one (self–pay). Table 3–12 provides a partial decomposition of the data. This calculation procedure is not efficient for large problems. Rather, it seeks to create an understanding of the purpose and logic behind each step in the analysis.

The data block at the far left of Table 3–12 lists the observations. Next, values for the grand mean, method, and block derivations are provided. They are followed by the compliance rates predicted for each combination of levels of the block and method variables. The right–hand block of data lists the residuals.

To form the block and method deviations, take each of the means for the levels of the block and method and subtract the grand mean. Thus, the rows in the block deviations are given by

$$\bar{x}_i - \bar{\bar{x}} = 92 - 86 = 6$$

Similarly, the columns for the method deviations are

$$\bar{x}_j - \bar{\bar{x}} = 84 - 86 = -2$$

Calculation for the predicted values follows the model

$$\text{prediction} = \text{mean} + \text{block deviations} + \text{method deviations}$$

and, using our notation, by

$$\hat{x}_{ij} = \bar{\bar{x}} + (\bar{x}_i - \bar{\bar{x}}) + (\bar{x}_j - \bar{\bar{x}})$$

The percent compliance is predicted using the average for each row and the average for each column in Table 3–11. The average shown for each row represents levels for the block effect, and the average of each column represents levels for the method effect. To predict compliance, using the postulated cause and effect relationship, an appropriate level of the block effect and the method effect are added and the grand mean is subtracted. The prediction for the typical self–pay patient's compliance to physicians would be 86 + (92 − 86) + (84 − 86) or 90, or simplifying, by

$$\hat{x}_{1A} = 92 + 84 - 86 = 90$$

Table 3-12. Decomposition of Data With Blocking And Several Intervention Programs

x_{ij} Observations				$\bar{\bar{x}}$ Grand Mean				$\bar{x}_i - \bar{\bar{x}}$ Block Deviation				$\bar{x}_j - \bar{\bar{x}}$ Method Deviation				$\hat{x}_{ij} = \bar{x}_j + \bar{x}_i - \bar{\bar{x}}$ Prediction				$x_{ij} - \hat{x}_{ij}$ Residuals			
89	88	97	94	86	86	86	86	6	6	6	6	-2	-1	3	0	90	91	95	92	-1	-3	2	2
84	77	92	79	86	86	86	86	-3	-3	-3	-3	-2	-1	3	0	81	82	86	83	-3	-5	6	-4
81	87	87	85	86	86	86	86	-1	-1	-1	-1	-2	-1	3	0	83	84	88	85	-2	3	-1	0
87	92	89	84	86	86	86	86	2	2	2	2	-2	-1	3	0	86	87	91	88	-1	5	-2	-4
79	81	80	88	86	86	86	86	-4	-4	-4	-4	-2	-1	3	0	80	81	85	82	-1	0	-5	6

Vector	T	M	B	G	P Regression M + G + B	R
ss	148,480	147,920	264	70	8	226
df	20	1	4	3	8	12

To form the residuals, each cell in the observation data block is subtracted from each cell in the predictor data block. For example, the upper–left–hand cell of the observations (self–pay patients' compliance with physicians) is 89. The predictive model suggests that this value should be 90. Therefore, the residual is 89 − 90 or −1 as shown in the upper–left–hand corner of the data block for residuals.

The calculation for the sum of squares is carried out by squaring each entry in the data block in Table 3–12 and adding their elements. There are four sources of variation: the block effect, the method effect, the residual, and the mean. The total sum of squares is equal to the block sum of squares plus the method sum of squares plus the residual sum of squares, plus the mean sum of squares.

The degrees of freedom for each data block can be visualized. To calculate the sum of squares for the method effect, the means due methods are subtracted from a grand mean. Given the means for three of the methods and the grand mean, the mean for the fourth method can be deduced: thus, 1 degree of freedom is lost. The degrees of freedom for the method effect is 3. The same logic is used for the block effect. The calculation process is identical. The degrees of freedom for the block effect is 4. The mean absorbs the additional degree of freedom.

The degrees of freedom for the residual is often found by subtraction. The degrees of freedom for the mean, the block effect, and the method effect are subtracted from the number of observations, or the total degrees of freedom in the data. The residual for the data in Table 3–11 has 12 degrees of freedom (20−4−3−1).

Determining the residual degrees of freedom by an alternative procedure can be insightful. Four means were needed to describe the method effects, so 4 degrees of freedom must be lost from the total of 20 available. The same applies to the block effect, and 5 more degrees of freedom would be lost, for a total of 9. Eight degrees of freedom are subtracted from the total, to avoid double counting. Only 12 of the total of 20 pieces of data that describe the residual are independent. To visualize residual degrees of freedom, note that the sum of any row or any column in the block of residuals in Table 3–12 must be zero. Both the rows and the columns have 1 less degree of freedom than entries that are shown. Draw a line through one row and one column, to account for these dependencies, and count the remaining entries.

The mean squares in analysis of variance table are calculated by dividing each entry's sum of squares by its degrees of freedom. Each mean square also represents the variance of a particular effect. The F ratio is formed by the mean square, associated with a particular effect, divided by the mean square for the residual. The analysis of variance table for the data in Table 3–12 is the following:

Source	SS	d.f.	ms	F ratio
Block	264	4	66.0	3.51
Method	70	3	23.3	1.24
Residual	226	12	18.8	
Mean	147,920	1		
Total	148,480	20		

Each F ratio is compared to its critical value. For the block effect $F_c = F_{4,12,.05} = 3.26$, and the method effect $F_c = F_{3,12,;.05} = 3.49$. If the calculated F ratio is larger than the critical value, the method effect is significant. The interventions did not have an important effect. In the example shown, the method effect was not significant. As anticipated, the block effect influenced compliance rates.

A Geometric Interpretation of the Effects

The analysis of variance can be illustrated geometrically, as shown

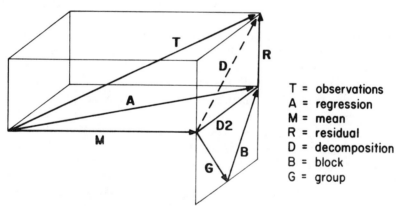

T = observations
A = regression
M = mean
R = residual
D = decomposition
B = block
G = group

G & B provide one additional split of the sum of squares

Figure 3.7 GEOMETRIC REPRESENTATION OF THE ANOVA

in Figure 3–7. As before, T represents the total (sum of squares), R represents the residual, and A the regression (model) sum of squares. The property of additivity is insured by the right angle between the vectors A and R. This permits a breakdown of the total sum of squares into two components: the regression and the residual. The regression is further broken down into D2 and the mean, where D2 is composed of the G (group effect) and B (the block effect).

When analyzing data retrospectively, a Multiple Regression approach is often used. A criterion used by multiple regression is the amount of variance in the data explained by the regression equation A divided by T. The percent variance explained is called "regression coefficient" or the "coefficient of multiple determination."

Prospective data collection schemes permit the evaluator to separate components of the regression to consider each individually. The breakdown breaks out the mean and decomposition component (D2). The decomposition component (D2) can be further broken down into the treatment effect (G) and the block effect (B). Thus, prospective data collection schemes permit the evaluator to study the effect of each variable. Multiple Regression can only directly assess the relationship as a whole.

Interpretation of the Results

The analysis of variance table is used to interpret the evaluation results. First, the evaluator determines whether the intervention program produced a result. In the current example none of the interventions had an effect on compliance, when mode of payment was blocked. If the results had been significant, confidence intervals would be calculated for each method to describe how particular types of interventions altered patient compliance rates. The importance of these effects would be judged by considering the costs of each intervention. The administrator compares the rate of compliance in each intervention with its costs to judge the value of each intervention.

The random block analysis points out several important decision points in an evaluation study. First, the evaluator must carefully construct the cause and effect relationship (or model) which indicates how performance measures are though to be related to the interventions. The relationship is expanded to include intervening factors that seem likely to influence performance. In this example, patient's susceptibility to instructions, defined by patient's mode of payment, was used as the block variable. The evaluator could have blocked for the day of the week, patient problem, or other factors. Next, the evaluator must consider the trade-off between sensitivity and validity. Several block variables may have important effects. But adding block variables dramatically increases the data demands. For example, adding five kinds of patient problems as an additional block would increase the data demands fivefold.

Observations represent samples drawn from naturally occurring populations and populations created by the evaluation. The intersection of each row and column in Table 3-11 identifies a particular population. The population of self–pay patients was sampled in the evaluation. Another population was created by randomly assigning patients who fall in each payment mode to one of the interventions. The observation is the mean of a sample drawn from that population. For instance, the average response of self–pay patients to physicians was 89. The sample size of an evaluation study is the number of samples drawn for each population times the number of populations considered.

The decision rule used to draw conclusions in evaluation studies is based on variances. Variances are composed of sums of squares adjusted by the degrees of freedom in the samples drawn from a population. As the number of samples increase, the denominator in this relationship becomes smaller and the F ratio increases. So every entry in the analysis of variance table is affected when the residual or error variance gets large. Large residual variances increase the chance that inherent variability in the data will mask differences in the intervention programs. The evaluator must always trade off sensitivity and validity against the cost of data collection.

TESTS FOR MODEL ADEQUACY

The assumptions required in analysis of variance follow:

(1) *Independent:* Each observation used to compute the mean of a cell, shown in Table 3–11, is assumed to be independent. For instance, patients filling out questionnaires are assumed to be responding according to their experiences and not to be influenced by the comments of other patients.

(2) *Equal cell variance:* The variances for the data, at the intersection of any row and column (Table 3–11), are assumed to be similar. For example, the variance of patient compliance associated with self–pay patients who see physicians is assumed to be equal to the variance in patient compliance for Medicare patients who receive instructions from a nurse–practitioner.

(3) *Residuals:* The residuals are assumed to be independent and normally distributed, with a zero mean.

(4) *Cause and effect relationship or model:* The model must be correct for the analysis to be valid. The models presented in Chapter 3 assume additive effects.

Assumptions concerning the distribution of residuals and cell variances are robust. Departures from these assumptions must be extreme before the results become invalid. But when the model is incorrect, the analysis becomes meaningless.

Tests for model adequacy are indirect, examining the properties of the residuals. Draper and Smith plot residuals against the study variables in an evaluation study as a test of model adequacy.[8] Graph a in Figure 3.8 illustrates the desired pattern when residuals are plotted against another variable. A random pattern is required to validate the model. The spread or width of the random pattern is related to the size of the residual's variance.

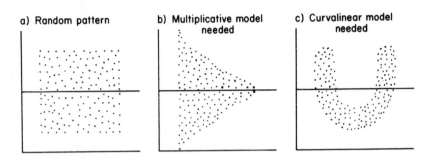

Figure 3.8 RESIDUAL PLOTS TO TEST MODEL ADEQUACY

Graph b in Figure 3.8 illustrates a plot where the residuals get smaller as some other variable increases. In this case the linear assumption is invalid and a multiplicative model is needed. A curvilinear model is required when the residuals follow a U–shaped relationship (graph c) as some other variable increases.

Typically, residuals are plotted against the block and the treatment variable, against observations, against the *order* in which the observations were recorded, and against the predicted values. To construct a plot of the residual and the block variable, associate the value of a particular residual with the corresponding value for block variable. To illustrate, the block effect is plotted against the residuals. The block effect of 6 is plotted against the residual values of $-1, -3, +2$, and $+2$ shown in Table 3–12. The result is shown on Figure 3.9. The other rows in the block deviations in Table 3–12 are also plotted against the corresponding row in the residual matrix. Plots of the method effect, predicted values, and still other variables are constructed in the same way.

Another important check can be made to see whether the residuals shifted during the study. The residuals could be plotted against the order in which the data were collected to detect whether learning effects and other changes over time occurred which can invalidate the analysis.

In summary, a critical assumption in the ANOVA is the model. The model's adequacy can be checked by plotting residuals against values of several variables. If these plots result in rectangular bands of data, the model or causal relationship is assumed to be valid. (Typically, computers provide these plots as an optional output of statistical analysis.)

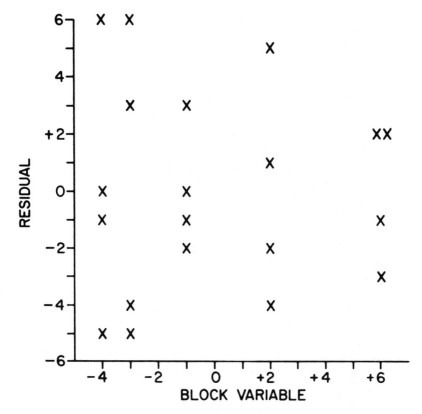

Figure 3.9 RESIDUAL PLOT FOR BLOCK FACTOR

EVALUATIONS WITH SEVERAL FACTORS,
EACH WITH SEVERAL LEVELS

In the previous example, the evaluation considered a causal relationship that had intervention program options and several levels of a block factor. The evaluator sought to explore the effects of the program options, independent of these block effects. Data were collected and categorized according to the occurrence of levels of a block variable. Often evaluations must block for more than two factors. In other cases, the evaluation project may seek to compare several policy options, each with several levels.

Data collection devices which can compare three of more factors, each with several levels, can be constructed. For instance, three factors, each with four levels, can be investigated by placing the data into 64 (4x4x4) strata. For example, data could be collected by randomly assigning patients with a given pay status and condition to one of the four interventions. This model is given by:

$$x_{ijk} = \bar{\bar{x}} + (\bar{x}_i - \bar{\bar{x}}) + (\bar{x}_j - \bar{\bar{x}}) + \bar{x}_k - \bar{\bar{x}}) + \epsilon$$

Each observation x_{ijk} is predicted by the grand mean, $\bar{\bar{x}}$, the deviations due to method, $\bar{x}_i - \bar{\bar{x}}$, and the deviations due to block factors, $\bar{x}_j - \bar{\bar{x}}$ and $\bar{x}_k - \bar{\bar{x}}$. The number of variables can be increased again, which would add a fourth factor to the relationship. If this variable also had four levels, the sample size would be 256 (4 × 4 × 4 × 4) times the number of samples drawn for each population, creating the need for considerable data.

Several designs (or data collection devices) have been proposed to reduce data demands. A "Latin Square" design is used to study the effects of three variables, each with several levels. For instance, sixteen strata are used to study the effects of three variables, each with four levels. Assuming four samples are drawn from each population, the data demands are cut from 256 (4 samples × 64 strata) to 64 (4 samples × 16 strata). To study four variables, a "Graeco Latin Square" can be used, with a similar reduction in the data requirements.

Latin Square and Graeco Latin Square designs are efficient, but have several undesirable features.[9] In particular, they cannot provide an estimate of interaction effects: the effectiveness of the practitioner when dealing with low–income (Medicaid) patients. Designs which allow the assessment of interactions terms while minimizing data requirements will be described in the next chapter.

NOTES

1. Additional information on blocking can be found in Box G.E.P., W.G. Hunter, and J. S. Hunter, *Statistics for Experimentors,* New York: Wiley, 1978.
2. Procedures described in this section were drawn from Box G.E.P., *et al., Statistics for Experimentors,* New York: Wiley, 1978 (Chapter 4, "Randomization and Blocking with Paired Comparisons").
3. *Ibid.,* p. 176.
4. *Ibid.,* p. 179.
5. Least significant difference (LSD) t tests for all pairs of levels in a variable are reccommended as the best way to select a preferred alternative when several must be compared. (Carmer S.G. and M.R. Swanson,"On Evaluating Ten Pairwise Multiple comparison Procedures," *J.A.S.A.* Vol 68, No 341, March 1973, pp. 66–74.) Comparing Confidence intervals for each option is similar to the pairwise procedure and conceptually easier to appreciate the decision rule that is used.
6. Evaluation studies should allow for a sample size of at least five times the number of strata. For instance, in the nurse–practitioner evaluation there were 4 options, 5 modes of payment, and 5 patient problems yielding (4 x 5 x 5) 100 strata. A sample size of 500 would be recommended. Thus, a minimum of 5 samples per strata or cell can be used as a crude rule of thumb. This rule is based on how an estimate of variance stabilizes as additional samples are drawn. See Box G.E.P.

and J.S. Hunter, "Multifactor Experimental Designs for Exploring Response Surfaces," *Annals of Mathematical Statistics*, Vol. 28, 1959, pp. 195–241, for details.

7. Procedures described in this section were drawn from Box G.E.P. *et al.*, *Statistics for Experimentors*, New York: Wiley, 1978. (See chapter 7, "Randomized Blocks & Two–way Factorials, p. 208–228.)

8. Draper, N. and H. Smith, Chapter 4, "The Examination of Residuals," in *Applied Regression Analysis*. New York: Wiley, 1966.

9. For a discussion of Latin Square and Graeco–Latin Square designs and their limitations, see Davies, O., *The Design and Analysis of Industrial Experiments*. New York, Hafner: 1967.

More Complex Evaluation Experiments

Happy is the man who has learned the cause of things, and has put under his feet fear, inexorable fate, and noisy strife...

Francis Bacon

Most evaluations consider or control several extraneous variables to give the findings of an evaluation a clearer meaning. As the number of block and policy variables[1] increases, the value of the data collection methods described in Chapter 3 declines. Because they must consider all levels of evaluation variables, the data demands become extensive, leading to costly evaluation projects. The data collection procedures discussed in this chapter permit a formal study of several variables and variable interactions while minimizing the amount of data that must be collected.

FACTORIAL EVALUATION EXPERIMENTS

The data collection plan in this chapter is specified by a "factorial design."[2] Factorials consider all combinations of high and low levels of the evaluation variables, permitting an assessment of the effects that result from *interactions* among these variables. This permits factorial arrangements to be efficient, collecting only the minimum number of observations.

Factorial designs collect data to explore how a system (or a person) responds to various treatments. The effects of several treatment variables are studied over a specified range for each variable. For instance, a patient's age and the time since the onset of symptoms may be important indicators of prognosis, given a diagnosis of ischemic heart disease. The evaluator hopes to draw conclusions that hold over a wide range of values for age and time since the onset of symptoms. This range is called the "operational region" of the study.

Factorial designs assume a linear relationship between the causal factors (independent variables) and the performance measure.[3] The magnitude of the slope of this line determines the importance of the relationship between the independent (cause) and dependent (effect) variables. The best estimate of a slope is obtained by sampling at the extreme points on the independent variable. For instance, if age is an important factor in compliance to medical instructions, an evaluator might sample the behavior of very old patients and patients as yet unaffected by the aging process. To explore the relationship between age and methods of presenting instructions, 60 to 65 year olds could be used to represent the second group and 80 to 85 year olds the first group. Samples taken at the extreme points along the independent variable (age) provide the best estimate of the slope of the line that represents the linear decrease in compliance associated with age. Factorial designs employ such a sampling process.

Two-level factorial designs are used when a linear relationship is assumed by the causal model. The two levels refer to the two points where data are collected to approximate the linear relationship.

Table 4-1.   Factorial Design in Two Variables

The Factorial Design

Yates Order	Weight x_1*	Diagnosis x_2	Design Matrix		Mortality Rate (Observations)
1	1000 grams	RDS	-1	-1	$y1$
2	3000 grams	RDS	1	-1	$y2$
3	1000 grams	SGA	-1	1	$y3$
4	3000 grams	SGA	1	1	$y4$

* within 100 grams

Geometric Representation

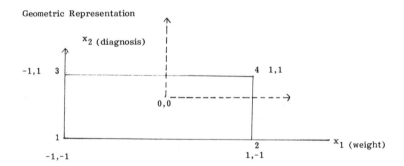

The experimental arrangement for a two level factorial design is shown in Table 4–1. In this example, birthweight (in grams) and diagnosis (two independent conditions) are used to estimate the expected survival of infants in a neonatology ward. Rather than collecting data over the range of diagnoses and weights, the evaluator samples at extreme points which define the operational region. In this example, the operational region is defined as weights of 1000 or 3000 grams (within 100 grams) and by a diagnosis of prematurity or respiratory distress syndrome (RDS). (See Figure 4.1.) The impact of two variables are tested: diagnosis and birthweight. A linear relationship between these variables and mortality is assumed.

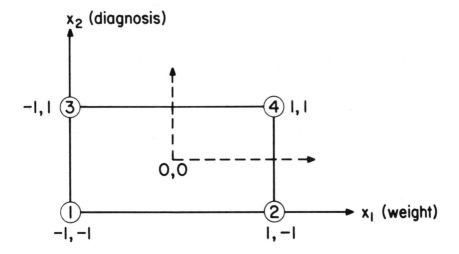

Figure 4.1 REPRESENTATION OF A FACTORIAL IN TWO VARIABLES

The independent variables (diagnosis and birthweight) illustrate that the factorial design can collect data defined in several ways. Birthweight is measured on a continuous scale. The factorial has the evaluator sample at two points along the scale which defines an infant's weight. Diagnosis has a binary or dichotomous scale. The levels for the diagnosis in a neonatology ward could be determined by ranking their approximate severity, as shown below:
(1) prematurity
(2) hyperbilirubinemia
(3) small for gestational age (SGA)
(4) patient ductus arterious (PDS)
(5) idiopathic respiratory distress syndrome (RDS)
(6) RDS and hyperbili

(7) RDS and PDA

(8) Bronchopulmonary displasia (BPD)

(9) meconium aspirations

Diagnoses with a particular interest can be selected, and sampling would be restricted to these categories.

Factorials can also sample an independent variable defined by integers. For instance, the APGAR score is made up of integers, running from 1 to 10, which are assigned to depict a newborn's general condition.[4] Sampling could be restricted to infants with scores of 1 and 5 if these APGAR scores represent a large portion of the newborns in a neonatology ward.

The independent variables are coded as shown in Figure 4.2. The scale of the "weight variable" is transformed to a coded scale where –1 represents the

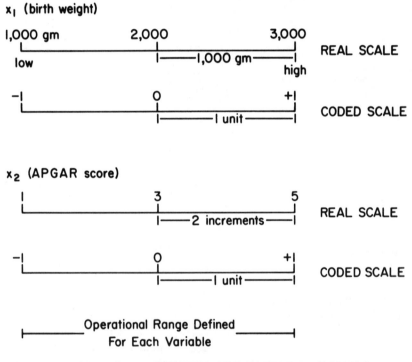

Figure 4.2 CODING ILLUSTRATION FOR FACTORIAL DESIGNS

low level of birthweight and +1 represents the high level of birthweight. The formula for this coding relationship is given by

$$x_n = \frac{x - [xmax + xmin]/2}{[xmax - xmin]/2}$$

The coding for the weight variable, where W is the baby's weight, is given by

$$x_W = \frac{W - (1000 + 3000)/2}{(3000 - 1000)/2} = \frac{W - 2000}{1000}$$

The coding for the APGAR score follows the same logic. The relationship is given by

$$x_A = \frac{(APGAR - (1 + 5)/2)}{(5 - 1)/2} = \frac{APGAR - 3}{2}$$

The diagnosis variable is coded by associating its low level, –1, with the more severe condition, RDS; and the high level, +1, with the less severe condition, prematurity. Figure 4.2 illustrates how the coding transforms the operational range for each variable. Two thousand grams for birthweight and 2 increments for the APGAR Score are transferred to a standard 1 unit. For dichotomous variables, –1 and +1 are associated with the categories of interest.

The design matrix (Table 4–1) defines several strata or populations. Observations are drawn from each strata. (These strata are often called contrasts.) When two variables are considered in a factorial design, four strata are observed, two levels raised to the power of two variables. For a two–level design, the general relationship between observations and number of variables is given by

$$2^k = n \qquad \text{where } k = \text{ number of variables}$$
$$n = \text{ number of observations}$$

The design matrix is constructed by writing down the pattern shown in Table 4-1. This pattern results in what is called "Yates Order," after its originator. The settings for first variable begin with –1 and alternate between the high and low values. The second variable begins with the value of –1 in the first two positions followed by +1 in the last two positions. This pattern represents all combinations of two variables with two levels (2 x 2). Observations are taken for each combination of levels defined by the Yates Order.

Conceptually, a factorial design generates data which are used to construct a response surface.[5] The response surface describes how a measure of effectiveness increases (or decreases) with changes in the independent variables. A plane is constructed from the means of several observations taken at each of the four possible settings for variables x_1 and x_2. The model describing the cause and effect relationship for this data collection procedure is shown below.

$$\text{Response} = \begin{array}{c} \text{average} \\ \text{response} \end{array} + \begin{array}{c} \text{linear} \\ \text{effects} \end{array} + \begin{array}{c} \text{interaction} \\ \text{effects} \end{array} + \epsilon$$

Following the notation to be used in this chapter, the relationship for a two–variable model is given by

$$y = b_0 + b_1x_1 + b_2x_2 + b_{12}x_1x_2 + \epsilon$$

where b_0 = average of the observations
b_1 = slope of variable x_1
b_2 = slope of variable x_2
b_{12} = warp, twist, or slant
in the plane

Figure 4.3 illustrates some hypothetical response surfaces in two variables.

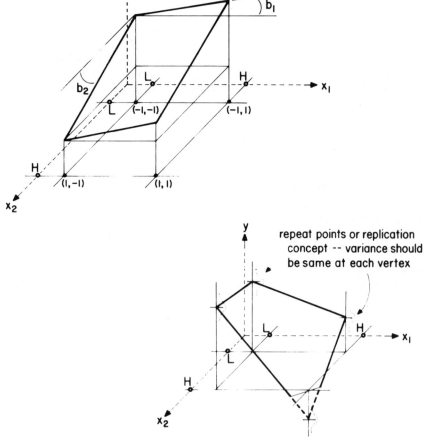

Figure 4.3 RESPONSE SURFACE FOR A FACTORIAL DESIGN

The parameter b_0 represents the grand mean of the data. The grand mean can be visualized as a flat plane that bisects the response surface, a fixed distance from the plane x_1x_2. b_1 represents the slope on variable x_1 and b_2 represents the slope on variable x_2. In the upper diagram in Figure 4.3, the slope on x_1 is increasing, whereas the slope on x_2 is decreasing. This means that as the variable x_1 increases (from the low setting to the high setting), the response (y) also increases. However, as variable x_2 increases from the low level to the high level, the response decreases. The interaction term is close to zero. Thus the plane has no appreciable tilt or warp. The response surface specifies the expected response predicted by knowing the values of x_1 and x_2. In this example, to maximize the response, variable 1 would be set at its high level, and variable 2 set at its low level.

A somewhat more complex response surface is shown at the bottom of Figure 4.3. In this illustration, the interaction term (x_1x_2) distorts the response surface at high values of x_1 and x_2, making the predicted response become negative. Evaluation data is used to construct a response surface for the system (person) under study so predictions about responses can be made for points that fall within or near the operational region of the study variables.

For three or more variables the response surface becomes more complex and difficult to picture. However, the same principles apply. Responses are predicted over the range of variables that were studied. A linear or proportional response is assumed as variables change from their low levels to their high levels.

Following the equal variance assumption, the variance among the repeat observations, for particular variable settings, should be the same. The other assumptions discussed in Chapter 3 also apply. In particular, it is assumed that the observations are independent, that prediction errors (the residuals) are independent normally distributed random variables with a zero mean, and that a linear model provides a reasonable approximation of the relationship between each variable and the response.

FACTORIALS IN THREE VARIABLES

Assume that an administrator in a for-profit chain of hospitals is charged with improving profits in the chain's cafeterias. The administrator seeks the advice of experts in restaurant management to determine a list of factors that may stimulate sales and thus profits. Assume that menu, music, and number of food items are suggested. The food option can be defined in several ways. A fast-food franchise like McDonald's could be sought, a delicatessen could be started, or the food selections in the cafeteria could be altered. Food items could be defined as the variety of food offered (e.g., the aggregate number of beverages, salads, entrees, and desserts offered). Several music types could be provided (country, classical, folk, or rock), or music could be defined in terms of its obtrusiveness, measured by its loudness. The response of the system (profit in the cafeteria) is to be studied when treatments are applied which alter food, music, and menu options.

Definition of Contrasts (strata)

An experimental arrangement used to test the effects of music loudness, food items, and food options is shown in Table 4-2. A linear relationship

Table 4-2. 2 Level Factorial Design in Three Variables

YATES ORDER	Food Options x_1	Music Loudness x_2	Beer Varieties x_3	Design Matrix	Profits (Observations)
1	McDonalds	10 db	1 local	-1 -1 -1	y_1
2	Deli	10 db	1 local	1 -1 -1	y_2
3	McDonalds	50 db	1 local	-1 1 -1	.
4	Deli	50 db	1 local	1 1 -1	.
5	McDonalds	10 db	5 imports	-1 -1 1	.
6	Deli	10 db	5 imports	1 -1 1	.
7	McDonalds	50 db	5 imports	-1 1 1	.
8	Deli	50 db	5 imports	1 1 1	y_8

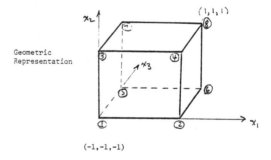

Geometric Representation

$(1, 1, 1)$

$(-1, -1, -1)$

between each variable and the measure of effectiveness (profit) is assumed. Each of the variables under study (music, food, items) are treatments which will be manipulated during the evaluation. The music system's loudness has a continuous scale. The system's loudness can be set using a decibel indicator. Food items are integers, depicting various combinations of items that can be made available. In this example a limited number of items will be compared to an extended range of items. The food option is a dichotomous variable: a McDonald's franchise or a deli.

The coding for the variables in Table 4–2 is shown below:

$x_1 = -1$: McDonald's
    $+1$: deli
$x_2 = (M - 30)/20$
$x_3 = -1$: Limited (5 beverages, no salads, 4 entrees, no desserts)
    $+1$: Extended (10 beverages, 2 salads, 8 entrees, 2 desserts)

The Data Collection Approach

The *design matrix,* shown in Table 4–4, specifies how the data will be collected. Switching from a McDonald's franchise to a deli at regular intervals is clearly infeasible. The needed data could be collected by offering both types of food on a trial basis, assuming that vendors offering each food option could be persuaded to provide food service for one year on a trial basis. Contracts with the food vendors would be written for a year. The first three months of the study would allow the vendors a "shake–down" period to initiate service. In the next month, data would be collected in both the deli and the McDonald's food outlets. Observations 1, 3, 5, and 7 would be collected in the McDonald's food service. Observation 1 determines the profit y_1, (revenue less operating costs) over a period of one month when music is set at its low level with a "limited" number of food items available in the McDonald's food area. For observation 3, the music volume in the McDonald's food service area is turned up, retaining the limited menu. Observation 5 determines profit (y_5) in the McDonald's food service after the music volume is reduced with an extended list of food items added; and observation 7 maintains the extended menu and turns up music volume and measures the McDonald's profit (y_7) for the month. The deli would be operated at the same time, collecting data to measure profits for variable settings defined by observations 2, 4, 6, and 8. To control for a variety sequence effects, observations 1, 3, 5, and 7 and 2, 4, 6, and 8 are taken in a random order.

Both McDonald's and the deli are operated at the same time. The availability of both food options allows customers to choose, incorporating demand factors into the profit measures. But collecting the data over a four–month period may introduce sequence effects: one type of food may be tried, and then another. A second set of data is often collected to determine the precision that profit was measured in each stratum, defined by the Yates Order. Observations for each of the 8 variable settings would be collected a second time. This creates an eight–month study, with three months for start–up and one month for analysis.

Constructing the Design Matrix

The pattern in the design matrix can be constructed in two ways. The contrasts can be represented geometrically by a cube, shown in Figure 4.4. The vertices of the cube define each of the eight observations which represent all combinations of the three variables, each with two levels. The numbers of the vertices of the cube correspond to the Yates Order, used to number the observations in the design matrix. Note how the vertices in the cube correspond to those observations in the design matrix in the same way that the

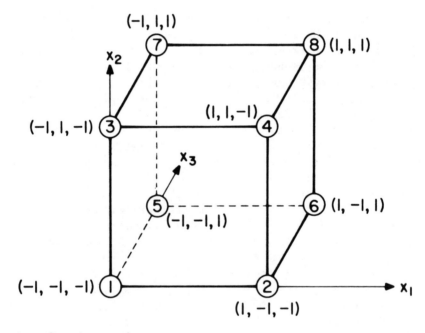

1····8 yates order

Figure 4.4 GEOMETRIC REPRESENTATION OF A FACTORIAL IN THREE VARIABLES

vertices in the squares for two variables corresponded to the observations in the design matrix in Figure 4–1.

The pattern in the design matrix can be created by following a simple rule. The first column in the design matrix is constructed by beginning with the low level and alternating −1, +1, −1, +1, etc. The total number of observations is always an even number, determined by raising two levels to a power corresponding to the number of variables tested. The second column of data has two observations at the low level followed by two at the high level, with the pattern repeating −1, −1, +1, +1, etc. The third column has four observations at the low level followed by four observations at the high level. Yates Order "one" requires data to be collected with each variable set at its low level. The profit (revenues less cost) would be determined with a McDonald's food service, the music set at 10 decibels, with limited menu.

The conceptual relationship between the levels of the variables in the design matrix and the geometric representation of the variables should be carefully studied. It is often helpful to identify the variable settings associated with each vertex of the cube shown in Figure 4–4 and relate them to the corresponding Yates Order number to verify that the settings are the same. For example, vertex one represents the low level for each variable and corresponds to Yates Order One. Vertex 8 would represent the high level of each variable and corresponds to Yates Order 8.

The distance between any two vertices is measured by the coded intervals. Recall that each variable was transformed and centered at zero. Moving from zero to the point where observations are taken corresponds to *one* unit for each variable. The variable coding simplifies the calculations and is helpful in visualizing how the computations are carried out. Careful inspection of the coded variables should point out that all combinations of the variables have been considered. Also note that the axis for the independent variable must run through the center of the cube.

Analysis Procedure

A factorial design assumes that the cause and effect relationship is made up of main effects and interactions among these variables. The predictive relationship for the example can be written as follows:

total		average		linear effects due		interactions		
profit	=	profit	+	to music, menu,	+	between all	+	error
				& food policy		combinations		
				variables		of the policy		
						variables		

And, in the notational form used in this example, the relationship is given by

$$y = E_0 + E_1x_1 + E_2x_2 + E_3x_3 + E_{12}x_1x_2 + E_{13}x_1x_3 + E_{23}x_2x_3 + E_{123}x_1x_2x_3 + \epsilon$$

where y = response (profit)

x_i = policy variable i

E_i = the effect of variable i (a main effect)

E_{ij} = the joint effect of variables i & j (a two–way interaction)

E_{ijk} = the joint effect of variables i, j, & k (a three–way interaction)

ϵ = error

Assume that the data shown in Table 4–3 were collected for the evaluation

Table 4–3: Sample Data For A Three Variable Factorial Design For The Cafeteria Example

Yates Order	Food x_1	Music x_2	Menu x_3	y_a	y_b	y_i
1	-1	-1	-1	4,200.	4,600.	4,400.
2	1	-1	-1	4,600.	4,200.	4,400.
3	-1	1	-1	3,500.	4,300.	3,900.
4	1	1	-1	3,800.	4,600.	4,200.
5	-1	-1	1	3,900.	4,100.	4,000.
6	1	-1	1	5,000.	4,800.	4,900.
7	-1	1	1	4,100.	3,700.	3,900.
8	1	1	1	4,700.	4,100.	4,400.

experiment. To interpret, when the music, menu, and food variables were set at their low levels, average profits were $4,200 and $4,600, for an average of $4,400 over the two–month period. Thus $4,400 is the average response for

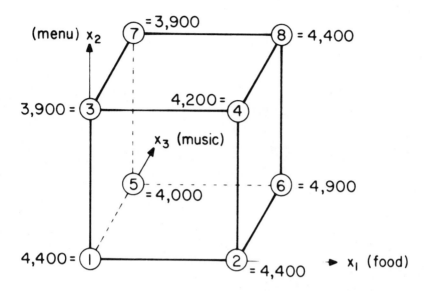

Figure 4.5 GEOMETRIC REPRESENTATION OF
SAMPLE DATA

observation one. Each response can be keyed to the cube, providing a geometric representation as shown in Figure 4.5.

Figure 4.6 provides a graphic illustration of how the *main effects* in the factorial design can be calculated.[6] The shaded sides of the cube represent all responses associated with the food variable set at its high and low levels. To assess the effect of the food options, all the vertices associated with the plane on the left, the low level, are subtracted from those at the right, the high level. This calculation is carried out below.

Food (x_1)

$$
\begin{array}{llll}
(2 - 1) = 4{,}400 & 4{,}400 = & 0 \\
(4 - 3) = 4{,}200 & 3{,}900 = & 300 & 1{,}700/4 = 425 \\
(6 - 5) = 4{,}900 & 4{,}000 = & 900 \\
(8 - 7) = 4{,}400 & 3{,}900 = & 500
\end{array}
$$

The top and the bottom faces of the cube represent the average profit associated with music set at its high level and its low level. To assess the effect of music, the average responses associated with the low levels (the bottom plane) are subtracted from the responses at the high level (the top plane). The

Main Effect (E_1)

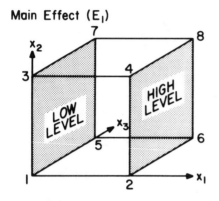

Interaction Effect (E_{12})

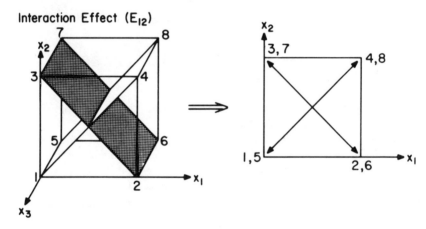

Figure 4.6   GEOMETRIC APPROACH IN THE COMPUTATION
OF EFFECTS

Adapted from Box, G.E.P., et al., *Statistics for Experimentors,* Wiley, New York, p. 312, (1978).

main effect for menu is computed in the same way. The main effects were found to be

E₁ (FOOD)   =   425
E₂ (MUSIC) = −325
E₃ (MENU) =   75

These effects show that profits were increased by \$425 per month by the deli food service. (This effect would be negative if the McDonald's franchise stimulated greater profit because the McDonald's option was associated with the low level in the design.) Profits declined by $325 per month when music was changed from a low to a high level and a small increase in monthly profit ($75) followed the introduction of an extended menu.

To compute the two–factor *interaction effects* the cube is collapsed on one variable so the joint impact of the remaining two variables can be assessed. Interaction effects are computed by holding all factors not involved in the interaction constant and computing the cross product. Eliminating variable x_3 collapses the cube into the plane x_1x_2, which permits the interaction x_1x_2 to be calculated. In the plane x_1x_2, vertices 1 and 5 appear at the same point as do vertices 2 and 6, 4 and 8, and 3 and 7. To compute the interaction effect, the responses associated with the high level of one factor and the low level factor of the other are subtracted from the responses associated with the low level and the high level of these same factors. Using the numbers of the vertices as aids (see Figure 4.5), the effect associated with the two-factor interaction x_1x_2 is computed by

$$E_{12} = \tfrac{1}{4}[(1 + 4 + 5 - 8) - (2 + 3 + 6 + 7)]$$

Substituting for the responses yields

$$E_{12} = \tfrac{1}{4}[(4,400 + 4,200 + 4,000 + 4,400) - (4,400 + 3,900 + 4,900 + 3,900)] = 25$$

Using the same approach gives

$$E_{13} = 275$$
$$E_{23} = 25$$

Interaction effects occur when the responses change comparing the high level of one factor and the low level of another to the high level of the second factor and the low level from the first. In this example, only the E_{13}, the food–beer interaction, seems important. To explore the magnitude of this effect a two–way table of means is constructed.

		McDonald's Food	Deli
Menu	limited	4,150	4,300
	extended	3,950	4,650

The extended menu and the deli acted together to produce from $350 to $700 additional monthly profits.

Figure 4 7 provides a guide to identify potentially important main effects

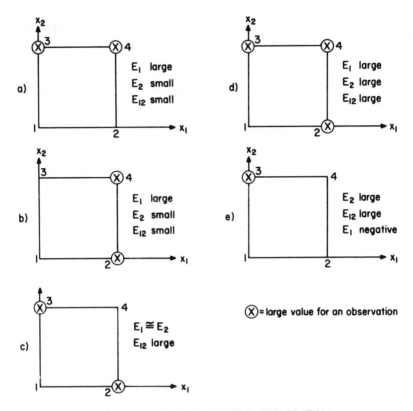

Figure 4.7   IDENTIFYING EFFECTS THAT MERIT EXPLORATION

and two–way interactions by inspection. In diagram (a), the response at Yates Points 3 and 4 is "large." The high levels on variable x_2 must be larger than its low levels, making E_2 potentially important. Both the high level and the low level of variable x_1 have one of the large responses, so their effect cancels. E_1 is likely to be small. Interactions are computed by the cross product $(1 + 4) - (2 + 3)$. The large values cancel, suggesting that the interaction term E_{12} is small. Diagram (b) creates a situation where E_1 is potentially important, but E_2 and E_{12} are not. In diagram (c), the interaction is important because large response values occur on the diagonal, but the main effects are unimportant. This seldom occurs in practice. Diagrams (c) and (d) illustrate typical situations where interactions tend to occur: three or just one of the responses are comparatively large.

The three–factor interaction is shown geometrically in Figure 4–8. There are two pyramids in the cube. The three–way interaction can be computed by subtracting the vertices of one pyramid from the other and averaging. In this

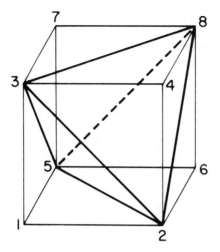

Figure 4.8   COMPUTING 3-WAY
INTERACTIONS

Adapted from: Box, G.E.P., et al.,*Statistics for Experimentors,* Wiley: New York, p. 312 (1978).

example, the three way interaction is found to be

$$E_{123} = \tfrac{1}{4}[(2 + 3 + 5 + 8) - (1 + 4 + 6 + 7)]$$
$$= \tfrac{1}{4}[(4,400 + 3,900 + 4,000 + 4,400) -$$
$$(4,400 + 4,200 + 4,900 + 3,900)]$$
$$= 175$$

The highest average profit of $4,900 occurs with observation 6 (Yates Order 6). The next highest level of profit is $4,400, suggesting that an increase in monthly profit of $500 was observed with deli food, an extended menu, and soft music.

The findings in this contrived example are typical. Two–way interactions seldom occur unless main effects of one of its factors are also important. Similarly, three-way interactions are seldom important unless two of the variables combine in a two–way interaction that is also important.

The significance (importance) of the observed differences is interpreted with an analysis of the variance in the data. The analysis of variance (ANOVA) table is constructed following procedures like those discussed in Chapter 3. The calculation formula for the sum of squares column, in the analysis of variance, is

$$ss = \tfrac{1}{4}nE^2 \qquad \text{where} \quad n = \text{number of observations}$$
$$E = \text{effect}$$
$$ss = \text{sum of squares}$$

The sum of squares for factor 1 is computed as

$$ss_1 = 16/4 \, (425)^2 = 722,500$$

In this example, there are seven decomposition factors, three main effects, three two–way interaction effects, and one three–way interaction. A sum of squares is computed for each variable. Because there are two levels, each variable in a factorial design always has 1 degree of freedom. One degree of freedom is used up for each main effect, each two–way and three–way interactions, and the grand mean, for a total of 8. The residual has 8 degrees of freedom (16 observations less the 8 used up by the model and the grand mean). The analysis of variance table for the data in Figure 4–5 is shown in Table 4.4.

Table 4.4
ANOVA for Cafeteria Example

Source	Code	SS	df	MS	F
Food	X_1	722,500	1	722,500	5.25
Music	X_2	422,500	1	422,500	3.07
Menu	X_3	22,500	1	22,500	.16
Food–Music	X_1X_2	2,500	1	2,500	.02
Food–Menu	X_1X_3	302,500	1	302,500	2.20
Music–Menu	X_2X_3	2,500	1	2,500	.02
Food–Music–Menu	$X_1X_2X_3$	122,500	1	122,500	.89
Residual		1,100,000	8	137,500	
Corrected Total		2,697,500	15		

The percent of the variance expanded by the model, called the "multiple correlation coefficient" or the "coefficient of multiple determination," is given by

$$R^2 = \frac{\text{Variation Explained In Model}}{\text{(Corrected) Total Variation}}$$

$$= (2,697,500 - 1,100,000)/2,697,500 = .592$$

This ratio can be tested by an F, given by $F_{7,15;.05}$ in this example. Because the R^2 measures the significance of the model, and not the variables in the model, it has limited value in an evaluation.

Interpretation

Thus F values in the ANOVA table are compared to critical values to detect their significance.

$$F_c = F_{1,8;.05} = 5.32$$
$$F_c = F_{1,8;.10} = 3.46$$

The food variable is significant at the .05 level and the music variable is nearly significant at the .10 level. The interaction effects that appeared to be so interesting were not statistically significant. (The residual variability in the study may have masked these effects.) This finding suggests that increased profits can be obtained with deli food and that soft music is preferable. Limited menu would be served, as no statistically significant preference for the extended menu was found. If the interactions had been important, the policy variables in the interaction would have to be moved in the appropriate direction *at the same time*. For instance, had the music–menu interactions been significant, soft music coupled with an extended menu would be necessary to insure the desired response: increased profit.

AN ANALYSIS PROCEDURE FOR LARGE EVALUATIONS

For large evaluation problems involving factorials with several variables, the geometric calculations of the data quickly become tedious. The design matrix provides another way to carry out the necessary calculations.

* Matched naturally occurring groups (e.g., neighborhood held centers). Physicians are matched to equate their initial views toward the medical record.

Table 4-5. Constructing the Calculation Matrix

Yates Order	Design Matrix			Calculation Matrix					Observations
	x_1	x_2	x_3	$x_1 x_2$	$x_1 x_3$	$x_2 x_3$	$x_1 x_2 x_3$	x_0	y_i
1	-1	-1	-1	(-1)(-1)=1	1	1	(-1)(-1)(-1)=-1	1	y_1
2	1	-1	-1	-1	-1	1	1	1	y_2
3	-1	1	-1	-1	1	-1	1	1	y_3
4	1	1	-1	1	-1	-1	-1	1	y_4
5	-1	-1	1	1	-1	-1	1	1	y_5
6	1	-1	1	-1	1	-1	-1	1	y_6
7	-1	1	1	-1	-1	1	-1	1	y_7
8	1	1	1	1	1	1	1	1	y_8

Analysis Procedure

The design matrix lists the coded values for each variable. These values specify settings for each variable which govern how the data will be collected. The calculation matrix is formed by multiplying columns in the design matrix to create each of the interaction terms in the predictive equation. The calculation matrix for a 2^3 factorial is shown in Table 4–5. To construct a column for the interaction term x_1x_2, all coded entries in the column x_1 are multiplied by the entries in the column x_2. This is shown in the x_1x_2 column in

Table 4–5. The column for the interaction term x_1x_3 comes from multiplying columns x_1 and x_3. x_0 represents the calculation column necessary to compute the grand mean.

The column associated with each variable in Table 4–6 is multiplied by the column of responses . For variable 1, the x_1 column is multiplied by the column of observations. The first response is subtracted from the second, the third from the fourth, the fifth from the sixth, and the seventh from the eighth, creating a vector of values

Table 4-6. Calculating the Value of Effects With the Design Matrix

	x_1	x_2	x_3	x_1x_2	x_1x_3	x_2x_3	$x_1x_2x_3$	y_a	y_b	Mean	$(y_a-y_b)_d$
1	-1	-1	-1	1	1	1	-1	4200	4600.	4400.	-400.
2	1	-1	-1	-1	-1	1	1	4600	4700.	4400.	400.
3	-1	1	-1	-1	1	-1	1	3500.	4300.	3900.	-800.
4	1	1	-1	1	-1	-1	-1	3800.	4600.	4200.	-800.
5	-1	-1	1	1	-1	-1	1	3900.	4100.	4000.	-200.
6	1	-1	1	-1	1	-1	-1	5000.	4800.	4900.	200.
7	-1	1	1	-1	-1	1	-1	4100.	3700.	3900.	400.
8	1	1	1	1	1	1	1	4700.	4100.	4400.	600.

Design Matrix
(Specifies how to
collect the data)   Observations
              Calculation Matrix
       (Specifies how to compute effects)

$$b_1 = [-1(y_1) + 1(y_2) - 1(y_3) + 1(y_4) - 1(y_5) + 1(y_6) - 1(y_7) + 1(y_8)]/8$$
$$b_1 = [-4,400 + 4,400 - 3,900 + 4,200 - 4,000 + 4,900 - 3,900 + 4,400]/8$$
$$b_1 = 212.5$$

b_1 specifies the slope of the relationship between variable 1 and its effect. Using the same approach, slopes for two- and three-factor interactions are calculated by

$$b_{12} = (4,400 - 4,400 - 3,900 + 4,200 + 4,000 - 4,900 - 3,900 + 4,400)/8 = 12.5$$
$$b_{123} = (-4,400 + 4,400 + 3,900 - 4,200 + 4,000 - 4,900 - 3,900 + 4,400)/8 = 87.5$$

Each slope is calculated in the same way. The column representing the variable is multiplied by the column labeled observations. The grand mean is determined by adding all the observations, as implied by the column of ones labeled x_0.

To compute a slope, each entry in the calculation matrix is multiplied by the responses and the total is divided by the number of observations. Calculation equations for b_{12}, b_{123} and b_0 are given by

$$b_{12} = (y_1 - y_2 - y_3 + y_4 + y_5 - y_6 - y_7 + y_8)/8$$
$$b_{123} = (-y_1 + y_2 + y_3 - y_4 + y_5 - y_6 - y_7 + y_8)/8$$
$$b_0 = (y_1 + y_2 + y_3 + y_4 + y_5 + y_6 + y_7 + y_8)/8$$

The geometric approach provided different results. It computed a value for each variable in its original scale units. Multiplying the vectors in the calculation matrix by the observations requires division by the total number of contrasts to scale the grand mean properly. As a consequence, the effect E is equal to two times the slope b in these calculations. This is shown graphically in Figure 4–9. The slope, b, is calculated by a ratio of the rise, y divided by the increment, x, or $b = y/x$. In this example the rise y is equal to E, the magnitude of the effect, and the increment x is two standard units so the relationship becomes $b = E/2$. The ANOVA table is made up of these rescaled "b" or regression values which are used to study the effects associated with a particular variable.

The residual or error sum of squares can be calculated using a short cut when there are two repeat values or one replication for each combination of variables. For Yates Order One, with each variable set at a "low" level, profits of 4,200 and 4,600 were observed. In a well–controlled experiment, with little measurement error, these responses would be nearly the same. The difference between the responses is an indicator of error. The residual sum of squares can be computed from the squared differences in responses collected with the variables set at a particular level.[9]

Yates Order	y_a	y_b	d_i	d_i^2
1	4,200	4,600	−400	160,000
2	4,600	4,200	400	160,000
3	3,500	4,300	−800	640,000
4	3,800	4,600	−800	640,000
5	3,900	4,100	−200	40,000
6	5,000	4,800	200	40,000
7	4,100	3,700	400	160,000
8	4,700	4,100	600	360,000

$\sum_i d_i^2 = 2,200,000$

ss residual $= \frac{1}{2} \Sigma d_i^2 = \frac{1}{2} \ 2,200,000 = 1,100,000$

The ANOVA calculations are the same as those in the geometric approach.

$ss_i = \frac{1}{4} \ n \ (E_i)^2 = \frac{1}{4} \ n \ (2b_i)^2 = nb_i^2$

The ANOVA calculations and conclusions based on the slope, b, are identical to those based on the effect, E.

Interpretation

The parameters in the causal relationship (the b's or the E's) represent the "importance measures" for each variable. Confidence intervals can be constructed around these parameters to interpret them for managerial decision

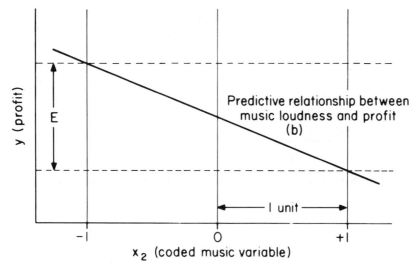

E = value of the effect
b = slope of the regression line for that effect

Figure 4.9 RELATIONSHIP BETWEEN E AND b

making. The parameter variance in a factorial design is given by

$$V(\text{effect}) = \frac{4s^2}{r2^k}$$

where s^2 is the residual, or error variance
r is the number of replications
k is the number of variables
V(effect) is the variance for a given effect

For a three variable factorial
    $V(\text{effect}) = s^2/4$
the standard deviation of each effect is given by
    $SD(\text{effect}) = s/2$
In the example
    $SD(\text{effects}) = (137,500)^{.5}/2 = 370.81/2 = 185.4$
and for the regression parameters
    $SD(b) = s/4 = 92.7$
The range, defined by two standard error limits, for each parameter in the
model is given in Table 4–7.

Table 4-7.
Confidence Intervals for Effects in Cafeteria Example

	geometric (E or Effects)			regression (b or slopes)		
x_1	425	±	370	213	±	185
x_2	−325	±	370	−163	±	185
x_3	75	±	370	38	±	185

FRACTIONAL FACTORIAL EVALUATION EXPERIMENTS

Factorial evaluation experiments demand consideration of all combinations of variables. Several explanatory variables will dramatically increase the number of required observations. Several hundred observations are often required. For example, a full factorial with seven variables would require 256 (2 — 27) observations, with two replications per contrast. With four replications per contrast, 512 observations are needed.

The Fractional Factorial Design was devised to reduce these data requirements.[10] They can be useful when a large number of variables may have an impact and little is known about the importance of these variables, and thus no basis exists to rule out any of the variables. For example, a for–profit hospital corporation seeking to explore the impact of management contracts on the unit costs of hospital purchasing must control or block for several variables. Participating hospitals are likely to differ in terms of their size (measured by number of beds), the services they offer, the composition of the medical staff, including the number with joint hospital privileges and board certification status in particular specialty areas, dollar investment in tertiary care services, the relative scarcity of beds in the community in which each hospital resides, and the availability of skilled personnel in the community.

Fractional factorial designs permit an evaluation of a large number of variables. A confounding pattern is selected that is best for a particular study. The evaluator deliberately mixes some main effects and higher order interactions will have little explanatory power. This allows the evaluator to screen for the effects of particular variables. But the effects of variables are confounded, or mixed, with higher order interactions, so their impact must be studied indirectly. The advantage of fractional factorial designs is the reduction in the data demands, whereas their limitation is the confounding that must be introduced in the estimation of each variable's effect.

Fractional factorial designs also provide a framework for carrying out sequential evaluation projects. When the costs of an observation are very high or when the evaluator is limited in number of observations that can be taken at any point in time, sequential experimentation is very useful. A half fraction can be run at one point in time, followed by the remaining observations at a later point. By combining the two sets of observations the full factorial is obtained. A quarter fraction and still smaller fractions can be run in larger data–collection efforts. For example, a financial manager of a multihospital corporation may be interested in studying the impact of various budgeting procedures in comparable hospital departments. The treatment variable includes the two budgeting options. Other variables could define differences in the departments such as their projected volume of activity, managerial skills, and past performance in cost control. It may be easier to justify an evaluation that assesses these variables with sequential data collection. Initially four departments (two high–volume and two low–volume) prepare two budgets, using both budgeting approaches. (The order in which the budgeting approach was carried out by each department must be randomized.) To minimize disruption in the hospitals, four departments would participate in the first phase of the evaluation. Four more departments would participate at a later point in time. Ultimately the evaluator can build an information file that will be totally diagnostic, representing a full factorial in the variables to be assessed.

In some evaluation studies, specific combinations of the variable levels cannot be realized. For example, to predict the number of nursing hours required in a neonatology unit, information describing the infant's gestational age, body weight, and diagnosis may be required. However, the diagnosis "Aspirations" never occurs for small babies (between 750 and 2,500 grams). On the other hand, "Hylane Membrane" disease never occurs in babies above 3,000 grams. Thus, some combinations of diagnosis and body weight are physically impossible and never occur. Fractional factorial designs provide patterns that can permit data collection which avoids impossible combinations of the variables, extrapolating between combinations of the variable that *can* be realized.[11]

The 2^{3-1} Fractional Factorial

Data Collection Approach

The simplest fractional factorial design is shown in Table 4–8. Four contrasts are required. To study the third variable, observations are taken using the interaction term in the calculation matrix, x_1x_2, to specify the settings for variable x_3 as shown in Table 4–9. The third variable is deliberately confounded with an interaction term. So the design matrix for the 2^{3-1} fractional factor design specifies settings for the variables by using the interaction term in a 2^2 factorial. Three factors can be studied in four tests (with

Table 4-8.   The 2^{3-1} Fractional Factorial Design

x_1	x_2	x_1x_2			x_1	x_2	(x_3) x_{12}	x_0
-1	-1	(-1)(-1)	1		-1	-1	1	1
1	-1	(1)(-1)	-1	=>	1	-1	-1	1
-1	1	(-1)(1)	-1		-1	1	-1	1
1	1	1	1	1	1	1	1	1

Design Matrix

Calculation Matrix

Effect x_3 is confounded with x_1x_2

a known variance), a very efficient evaluation experiment.

The geometric relationship between the half fractional and the full fraction is shown in Figure 4.10. The observations in the half fraction correspond to observations 2, 3, 5, and 8 in the 2^2 design. For a sequential evaluation, observations associated with the Yates Order 2, 3, 5, and 8 can be collected initially. The remaining observations (1, 4, 6, 7), which correspond to the other half fraction, could be collected at some later point in time.

Analysis Procedure

The confounding pattern can be identified in two ways. The model is always based on the lower order design. For instance, the model for 2^{3-1} design is based on a 2^2 design and given by

$$y = \hat{b}_0 + \hat{b}_1x_1 + \hat{b}_2x_2 + \hat{b}_3x_3 + \epsilon$$

where $\hat{b}_i$ represents an estimate of effect i. The confounding relationship is given by I = 123, because variable 3 is mixed with variable 12. The parameters measured in a 2^{3-1} are

$$\hat{b}_0 = b_0 + b_{123}$$
$$\hat{b}_1 = b_1 + b_{23}$$
$$\hat{b}_2 = b_2 + b_{13}$$
$$\hat{b}_3 = b_3 + b_{12}$$

Table 4-9.   Relationship Between Half and Full Fractions

2^2 Fraction				2^3 Fraction							
x_1	x_2	$x_1x_2{=}x_3$		x_1	x_2	x_3	x_1x_2	x_1x_3	x_2x_3	$x_1x_2x_3$	x_0
-1	-1	1	1	-1	-1	-1	1	1	1	-1	1
1	-1	-1	2	1	-1	-1	-1	-1	1	1	1
-1	1	-1	3	-1	1	-1	-1	1	-1	1	1
1	1	1	4	1	1	-1	1	-1	-1	-1	1
			5	-1	-1	1	1	-1	-1	1	1
			6	1	-1	1	-1	1	-1	-1	1
			7	-1	1	1	-1	-1	1	-1	1
			8	1	1	1	1	1	1	1	1

Confounding relationship

3 = 12   or   123

Parameters that can be estimated

mean + 123
1 + 23
2 + 13
3 + 12

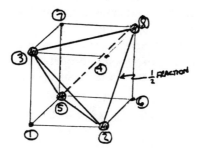

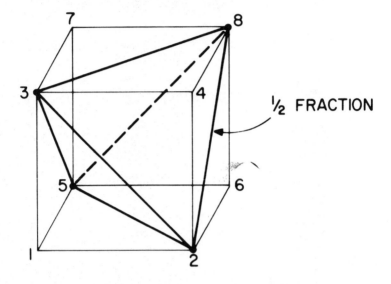

Figure 4.10 GEOMETRIC RELATIONSHIP BETWEEN THE HALF & FULL FRACTION IN A 2^{3-1}

The confounding relationship can be verified by inspecting the columns in the calculation matrix in Table 4–9. Note that for observations 2, 3, 5, and 8 in the 2^3 factorial, column x_1 and column x_2x_3 are identical. Also, column x_2 and column x_1x_3, column x_3 and column x_1x_2, and columns x_0 and $x_1x_2x_3$ are identical for these observations. The design cannot determine whether x_i or x_{ij} has been measured, so the effects of these variables are confounded or mixed. Similarly, x_0 is mixed with the high level of x_{123}.

Fractional factorial designs assume that a proportional or linear relationship among variables provides an adequate approximation of the response surface. The model is written in terms of the confounded factors as

$$y = (b_0 + b_{123})(x_0 + x_1x_2x_3) + \hat{b}(x_1 + x_2x_3) + \hat{b}_2(x_2 + x_1x_3)\,\hat{b}_3(x_3 + x_1x_2) + \epsilon$$

where
$$\hat{b}_1 = b_1 + b_{23}$$
$$\hat{b}_2 = b_2 + b_{13}$$
$$\hat{b}_3 = b_3 + b_{12}$$

The analysis of variance is givén by

Source	Source Code	SS	df
Variable 1	$x_1 + x_2x_3$	$n\hat{b}_1^2$	1
Variable 2	$x_2 + x_1x_3$	$n\hat{b}_2^2$	1
Variable 3	$x_3 + x_1x_2$	$n\hat{b}_3^2$	1
Mean	$x_0 + x_1x_2x_3$	$n\hat{b}_0^2$	1
Residual		by subtraction	4
Total		Σy_i^2	8

Each of the parameters in the model estimates the value of a main effect and a two–way interaction. (Note that only four parameters can be interpreted by this ANOVA.) The fractional factorial design confounds (mixes) main effects and two–way interactions. By assuming that the two–factor interactions are zero, an estimate of each main effect can be made. With responses representing a month of cafeteria profits, a 2^{3-1} factorial provides an estimate of the effects of music, menu , and food in an eight–month interval, with two replications. The food effect (x_1) is confounded, or mixed, with the interaction effect associated with music loudness (x_2) and menu variety (x_3). The same is true for the other main effects: the music effect is mixed with the menu effect acting in conjunction with food options, and the effect of the menu is mixed with the combined effect of music and food options.

The 2^{4-1} Fractional Factorial

Data Collection Approach

A 2^{4-1} fractional factorial design in Table 4–10 uses 16 observations to study four variables, each with two levels, with 2 observations per contrast. Using the example of the cafeteria, the administrator may study how combinations of three variables, (food, music, and menu options), and fourth variable, hours of service, influence profits. (In this example, the low level for hours of service could be defined by breakfast and lunch hours only, and the high level by continuous service, such as 6:00 AM to midnight.) The menu and music as well as the hours of service can be altered at monthly intervals for each food service. Using a fractional factorial, the study can be completed in eight, rather than sixteen months.

Observations 1, 4, 6, and 7 are collected for McDonald's, and 2, 3, 5, and 8 for the deli. One observation from each set would be obtained at the same time. The data collection plan for one of the months is given by observation

Table 4-10: The 2^{4-1} Fractional Factorial Design

Yates Order	x_1	x_2	x_3	$x_1x_2x_3=x_4$	x_1x_2	x_1x_3	x_2x_3	x_0
1	-1	-1	-1	-1	1	1	1	1
2	1	-1	-1	1	-1	-1	1	1
3	-1	1	-1	1	-1	1	-1	1
4	1	1	-1	-1	1	-1	-1	1
5	-1	-1	1	1	1	-1	-1	1
6	1	-1	1	-1	-1	1	-1	1
7	-1	1	1	-1	-1	-1	1	1
8	1	1	1	1	1	1	1	1

x_1 music (-1 is 10db; +1 is 50 db)

x_2 menu (-1 is limited; +1 is extended)

x_3 hours of service (-1 is limited; +1 is continuous)

x_4 food options (-1 is McDonald's; +1 is the deli)

Confounding Relation

$$x_4 = x_1x_2x_3 = 1234$$
$$I = 1234$$

1 [−1, −1, −1, −1] and observation 2 [1, −1, −1, 1]. Interpreting for observation 1, soft music, limited menu, and limited hours of service would be offered in the McDonald's outlet and somewhat louder music, limited menu,

and hours of service in the deli. Customers could choose, and profits would be computed for the month for both the deli and McDonald's.

In the second month, observations 3 and 4 could be collected. For the deli (observation 3), the music would be turned down, an expanded menu adopted, and limited service maintained. The McDonald's food service (observation 4) would turn up the music volume, expand the menu, and continue with limited service. Observations 5, 6, 7, and 8 are interpreted in the same way. The music is turned up or down, menu items added or deleted, and hours of service expanded or contracted. At some point in the eight–month interval, each combination of variables would be repeated. (To control for sequence effects, the order would be randomized.)

Analysis Procedure

Table 4–10 describes the ideal data collection arrangement for a 2^{4-1} fractional factorial design. The fourth variable is confounded with the three–way interaction. The confounding relationship is 1234. As a result, each main effect is mixed with a three–factor interaction (1 with 234, 2 with 134, 3 with 124, and 4 with 123). Each two–factor interaction is mixed with one other two–factor interaction. The interaction term x_1x_2 is mixed with x_3x_4, x_1x_3 mixed with x_2x_4, and x_2x_3 mixed with x_1x_4. The cause and effect relationship that accounts for this confounding pattern, is given by

$$y = \hat{b}_0 + \hat{b}_1x_1 + \hat{b}_2x_2 + \hat{b}_3x_3 + \hat{b}_4x_1x_2x_3 + \hat{b}_{12}x_1x_2$$
$$+ \hat{b}_{13}x_1x_3 + \hat{b}_{23}x_2x_3 + \epsilon$$

$$\text{where} \quad \hat{b}_0 = b_0 + b_{1234}$$
$$\hat{b}_1 = b_1 + b_{234}$$
$$\hat{b}_2 = b_2 + b_{134}$$
$$\hat{b}_3 = b_3 + b_{124}$$
$$\hat{b}_4 = b_4 + b_{123}$$
$$\hat{b}_{12} = b_{12} + b_{34}$$
$$\hat{b}_{13} = b_{13} + b_{24}$$
$$\hat{b}_{23} = b_{23} + b_{14}$$

The analysis of variance is given in Table 4–11.

Note that the sum of squares for each main effect is mixed with a three–way interaction, the sum of squares for each two–way interaction is mixed with another two–way interaction, and the sum of squares for the four–way interaction is mixed with the mean.

Table 4-11.   Anova For the 2^{4-1} Fractional Factorial Design

Source	Code	ss	df
Variable 1	$x_1 + x_2 x_3 x_4$	nb_1^2	1
Variable 2	$x_2 + x_1 x_3 x_4$	nb_2^2	1
Variable 3	$x_3 + x_1 x_2 x_4$	nb_3^2	1
Variable 4	$x_4 + x_1 x_2 x_3$	nb_4^2	1
Variable 12	$x_1 x_2 + x_3 x_4$	nb_{12}^2	1
Variable 13	$x_1 x_3 + x_2 x_4$	nb_{13}^2	1
Variable 23	$x_2 x_3 + x_3 x_4$	nb_{23}^2	1
Mean	$x_0 + x_1 x_2 x_3 x_4$	nb_0^2	1
Residual		by substraction	8
Total		Ey_i^2	16

If any of the variables are significant, the evaluator works backward to deduce which merit further study. For example, if variable 1 turns out to be significant, either the main effect (x_1) or the three–way interaction ($x_2 x_3 x_4$) could have been responsible. The evaluator can often rule out three–way interactions, unless they have a particular meaning in a postulated cause and effect relationship. When variable 12 is significant, either $x_1 x_2$ or $x_3 x_4$ could be the cause. To interpret, if x_3 and x_4 were insignificant and if the main effect x_1 (or x_2) had significance, the $x_1 x_2$ interaction term merits further study. Fractional factorial designs are often called screening designs because they allow the evaluator to select variables that should be considered in a follow–up evaluation.

Other Fractional Factorials

A 2^{5-1} fractional factorial design is illustrated in Table 4–12. As before, the ideal half fraction is formed by confounding the fifth variable with a highest order interaction term, in this case 1234. The design matrix, which specifies how to collect the evaluation data, includes the calculation column for the four–way interaction. A 2^{5-1} fractional factorial design corresponds with 2^4

Table 4-12: The 2^{5-1} Fractional Factorial Design

Yates Order	x_1	x_2	x_3	x_4	$x_1x_2x_3x_4=x_5$	x_1x_2	x_1x_3	$x_1x_2x_3$	x_0
1	-1	-1	-1	-1	1	1	1	-1	1
2	1	-1	-1	-1	-1	-1	-1	1	1
3	-1	1	-1	-1	-1	-1	1	1	1
4	1	1	-1	-1	1	1	-1	-1	1
5	-1	-1	1	-1	-1	1	1	-	1
6	1	-1	1	-1	1	-1	-		1
7	-1	1	1	-1	1	-1			1
8	1	1	1	-1	-1	1			1
9	-1	-1	-1	1	-1	1			1
10	1	-1	-1	1	1	-1			1
11	-1	1	-1	1	1	-1			1
12	1	1	-1	1	-1	1			1
13	-1	-1	1	1	1	1			1
14	1	-1	1	1	-1	-1			1
15	-1	1	1	1	-1	-1			1
16	1	1	1	1	1	1			1

Confounding Relationship $x_5 = x_1x_2x_3x_4$

$$I = 12345$$

factorial design and requires one half the observations of a full fraction. The confounding pattern for the 2^{5-1} fractional factorial design is $I = 12345$. The confounding pattern for the main effects is the following:

$$\hat{b}_i = b_i + b_{jklm}$$

For the two-way interactions:

$$\hat{b}_{ij} = b_{ij} + b_{klm}$$

and for the mean:

$$\hat{b}_0 = b_0 + b_{ijklm}$$

A 2^{7-4} fractional factorial design illustrates a "saturated design." 2^3 or eight observations are used to determine the effects of seven variables. All of the calculation columns in a 2^3 must be used to specify the seven variable settings. The confounding relationship becomes quite complex, as shown in Table 4–13.

Table 4-13.   Saturated Designs (The 2^{7-4})

YATES	x_0	x_1	x_2	x_3	4 " $x_1 x_2$	5 " $x_2 x_3$	6 " $x_1 x_3$	7 " $x_1 x_2 x_3$
1	1	-1	-1	-1				
2	1	1	-1	-1				
3	1	-1	1	-1				
4	1	1	1	-1				
5	1	-1	-1	1				
6	1	1	-1	1				
7	1	-1	1	1				
8	1	1	1	1				

Defining Relation: I = 124 = 235 = 136 = 1237

Generating Relation: (indicates all the confounding for effects)

= 1345 = 2346 = 347 = 1256 = 157 = 267 = 1456 = 2457

= 3567 = 1467 = 1257

= 124 = 235 = 136 = 1237

factor $b_1 = b_1 + b_{24} + b_{36} + b_{57} + b_{237} + b_{345} + b_{256} + b_{456}$

$+ b_{467} + b_{257} +$ higher order interactions

Taking all combinations of the defining relation yields the generating relationship which specifies the confounding pattern. The confounding pattern indicates how the effects of the variables are mixed. For instance, the effect of b_1 is mixed with the two–way interactions 24, 36, 57, and as well as three– and four–way interactions 237, 2345, 256, 467, and 257. To determine confounding pattern for variable 2, cross out 2 in the confounding relationship and record the remaining numbers. For instance, if I equals 1234, *eliminate* the variable 2 to find that 2 is confounded with 134. The same logic applies for the more complex confounding relationships.

Summary

Fractional factorial designs offer the evaluator considerable flexibility in carrying out an evaluation. First, the variables that will be mixed are determined to reduce the data requirements. In sequential evaluation projects, the data collection is split into fractions, to permit an orderly collection of data. At the end of the study, the data are assembled to explore the effects of each variable and variable interactions. Finally, there are instances where specific combinations of the levels of variables are not defined. An approximation of the response surface can be obtained by selecting a data collection pattern that avoids the undefined combination of the evaluation variables.

TESTS FOR MODEL ADEQUACY

Throughout Chapter 3 and Chapter 4, a linear model has been assumed. If the linear relationship between the cause and effect variables is not correct, the ANOVA procedures can be invalid. Thus far, the test of model adequacy has been limited to plots of the residual against corresponding levels for several variables. Residuals were plotted against levels of the independent variables, the treatment effects, the block effects, time (order in which data were collected), and the like. If these plots had no pattern, manifesting a band of data, the postulated cause and effect relationship (model) was assumed to be valid. If a trend or a pattern was observed, one or more factors may have been omitted or the assumed linear relationship among the variables may be suspect.

Draper and Herzberg suggest another method of determining model adequacy, called a "lack of fit" test.[12] The lack of fit test characterizes the quality of evaluation findings. If the lack of fit test is insignificant, higher credence is placed on the ability of the variables in the study to explain the merits of managerial interventions. This reduces the uncertainty associated with the evaluation results, and decision makers can confidently manipulate policy variables to optimize some result.

The lack of fit test compares pure error, errors that stem from random variations, with an indicator of model inadequacy. The lack of fit sum of squares is obtained by subtracting pure error sum of squares from the residual.

The residual is calculated by taking the total sum of squares and subtracting the sum of squares associated with the model or regression. The ANOVA procedure decomposes the residual into two components: "pure error" and "lack of fit." The lack of fit sum of squares is compared to the pure error with an "F" test in an ANOVA table. An "F" test is applied to test for model adequacy in the same way as it used to determine the significance of variables.

To carry out the necessary computations the residual is broken down into two components, shown graphically in Figure 4.11. Recall that the residual

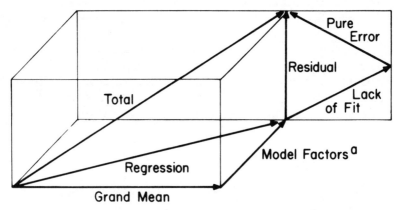

a) Model vector broken down further into all main effects and higher order interactions

Figure 4.11 GEOMETRIC REPRESENTATION OF THE MODEL ADEQUACY TEST

is the unexplained variation that remains after the sum of squares for each term in the model has been subtracted from the total sum of squares. Using the same logic, lack of fit is the unexplained variation that remains after pure error or measurement error has been removed from the residual. The residual is determined by subtracting the model sum of squares from the total sum of squares. The residual identifies the unexplained variation in the data after all the variations associated with the model, often called the regression, have been removed. Pure error is the variation in responses when variables have been set at particular levels, indicating measurement error. Lack of fit is obtained by subtraction. It represents unexplained variation in the responses after pure error (or measurement error) is removed.

There are three steps in the calculation procedure which can be summarized as follows:

(1) ss residual = total ss less regression (based on the model)
(2) ss pure error = the variance around replicate data points or $\Sigma_i (y_i - \bar{y})^2$
       for these points
(3) ss lack of fit = residual ss less pure error ss

The F statistic is formed by the sum of squares (ss) for the lack of fit divided by the sum of square for pure error, each adjusted by their degrees of freedom.

Test of Model Adequacy Using Center Points

Responses of a system under study can be collected when each variable is set at the coded center point of its operational region. The variation in these responses is used to calculate the pure error sum of squares.

A three-variable design with centerpoints is shown on Figure 4.12.

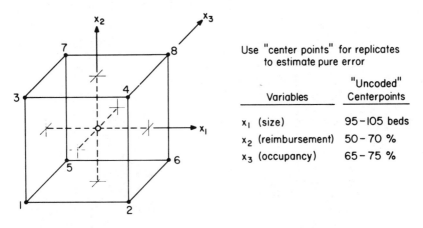

Use "center points" for replicates
to estimate pure error

Variables	"Uncoded" Centerpoints
x_1 (size)	95 – 105 beds
x_2 (reimbursement)	50 – 70 %
x_3 (occupancy)	65 – 75 %

Figure 4.12 GEOMETRIC RELATIONSHIP OF A CENTER POINT DESIGN

Additional responses are collected for each variable, set at the coded value zero. For example, a study of per diem costs in nursing homes could explore the influence of variables such as size (number of beds), percent of revenues derived from Medicaid reimbursement, and percent occupancy. The size variable had a low level of 40 to 60 beds and a high level of 140 to 160 beds. Medicaid reimbursement had a low level of 20 to 40 percent and a high level of 80 to 100 percent. A low level of occupancy would be 30 to 40 percent and a high level, 90 to 100 percent. The design matrix and calculation matrix are shown in Table 4-14.

Table 4-14. A Test For "Model" Adequacy Using Centerpoints

YATES ORDER	x_1	x_2	x_3	x_1x_2	x_1x_3	x_2x_3	$x_1x_2x_3$	x_0	(Per Diem Cost) OBSERVATIONS
1	-1	-1	-1	1	1	1	-1	1	Y_1
2	1	-1	-1	-1	-1	1	1	1	Y_2
3	-1	1	-1	-1	1	-1	1	1	Y_3
4	1	1	-1	1	-1	-1	-1	1	Y_4
5	-1	-1	1	1	-1	-1	1	1	Y_5
6	1	-1	1	-1	1	-1	-1	1	Y_6
7	-1	1	1	-1	-1	1	-1	1	Y_7
8	1	1	1	1	1	1	1	1	Y_8
9	0	0	0	0	0	0	0	1	Y_9
10	0	0	0	0	0	0	0	1	Y_{10}
11	0	0	0	0	0	0	0	1	Y_{11}
12	0	0	0	0	0	0	0	1	Y_{12}

Design Matrix
(Variable Settings)

Calculation Matrix (Multiply column by
observations to complete the effects)

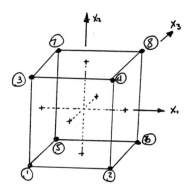

Use "Center Points" for Replicates
to estimate pure error

Variables	"Uncoded" Centerpoints
x_1 (size) :	95 - 105 beds
x_2 (reimbursement):	50 - 70%
x_3 (occupancy) :	65 - 75%

Table 4-15. Anova Table to Test Model Adequacy

Source of variation	ss	df	ms	F ratio
Pure Error	$E(y_i-\bar{y})^2$ = PESS	4- 1=3	PESS/3	(LFSS/1)/(PESS/3)
Lack of Fit	Residual- PESS=LFSS	1	LFSS/1	
Residual	Total SS- Model SS	4	(PESS+ LFSS)/4	

Analysis Procedure

The effects are computed by multiplying the code for each variable of interaction by the observations. Calculation for the "size" effect is given by

$$b_1 = [- y_1 + y_2 - y_3 + y_4 - y_5 + y_6 - y_7 + y_8 + 0 \, (y_9 + y_{10} + y_{11} + y_{12})]/8$$

for the "size–reimbursement" interaction

$$b_{12} = [y_1 - y_2 - y_3 + y + y_5 - y_6 - y_7 + y_8 + 0 \, (y_9 + y_{10} + y_{11} + y_{12})]/8$$

and for the grand mean

$$b_0 = (y_1 + y_2 + y_3 + y_4 + y_5 + y_6 + y_7 + y_8 + y_9 + y_{10} + y_{11} + y_{12})/12$$

The analysis of variance table is built from calculations which were described previously. The additional elements for the ANOVA table are computed by

$$\text{Pure Error (Sum of Squares)} = \sum_{i=1}^{4} (y_{8+i} - \bar{y}_{8+i})^2$$

$$= y_9^2 + y_{10}^2 + y_{11}^2 + y_{12}^2 + (y_9 + y_{10} + y_{11} + y_{12})^2/4$$

$$\text{Residual (Sum of Squares)} = \sum_{i=1}^{12} y_i^2 - (\text{regression ss})$$

Lack of fit sum of squares (LFSS) = Residual sum of squares (RSS) − pure error sum of squares (PESS)

The ANOVA table for this example is shown in Table 4–15.

The analysis of variance table is used to test the significance of the lack of fit. Significance is determined in the same manner as it was for main effects and interactions. The ratio $(\text{LFSS}/1)/(\text{PESS}/3)$ is tested against $F_{1,3;.05}$. If the ratio of lack of fit and pure error is insignificant (small), the model is assumed to be adequate. The lack of fit and the pure error variances are then pooled back into the residual variance and used to test significance of each main effect and interaction in the model under study. (A less conservative test would use the pure error variance to form the F ratios.) If the model was found to be adequate, the variables in the model would be tested as shown in Table 4–16.

Table 4-16. Anova Table to Test Effects

Source of Variation	ss	df	ms	F Ratio
Model: x_0 (grand mean)	$12\hat{b}_0^2$	1	$12b_0^2$	
x_1	$8b_1^2$	1	$8b_1^2$	$8b^2$/residual M.S.
x_2	$8b_2^2$	1	$8b_2^2$	"
x_3	$8b_3^2$	1	$8b_3^2$	"
x_1x_2	$8b_{12}^2$	1	$8b_{12}^2$	"
x_1x_3	$8b_{13}^2$	1	$8b_{13}^2$	"
x_2x_3	$8b_{23}^2$	1	$8b_{23}^2$	"
$x_1x_2x_3$	$8b_{123}^2$	1	$8b_{123}^2$	"
Pure error	$E(y_i - \bar{y})^2$ = PESS (4-1) = 3		PESS/3	
Lack of Fit	RSS-PESS=LFSS	1	LFSS/1	(LFSS/1)/(PESS/3)
Residual	total ss – model ss	4	Residual MS= (PESS+LFSS)/4	
Total	Ey_i^2=model ss	12		

The analysis of variance table is used to test the significance of the lack of fit. Significance is determined of the same manner as it was for main effects and interactions. The ratio (LFSS/1)(PESS/3) is

Interpretation of Results

When the ratio of lack of fit to pure error is large, the model is found to be *inadequate*. The response (per diem costs) was assumed to be linearly related to size, Medicaid reimbursement rates, or occupancy. A significant lack of fit suggests that cost was not linearaly related to these variables. Thus the relationship between, say, per diem costs and size may have curvature. Maximum (or minimum) cost occurs with intermediate–sized nursing homes. The ANOVA conclusion to encourage large homes may be invalid.

Typically, the linear relationship provides a good approximation between policy variables and a measure of effectiveness. For example, assume that an "S" curve represents the true relationship between size and per diem costs (Figure 4.13). Initially, costs are insensitive to the size of the home, but rapidly decrease, when size is midway in operational range, only to level off near the top of the range. Four observations are needed (a four–level design) to estimate the parameters in a "S" relationship. However, in Figure 4.13 the linear

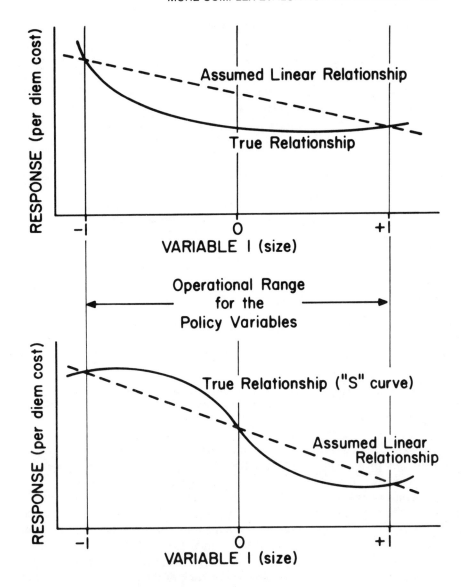

Figure 4.13 CENTER POINT LOGIC

relationship and the S curve provide the same policy guidance to the decision maker. Each indicates that increasing size will decrease cost. A precise model was not needed to draw the correct policy inference.

Distinction between Center Points and Repeat Observations

Repeat observations *do not* provide a lack of fit test. This section illustrates the similarity and differences in the data collection and analysis procedures for repeat observations and center point data. A three–factor design with replications for each contrast is shown in Figure 4–14. Each contrast defines a population to be sampled. To get a better sample of each population,

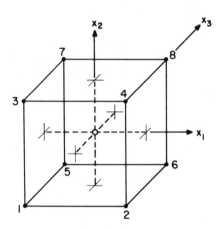

n samples at each point in
  the observation space

Contrast # I
  size, 40 to 60 beds
  reimbursement, 20 to 40 %
  occupancy, 60 to 70 %

Contrast # 2
  size, 140 to 160 beds
  reimbursement, 20 to 40 %
  occupancy, 60 to 70 %

Figure 4.14   TESTS FOR MODEL ADEQUACY WITH REPEATED POINTS

replications for each position in the Yates Order can be taken. For instance, in contrast 1, the per diem costs for a sample of nursing homes that have 40 to 60 beds, 20 to 40 percent Medicaid reimbursement, and 60 to 70 percent occupancy are collected. n represents the sample size at each point.

In the example shown in Figure 4–14, assume that n = 2, two observations were taken for each contrast. The error is calculated by summing the squared differences for the two observations taken for each of eight combinations of the variables. The sum of squares is equal to one–half the sum of these deviations squared. The degrees of freedom for the pure error sum of squares is 8. One degree of freedom is used up for each of the eight combinations to compute the mean. The calculation is given by

$$\text{error sum of squares} = \sum_{i=1}^{8} d_i^2 / 2$$

where $d_i = y_a - y_b$, the two observations taken at Yates Order i.

When $n = 3$ or more, the error is computed at each point in the Yates Order using the standard variance computation procedure, given by

$$\text{error sum of squares} = \sum_{i=1}^{8} \sum_{j=1}^{n} (y_{ij} - \bar{y})^2$$

$$= [(y_{1,12} + \ldots + y^2_{n,1} - n \text{ (mean of observations at Yates Order 1)}]^2$$

$$+ \ldots + (y_{1,8}^2 + \ldots + y_{n,8}^2) - n \text{ [mean of observations at Yates Order 8]}^2$$

where $y_{1,8}$ is the first observation for Yates Order 8 and $y_{n,8}$ is the last observation taken for Yates Order 8. In this example, error is equal to the residual, *not* pure error. Figure 4.15 illustrates why this statistic can not detect the appropriateness of a linear assumption. If a curved relationship exists between size and cost it would *not* be detected, because each sample is drawn at the end point of the operational range.

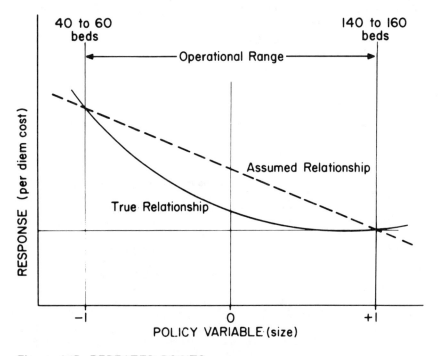

Figure 4.15   REPEATED POINTS

A replication approach is used to improve the estimates of the effects of each variable in the model. Each contrast in an evaluation experiment represents a population. For example, costs may vary which stem from nursing homes with low occupancy and low Medicaid reimbursement (Yates Order 1, Figure 4–15). As the number of replications increases, better estimates of the way this population responds to the treatment variables are obtained.

SUMMARY

Tests of model adequacy are conducted by decomposing the residual into a pure–error and lack–of–fit components. Pure error is the variation in system responses, such as cafeteria profits, when treatment variables are held at particular settings. Pure error can be calculated using center points for each contrast. Center points can detect linear model inadequacy. Replication tests for the effects of missing variables. When both center points and replications are used, important insights into sources of model inadequacy can be gained. For example, if a lack–of–fit pure–error ratio based on center points is insignificant and the variables tested in the ANOVA (with replication) are also insignificant, the inadequacy is due to missing variables not the linearity assumption. Other comparisons provide additional insights.

The lack–of–fit test characterizes the quality of evaluation findings. If the lack–of–fit test is insignificant, higher credence is placed on the ability of the variables in the study to explain the merits of managerial interventions. This reduces the uncertainty associated with the evaluation results and decision makers can confidently manipulate policy variables to optimize some result.

Notes

1. Variables subject to control by the administrator who sponsors the evaluation are called "policy variables." They define treatments, variables that are manipulated in an evaluation to study their policy significance. Variables under the control of others, or those acting as constraints, are termed "block variables." Block variables often define strata or populations the evaluation will sample.
2. Cochran, W.G. and G.M. Cox, Factorial Experiments in *Experimental Designs*. New York: Wiley, 1957.
3. Most evaluation projects seek to determine if particular relationships exist and do not fully explore the nature of the relationship between the independent and dependent variables.
4. For a definition of the APGAR score, see Note 24, Chapter 1.
5. For a complete discussion of response surface methods, see Box, G.E.P.,[11] The Determination of Optimum Conditions,[11] in O. Davies (ed.) *Design and Analysis of Industrial Experiments*. New York: Hafner, 1967 (revised edition) and Box G.E.P. *et al.*, "Response Surface Methods," in *Statistics for Experimentors*, New York: Wiley, 1978.

6. These computational procedures were drawn from Box, G.E.P. and N.R. Draper, "The 2^2 & 2^3 Factorial Designs." in *Evolutionary Operation,* New York: Wiley, 1969, and Box G.E.P., W.G. Hunter, and J.S. Hunter, "Factorial Designs at Two Levels," in *Statistics for Experimentors,* New York: Wiley, 1978.

7. Another way to compute the interaction term is by

$$E_{ij} = \tfrac{1}{2}[\text{average effect of variable j at the high level of factor i)}$$
$$- \text{ (average effect of variable j at the low level of factor i)}$$

8. The grand mean is often ignored, creating a "corrected total" as the bottom line in the ANOVA table.

9. The derivation is shown below:

$$s^2 = \frac{\Sigma x_i^2 - (\Sigma x_i)^2/n}{n-1} \quad \text{where: } x_i = x_1 + x_2$$
$$\Sigma x_i^2 = x_1^2 + x_2^2$$
$$n = 2$$

Substituting

$$s^2 = \frac{x_1^2 + x_2^2 - (x_1 + x_2)^2/2}{1}$$
$$= x_1^2 + x_2^2 - (x_1^2 + 2x_1x_2 + x_2^2)/2$$
$$= x_1^2/2 - x_1x_2 + x_2^2/2$$

Factoring

$$= \frac{(x_1 - x_2)^2}{2}$$

$$= \frac{\Sigma d_i^2}{2}$$

The pooled variance is given by

$$s\,\text{pool}^2 = \frac{s^2}{df} = \frac{\Sigma d_i^2}{2df}$$

where "df" is the degrees of freedom in the residual.

10. Box, G.E.P. and J.S. Hunter, "The 2^{k-p} Fractional Factorial Designs, Part I," *Technometrics,* August 1961, pp. 311–351.

11. When faced with these situations, multiple regression is often used. Regression considers *all* levels of the explanatory variable, and the associated response, found in some information file, to correlate the cause and effect variables. Regression may provide a misleading estimate of the importance of each causal factor. True causal factors may *suppress* or *distort* the variables under study, making unimportant variables seem important or masking the effects of variables that are important. Inconsistent data and the range of values for variables in the data file pose additional problems. For a discussion of the hazards of fitting happenstance data see "Modeling with Least Squares" in Box G.E.P. *et al., Statistics for Experimentors,* New York: Wiley, 1978.

12. Draper, N.R. and A.M. Herzberg, "On Lack of Fit," Technical Report No. 208. Madison: University of Wisconsin, Department of Statistics, June 1969.

CHAPTER 5

Quasi-Experimental Evaluation Methods

"[Methods] offer an asylum where no tyranny can penetrate."

Nietzsche

Evaluation compares measures of the effects of an intervention applied in an experimental group with these same measures observed in a control group. To make this comparison convincing, the experimental and control groups must have similar characteristics. For instance, negative income tax experiments measured the consumption behavior of low–income people who received direct income supplements (the experimental group) and compared them to a control group, people receiving welfare through food stamps, aid to dependent children programs, and the like.[1] To give this comparison meaning, the experimental and control groups were constructed so recipients in each group were similar in terms of their range of income, national origin, number of years on welfare, and other factors which may alter consumption behavior.

Randomly assigning people with similar characteristics to receive welfare benefits through a negative income tax and through traditional methods is the best way to construct these comparison groups. To illustrate, the names of people receiving welfare could be drawn from a pool of people with common characteristics (such as having income levels below a thousand dollars annually, being on welfare for ten years or more, and the like), and assigned to the experimental or control group by the flip of a coin. Some evaluations cannot use random assignment to form their comparison groups. This chapter describes several "quasi–experimental" data collection approaches which can be used to construct comparison groups when random assignment is impractical or unfeasible.

NOTATION

The factorial arrangement, described in Chapter 4, will be used to introduce the notation used in this chapter. In the example, shown in Table 5-1, two

Table 5-1.   Factorial Arrangement

MODEL:

$$\begin{array}{ccc} \text{measure} & = & \text{intervention program} & + & \text{measurement procedure} \\ \text{(objectives)} & & \text{(policy variable)} & & \text{(block variable)} \end{array}$$

PURPOSE: To assess and interpret the effects of a policy variable, a block variable, and the interaction between the policy and block variables,

EXPERIMENTAL ARRANGEMENTS:

Yates Order	Intervention Program	Measurement Procedure	Observation
1	R X	A	1
2	R (X)	A	2
3	R X	B	3
4	R (X)	B	4

NOTATION:

X:	signifies that Group 1 and Group 3 were exposed to an intervention program
(X):	signifies that Group 2 and Group 4 were exposed to the current practices or received a placebo
R:	indicates that the praticipants were randomly assigned to one of the groups
Blank:	control group not exposed to any stimuli
O:	observations taken or measured value for each (contrast) group

MEASUREABLE EFFECTS:

Program Effect:	01 & 03 > 02 & 04
Block Effect:	01 & 02 > 03 & 04
Interaction Effect:	01 & 04 > 02 & 03

factors are to be studied: an intervention program and a measurement procedure. Following the conventions established by Campbell and Stanley, X is used to signify the "experimental groups," or the comparison groups exposed to the intervention program.[2] In the example, groups one and three in Table 5-1 represent the experimental groups. (X) is used to signify the control groups. Comparison groups two and four in Table 5-1 are *not* exposed to the intervention program. Some evaluations expose control groups to a placebo, a program or activity with no inherent value which maintains the interest of participants. (X) is also used to signify a current practice or program. For example, X could designate a new bad-debts collection procedure by a hospital and the (X) could be used to signify the current practices used to collect bad-debt accounts. R indicates that the comparison groups were formed by a random process. For instance, to compare effects of the existing and a new bad-debt collection procedure, accounts could be assigned to the new process $\hat{X}$, or the current approach (X), by the flip of a coin. O represents the observations taken to measure the percent of bad debts recovered from each comparison group after one of the collection approaches has been attempted.

Several precautions are essential as the observations are taken. A blind measurement procedure is carried out so people with unpaid accounts are unaware that they are in the control group or the experimental group. Blind measurement insures that the observed rate of debt collection is due to the collection approach, and not associated with factors such as the specters which may be raised in the payee's mind when collection procedures are changed. Neither the participant nor the observer knows who is in the experimental group and who is in the control group in "double–blind" measurement. A double–blind measurement process controls for observers that have a stake in the outcome. For example, Rosenthal found that those advocating the new approach often look for desirable features in experimental groups and undesirable features in the control groups.[3] Double–blind measurement controls for these biases by using naive observers or by disguising the comparison groups.

Experimental designs are used to segregate the effects of block variables such as measurement procedures, and policy variables, often some form of intervention. Block variables help to control factors that may influence the intervention's effectiveness measures. Some common types of block variables are:

1. *Pretests* or other potentially obtrusive baseline observations.
2. Different *observers,* such as data recorders or those administering questionnaires.
3. Different *instruments,* like the response mode for survey questions.
4. *Several* (parallel) *measures,* such as "satisfaction" questions on a survey or counts of critical incidents.
5. *Time* factors, consistancy in measurement at different points in time.
6. *Participant* factors, like comparing the views of two or more classes of participants, such as physicians and administrators.

Baseline observations (called "pretests" in the education literature) may influence responses when participants in an evaluation study are asked to state their preferences or their opinions. The pretest or baseline measure often "suggests" the response desired, which may entice the participant to agree or to disagree. As shown in Table 5–2, the factorial arrangement can isolate the effects of baseline measurement by comparing the results of measurement process A with unobtrusive observations (measurement process B).

The type of instrument may also influence evaluation findings. For example, surveys can use "Likert Scales," and "Hackman items," or "anchored rating scales" (ARS).[4] Each response made may point to unique findings or conclusions. Consider, for example, a morale survey that seeks to detect work attitudes. A "Hackman item" would pose open ended questions. Respondents would write phrases which describe the reaction to questions like "When I work hard around here,"———.

A Likert scale would focus the question for a respondent, as shown below: "When I work hard, I'm rewarded":

Strongly Agree	Agree	Not Sure	Disagree	Strongly Disagree
( )	( )	( )	( )	( )

The ARS scale attempts to induce a finely tuned response:
"Are rewards tied to hard work?"

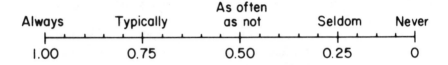

The respondents are asked to check the scale to signify their views.

The scales differ in terms of their power of discovery and their ability to measure respondent views. Hackman items can uncover new causal agents. For instance, when asked, "When I work hard around here," a respondent may indicate, "my friends won't talk to me." An ARS scale would miss this nuance. The ARS approach permits the evaluators to generalize views of reward–work linkages across large numbers of employees. This measure, when combined with other questions, permits a quantification of concepts like "organizational climate." Likert scales cannot be used for either discovery and extrapolation, and thus should be avoided. (A discussion of measurement issues appears in Chapter 7.)

Other factors that may influence measurement include the observer, the type of measure applied, the order measurements are taken, and the nature of the participants. Several examples of block factors are shown in Table 5–2. Data is collected for a factorial, all combinations of the policy and block variables. As discussed in Chapter 4, this arrangement permits an assessment of policy variables, block variables, and interactions between policy and block variables.

QUASI-EXPERIMENTAL DATA COLLECTION METHODS

Quasi–experimental data collection devices are used when the schedule of interventions and/or the schedule of measurements cannot be fully controlled.

Table 5-2.   Types of Block Variables Used to Explore Measurement Questions

EVALUATION ARRANGEMENTS:

Intervention Program

		X	(X)
Block	A	Group 1	Group 2
Variable	B	Group 3	Group 4

BLOCK VARIABLES:

base line	observers	types of measures	instrument
A = baseline measure	A = observer #1	A = behavioral	A = Likert Scale
B = no baseline measure	B = observer #2	B = projective	B = "BARS"

TIME SERIES REPRESENTATION   (with baseline measures as the block variable)

Yates Order

1	R	01	X	02
2	R	03	(X)	04
3	R		X	05
4	R		(X)	06

Quasi-experimental designs are used to construct comparison groups and to provide other types of baselines in constrained situations. These data collection devices should be used only when more powerful experimental designs cannot be applied. Chapter 6 compares the strengths and weaknesses of quasi-experimental and experimental data collection approaches.

There are three basic types of quasi-experimental data collection devices: matched groups, naturally occurring groups, and time-ordered performance data. *Matched groups* equate the profiles of comparison groups across a series of factors which may cause groups to behave or perform differently. For example, to compare the performance of various budgeting processes, the supervisors who construct the budgets can be matched in terms of past performance, years on the job, ranking by supervisors, and the like. *Naturally occurring groups* often represent independent organizations, work groups, or programs which, by virtue of their distinct origin or history, can be assumed independent. For example, HEW has established neighborhood health centers in various parts of the country. These centers tend to operate independently, with the possible exception of HEW's attempts to homogenize their administrative and patient care practices. As a result, neighborhood health centers are likely to exhibit independent behavior as long as the evaluation project does not touch on practices common to all centers. *Time-ordered performance data* track important performance indicators prior to and following an intervention program. By extracting trends, cycles, and other patterns in the data, the performance before and after the intervention can be compared. Quasi–experimental data collection designs use one or more of these principles (see Table 5–3).

Table 5-3.   Quasi - Experimental Data Collection Methods

1. Matched Groups (M)

2. Naturally Occuring Groups (N)

3. Time series of Time Ordered Performance Data
    –pick out trend effects before and after an intervention

4. Combinations of matched and naturally occuring groups, with and without randomization, and time series data

Matched Groups Designs

In matched group designs, each comparison group is constructed so its members have similar characteristics. A naturally occurring group can be used as a model. For example, an evaluator seeking to determine the impact of outpatient services on hospital utilization could describe the naturally occurring group that has used its outpatient services. This group is used to identify the characteristics of their clientele. Other groups are included in the evaluation if they are similar in terms of age; diagnosis; and ratio of Medicare, self–pay, and insured; and other factors. Matched groups are constructed to mimic the clientele of the evaluating organization, the hospital. In other situations, a particular mix of attributes may have policy significance. For instance, distributions of age and proportions of welfare and nonwelfare patients who correspond to the general population could be selected. The evaluator hopes to construct comparison groups whose utilization behavior may be typical in the population at large. Matched groups can be constructed to simulate the sponsor's current or anticipated clientele, or to match the characteristics or group whose behavior may have general interest, like low income service users.

Data Collection and Data Representation for "Matched Groups."

Data collection arrangements are shown in Table 5–4. The notation "M" preceding each comparison group designates a matched group. The format of a two–level, two–variable factorial shown in Table 5–1, is followed. In Table 5–4, the block variable is the type of survey instrument and the policy variable

Table 5-4.   Data Collection Arrangements For Matched Groups

PURPOSE: Isolate and interpret the effects of interventions, block variables
and block policy variable interactions, assuming the equivalency
of the comparison groups.

EVALUATION ARRANGEMENTS (Representation A)

		Intervention Program	
		X	(X)
		Group 1	Group 2
Block	Likert Scales	N*	M
Variable	Scales	Group 3	Group 4
		M	M

EVALUATION ARRANGEMENTS (Representation B)

Yates Order	Intervention Program	Block	Observation
Group 1	N X*	Likert	01
Group 2	M (X)	Likert	02
Group 3	M X	BARS	03
Group 4	M (X)	BARS	04

*   Group #1 is found in the field and groups 2, 3 and 4 are assembled
so their profiles match Group #1.   Alternatively, the profile of an
ideal or interesting group can be selected and the characteristics of
each group are made to conform with this profile.

MEASUREABLE EFFECTS:

Program Effect:	01 & 03 > 02 & 04
Block Effect:	01 & 02 > 03 & 04
Interaction:	01 & 04 > 02 & 03

is an intervention. Group number one is a naturally occurring one, based on
the characteristics of patients who use the outpatient services of the hospital
sponsoring the evaluation effort. Groups two, three, and four are similar,
matched according to important characteristics. If the matching process is
carried out with precision, the evaluation project can be both efficient and
precise. (Problems associated with matched groups will be discussed in
Chapter 6).

Analysis and Statistical Tests

The analysis for the quasi–experimental design shown in Table 5–4 follow the statistical procedures described in Chapters 3 and 4. To account for the policy variable, a paired t can be used as shown below:

Intervention Program	Current Practice	Difference (d)
01	02	$d1 = 01 - 02$
03	04	$d2 = 03 - 04$
⋮	⋮	⋮

The variance among the values of di would include both measurement error and the differences resulting from the survey instrument.

The ANOVA procedure can also be used. Given an estimate of variance or measurement error, this analysis can isolate the effects of the policy variable, the block variable, and their interaction. The analysis compares the variance between cells to the variance within columns, rows, and cross products. The data are formulated as shown below:

	Intervention	Nonintervention
Likert Scale	01	02
Bars Scale	03	04

In this case, the program effect would be determined by comparing observations two and four. If the variation between is significantly greater than the variation within, a significant program effect would occur. The same logic applies for the block and their interaction effects. The block effect, 01+02 less 03+04, and the interaction effect, 01+04 less 02+02, are compared to the residual or error. If the ratio is large, these effects appear to be important and their policy significance must be interpreted. (In this example, there are insufficient degrees of freedom for a statistical test unless 01 denotes the mean of a sample of a population defined by one of the four contrasts in Table 5–4. With several samples for each contrast, the residual becomes the pooled variance for observation sets 01, 02, 03, and 04.)

Naturally Occurring Groups

Naturally occurring groups provide a powerful way to simulate many of the requirements of an experimental design. Because each comparison group is isolated, its response to an intervention is likely to be independent. For example, HEW could initiate a new data collection procedure, an intervention, for its quality assessment (PSRO) organizations. A sample of the PSRO's throughout the United States could be selected to participate in the evaluation project. The response of physicians (a surrogate effectiveness measure) to the data demands of each procedure in each PSRO could be considered an

Table 5-5: Data Collection Arrangements for Naturally Occurring Groups

Purpose: To isolate and interpret the significance of policy and block variables and their interaction, assuming the independence of the naturally occurring comparison groups.

Representation A:

		INTERVENTION PROGRAM	
		X	(X)
Block	Baseline Observation	Group 1,2,3	Groups 4,5,6
	No Baseline Observation	Group 7,8,9	Group 10,11,12

Representation B:

Yates Order	Naturally Occurring Group	Program	Block	Observation
1	Group 1 [a]	N X	pretest	O1
1	Group 2	N X	pretest	O2
1	Group 3	N X	pretest	O3
2	Group 4	N(X)	pretest	O4
2	Group 5	N(X)	pretest	O5
2	Group 6	N(X)	pretest	O6
3	Group 7	N X	no pretest	O7
3	Group 8	N X	no pretest	O8
3	Group 9	N X	no pretest	O9
4	Group 10	N(X)	no pretest	O10
4	Group 11	N(X)	no pretest	O11
4	Group 12	N(X)	no pretest	O12

Measurable Effects:

Program effect: O1 to O3 & O7 to O9 > O4 to O6 & O10 to O12

Block effect: O1 to O6 > O7 to O12

Interaction effect: O1,O2,O3 and O10,O11,O12 less O4,O5,O6 and O7, O8,O9

[*a] random samples of physicians in each group (hospital) can be drawn to represent the population of physicians in each group (hospital).

independent observation. If the physician compliance rates are low for all PSRO's which used the new data collection procedure, problems concerning the physician's behavior would be predicted.

Data Collection and Representation

In Table 5–5, an evaluation project using naturally occurring groups is illustrated. The notation "N" is used to designate a naturally occurring group. In this example, twelve naturally occurring groups participated in the evaluation project. In six of these groups (1, 2, 3, 7, 8, and 9), an intervention was attempted, and in the remaining six (4, 5, 6, 10, 11, and 12), current practices were continued. In this case a baseline observation (the block variable) was used in groups 1 through 6, whereas no baseline observation was recorded for groups 7 through 12.

To illustrate, assume that a sponsor like a multihospital system sought to evaluate the acceptance of a new "physician compensation scheme" in contract–managed hospitals. Each comparison group is a single hospital. In hospitals 1, 2, 3, and 7, 8, 9, the new practice plan would be attempted which uses a sliding scale to charge physicians for overhead associated with hospital facility use. For instance, 30 percent of fees for the first $50,000, 20 percent on the next $50,000, and 10 percent on $100,000 and above would be charged in return for managing the physician's accounts, his billings and collections, office space and secretarial support, in addition to typical charges stemming from using hospital resources. In the remaining hospitals, the current compensation approach was continued whereby physicians maintained their own offices, staffs, do their own bill collection, and pay for hospital resources on a demand basis. In each of the 12 hospitals, a survey of physician satisfaction was carried out. In hospitals 1 through 6, this questionnaire was applied prior to the change in compensation procedures and following it. In hospitals 7 through 12, the questionnaire was used only at the end of the evaluation period.

Analysis and Statistical Tests

The analysis of the intervention's impact would be carried out in the same manner described for matched groups. The only difference between the evaluation information in Table 5–5 and the factorial in Table 5–1 is the origin of the comparison groups. Naturally occurring groups must be similar to avoid biasing the results. For example, if contract hospitals differed in terms of size or services offered, hospital size or service intensity may cause the observed differences in revenues or some other effectiveness measure, not the compensation program. However, by carefully selecting hospitals so the size range in hospitals 1, 2, and 3, are similar to hospitals 4, 5, 6, and 7, 8, 9 and 10, 11, 12, this problem will be minimal. In this evaluation example, the differences among hospitals are unlikely to influence the findings. The total number of patients admitted or the hospital revenue per patient, before–and–after the compensation program was initiated, could be used as measures of the program's success. As Webb and his colleagues point out, this type of measurement process is *unobtrusive*.[5] Precautions such as blind and double–blind arrangements, which keep the measurement process from interfering with the program, are unnecessary. When measurements are unobtrusive, performance differences in groups exposed and not exposed to pretests tend to reflect only measurement error. In this case, groups 7, 8, and 9 could be collapsed with groups 1, 2, and 3; and groups 10, 11, and 12 collapsed with groups 4, 5, and 6 (see Table 5–5). This will increase the sample size, which improves the estimate of the error variance.

The program effects are gleaned from the observations taken on groups 1, 2, 3, 7, 8, 9. (See representation A in Table 5–5.) When measures 01 to 03 and 07 to 09 are significantly greater than 04 to 06, and 010 to 012, the physician compensation program influenced satisfaction. As always, several measures are needed to fully evaluate an interaction. For instance, the evaluation could also measure changes in physician admitting behavior, following the new compensation program. The intervention would be called successful if the average physician's patient admission rates did not decline: the admission rates falling into the intervention and the nonintervention cells in Table 5–5 remained about the same. The block effect isolates the obtrusiveness of the measurement process by comparing indicators 01 to 06 with 07 to 012. The analysis of the data follows the principles of a factorial. The data are formatted for analysis as shown below:

	Intervention	No Intervention
Baseline	01, 02, 03	04, 05 06
No Baseline	07, 08, 09	010, 011, 012

The following conclusions can be drawn:

1. A block effect exists when 01 to 06 less 07 to 012 is several times greater than residual variance;
2. A program effect exists when (01 to 03 and 07 to 09) less (04 to 06 and 010 to 012) is several times greater than the residual variance;
3. An interaction effect exists when (01, 02, 03 and 010, 011, 012) less (04, 05, 06 and 07, 08, 09) is several times greater than the residual variance.

Time–Ordered Performance Data

When neither matched nor naturally occurring groups are feasible, tracking performance indicators over several time periods provides a useful evaluation format. The time series can be either single or multiple. A single time series tracks key performance indicators over some period of time before an intervention takes place, and for some period of time after the intervention. A multiple time series would track these same indicators in a matched or naturally occurring comparison group.

Data Collection and Representation

In Table 5–6, a format to record time–ordered performance data is shown.

Table 5-6.   Time Ordered Performance Data

Rationale

Time series data provides a visual display for evaluator to interpret and/or model to make relevant comparisons, after trends, cycles and other patterns, independent of the intervention, are removed.

Representation:

Yates Order	Program	Observation	
Group 1	(X)	01, 02 . . . 0i	
Group 1	X		0i + 1, 0i + 2 . . 0n
Group 2	MorN (X)	01, 02 . . . 0i	
Group 2	MorN (X)		0i + 1, 0i + 2 . . 0n

Illustration   (Group 1)

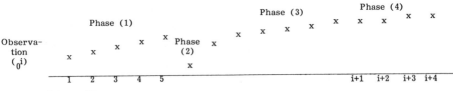

Intervention

Data Phases Shown:

Phase 1: slight performance improvement trend in the before data
Phase 2: sharp decline in performance as new system is introduced
Phase 3: learning phase, an exponential rise in performance
Phase 4: stable performance, slight improvement trend re-emerges

A single time series tracks the performance in the experimental groups (group 1 in Table 5–6) over a period of time, as shown in Figure 5.1. Typically, performance goes through several phases. By graphically displaying the movement of important performance indicators, trend and cycle effects not associated with the intervention can be visualized and extracted. To judge the effects of the intervention, performance before the intervention is compared to the stable performance phase.

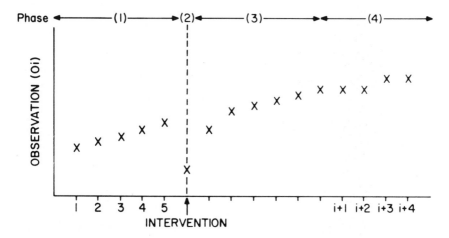

Data Phases Shown

1) Slight performance improvement trend before the intervention
2) Sharp decline in performance as new system is introduced
3) Learning phase, an exponential rise in performance
4) Stable performance, slight improvement trend reemerges

Figure 5.1   ILLUSTRATIVE TIMES SERIES DATA FOR AN EXPERIMENTAL GROUP

The illustration, shown in Figure 5.1, suggests a slight performance improvement trend prior to the intervention. This trend may be due to managers who continually attempt to improve their organization's efficiency or effectiveness, or they may be due to external forces, like inflation. At the point of intervention, an abrupt decline in performance is shown. This often occurs when new programs are established. Performance declines as key personnel learn operating procedures. Subsequently learning occurs which typically leads to rapid improvements in performances, often represented by an exponential relationship. Finally, the stable performance phase is reached where learning is complete. Again, normal fluctuations resulting from external and internal factors beyond the control of the evaluation sponsor will occur. To determine the effects of the interventions, the means of data sets 1 and 2 in Table 5–6 are compared after the trend effects have been removed.

Time–series data provide a visual display. The evaluator attempts to rationalize, interpret, or model the patterns in these data. Trends due to inflation and other factors, and cycles are removed so a before–and–after comparison can be made independent of these exogenous factors.

Analysis and Significance Tests

Statistical comparisons of before–and–after trends may be difficult to carry out and to interpret. When uncontrolled processes are known to operate as an evaluation is taking place, a subsidiary analysis can be used to remove the effects of this process. However, removing cycles, trends, and the like also remove some of the data's variability. As a result, the variance of the data can be understated. This increases the prospects that a significant difference between the before and after comparisons will be found, using standard statistical tests.

Covariance analysis and related techniques are often used to remove cycle and trend data. These approaches are essential when an uncontrollable process operated throughout a period when the time–series data were recorded. For instance, the benefits of a new teaching device will be confounded with intellectual growth of grade school children. A general improvement in performance occurs throughout the school year. To assess the effects of a new teaching, the covariant "student maturation" must be removed from the evaluation data.

A positive exponential may be used to model a learning curve, as most learning behavior seems to closely resemble this relationship or, for simplicity, a linear relationship may be assumed. In effect, analysis of covariance removes trend effects from data before applying ANOVA tests. To illustrate, assume that data depicting the performance of children in experimental and control groups are plotted, associating verbal achievement and their age in months, as shown in figure 5.2. Analysis of covariance computes the expected verbal score, using this relationship, and subtracts it from the observed verbal score. The deviations from expected achievement are analyzed by the usual statistical tests as a second step in the analysis procedure. To use covariance analysis, a well–developed empirical theory must be folded into the analysis to account for the shape of the time series.

Multiple Time Series

A multiple time series can be used to track time–ordered performance data

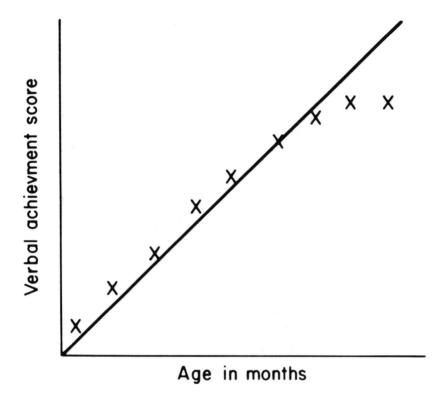

**Figure 5.2   An Example of Covariation Between Verbal
Achievement and Age**

in two comparison groups. Assuming the comparison groups have responded similarly to external factors, the differences in the patterns of performance indicators reflect the influence of the interaction program. A multiple time series is shown graphically in Figure 5.3 using data from group 2 in Table 5–6.

Data Collection and Representation

In the experimental group, time–series performance data are recorded before and after intervention as shown in Figure 5.3. In the control group, these same performance indicators are tracked over the same time period. Comparing the two sets of time–ordered performance data permits the evaluator to identify naturally occurring processes such as trends and cycles in

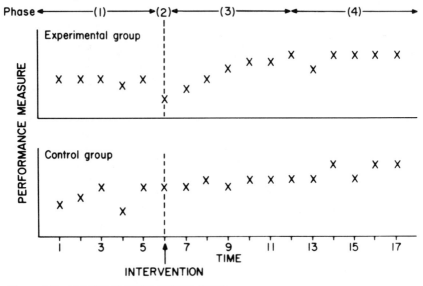

Figure 5.3 MULTIPLE TIME SERIES DATA

the data which occur independent of the intervention. An example might be seasonal fluctuation and institutional procedures which cause a decline in hospital occupancy on holidays or weekends. Comparing the experimental and control time series points out exogenous trends in the data, like inflation, and trends in the data that are associated with the intervention, like learning effects.

Analysis and Statistical Tests

Three comparisons are possible. First, the performance indicators in phases 1 and 4 for the experimental group can be compared (Figure 5.2). Next the performance measures, taken before the intervention, for a particular time interval are paired to block for trend effects. A paired t test can be used to test the equivalence of the comparison groups. Finally, the performance indicators after the learning phase can be compared to the same indicators collected during the same time period for the matched or naturally occurring group.

This comparison assumes that inflation and other exogenous factors influence the performance indicators in the comparison groups in the same way. The paired t test is again used to eliminate bias stemming from a trend effect by comparing performance of the experimental and control groups at each time interval data are recorded. This analysis is shown below:

Time Period	Intervention	Nonintervention	d
t1	O1E	O1C	d1 = O1E − O1C
t2	O2E	O2C	d2 = O2E − O2C
t3	O3E	O3C	d3 = O3E − O3C
⋮	⋮	⋮	⋮

O1E = performance for time period 1
in the experimental group
O1C = performance for time period 1
in the control group

This analysis blocks for trends in the evaluation data. If the difference, di, compared to its error is several times greater than zero the intervention may have policy significance.

The quality of inferences drawn from multiple–time–series performance data is strictly dependent upon the similarities of the comparison groups. If the groups are comparable, multiple–time–series performance data can be an insightful and very inexpensive way of carrying out a highly diagnostic evaluation of an intervention program. However, when the comparison groups differ along important dimensions, these differences between groups will be thoroughly mixed with the performance data. The effects of environment cannot be separated from the effects of the intervention program. The matching process must be very carefully executed to insure that comparison groups are comparable. For example, hospitals would be wise to work with sister institutions that have similar medical staffs, yearly admissions, revenues, bad debt experience, Medicare clientele, and the like. Hospitals could use one another as baselines for important studies. This sharing of information among organizations in comparable environments could dramatically reduce the cost of evaluation and improve the precision of evaluation findings.

SPECIALIZED QUASI–EXPERIMENTAL DESIGNS

A wide variety of data collection devices can be formed by using various combinations of matched groups, naturally occurring groups with and without partial randomization, and time–ordered performance data. To illustrate these points, several special purpose quasi–designs will be described. These designs illustrate a few of the data collection devices that can be constructed to fit the needs of an evaluation project.

Switchback Designs

In Table 5–7, a switchback design is illustrated. This data collection procedure is often used to dissociate the effects of an intervention program from some indigenous processes, such as on–the–job learning, from information acquired in an orientation program. The intervention is initiated, followed

Table 5-7. Switch Back Designs

DESIGN A   (Same group throughout, with i members)

Purpose: to test for permanency of the effects of intervention program

Program	Time	Observation
X_1	t_1	01_i
(X)	t_2	02_i
X_2	t_3	03_i

Measureable Effects

X effective if: $03 - 02 > 02 - 01$

DESIGN B   (Comparison Groups)

Purpose: to test for permanency of program effect while controlling for independent learning effects.

Time Series

(Group A)	R	X1	(X)	X2	(X)	01	02	03	04
(Group B)	R	(X)	X1	(X)	X2	05	06	07	08
(Time Period)		t1	t2	t3	t4	t1	t2	t3	t4

Measureable Effects

X effective if: $01 > 05,\ 06 > 02,\ 03 > 07,\ 08 > 04$

by a return to preintervention conditions, and then, in a subsequent time period, the intervention is initiated for a second time.

Data Arrangements

Data collection procedures for the switchback design are shown in Table 5-7. In design A, the program X is initiated in time period t1, and observations of performance are taken. In these designs, time series observations are often essential. 01_i indicates the ith time series observation taken during the first time interval. In the second time interval, preintervention conditions are established. Observations 02_i (also in a time series form) are recorded. Finally, the intervention is reestablished in time period 3, and the final set of observations (03_i) are recorded. To illustrate, the effects of a nurse orientation program in a hospital are often confounded with on–the–job learning. The switchback design can dissociate the effect of the orientation program from information a nurse can acquire on the job. The program could be initiated (in part) during time period 1. During time period 2 the indigenous process of information acquisition would supplant formal presentations. In time period 3, the orientation program is completed. If information acquisition rate declines during time period 2, and increases again in time period 3, compelling support for the orientation program can be provided.

To further control for factors that influence information acquisition, recently hired nurses could be randomly divided into two groups. Data would be collected as shown in Design B, Table 5-7. X1 and X2 represent the first and second portion of the orientation program and (X) represents on–the–job information acquisition. This data collection scheme controls for the rate of early information acquisition, which typically far exceeds the rate of information acquisition in later time periods.

Data Analysis

Performance tests in Design A are similar to those described in the time series design. It is expected that the performance 03 will exceed 01, in Table 5-7, when learning and other natural processes occur along with the intervention (orientation) program. However, if performance indicators 01 and 03 are greater than performance indicators 02, using a paired or independent t test, rationale for program adoption is established. The data are analyzed as shown below:

$02_i - 01_i$ = on–the–job information acquisition rate
$03_i - 02_i$ = orientation program information acquisition rate

Should $02 - 01$ indicate a decline in the rate of information acquisition, the orientation program may have been a useful source of reinforcement. If $03 - 02$ indicates a jump in information acquisition, the benefit of the orientation program is established. The data are analyzed, using a t test, as shown below:

On-the job information acquisition	Information acquisition due to orientation program	di
$02 - 01$	$03 - 02$	$(02 - 01) - (03 - 01)$
$\vdots$	$\vdots$	$\vdots$

An independent t test (discussed in Chapter 3) can be used to compare information acquired from the orientation program with information acquired on the job for each person. A paired t can be used to block for individual differences.

Design B controls for time-dependent information acquisition effects. These effects can be analyzed by a paired t test, as shown below:

Time	Information acquisition during program	Information acquisition on the job	di
t1	01_i	05_i	$01 - 05$
t2	06_i	02_i	$06 - 02$
t3	03_i	07_i	$03 - 07$
t4	08_i	04_i	$08 - 04$

This analysis blocks for learning effects. If the statistic d over its variance is nonzero, the program effects merit exploration. An ANOVA analysis procedure can be used to include the effect of different ordering of the program on groups A and B.

SOURCE OF INFORMATION

	On the job	Orientation program
1	$[(02 - 01) + (04 - 03)]^1$	$[01 + (03 - 02)]^1$
2	$[(02 - 01) + (04 - 03)]^2$	$[01 + (03 - 02)]^2$

GROUP A $\vdots$ $\vdots$ $\vdots$

1	$[05 + (07 - 06)]^1$	$[(06 - 05) + (08 - 07)]^1$
2	$[05 + (07 - 06)]^2$	$[06 - 05) + (08 - 07)]^2$
GROUP B :	:	:

$[(02 - 01) + (04 - 03)]$i is on–the–job information acquired by person i in Group A. This scheme permits an assessment of presentation or order effects (Group A vs. Group B), the program's effect, and the learning–order effects interaction.

Remission and Longitudinal Designs

In some evaluations it is difficult to separate the effects of an intervention program from obscure changes that occur in those exposed to the intervention. For example, when assessing the merits of a cancer treatment it is often difficult to relate the shrinkage of tumors with particular types of treatment like radiotherapy or chemotherapy. Changes in a tumor's size follow complex natural processes not fully understood. As a result, changes in the size of a tumor may have been caused by the treatment, by natural processes, or by both.

These same problems also occur whenever an intervention program evokes strong psychological responses from people. For instance, giving sugar pills (placebos) to those experiencing great pain often relieves the pain. (Consequently, the claims made for aspirin and similar pain relievers should be received with considerable skepticism.) In the same manner, the symbolic power of an intervention program may influence the perceptions of its clients.[6] The program may have no identifiable benefit, but its beneficiaries may be comforted by its attempts on their behalf. For example, Head Start continued to receive strong support from its clients after an evaluation by Westinghouse Learning Corporation concluded the program had no demonstrable benefits.[7]

Data Collection

Remission designs attempt to isolate internal changes in an intervention's target group. This design is shown in Table 5–8. Program recipients are randomly divided into three groups. Measurements are taken in the first group (time period 1) and compared to measurements taken in the second group (time period 2) prior to an intervention. The last group receives the intervention. Several measurements can be taken following the intervention to trace long–range effects.

Table 5-8. Remission Designs & Longitudinal Design

Purpose: test for indigeneous changes in target groups & long run effects

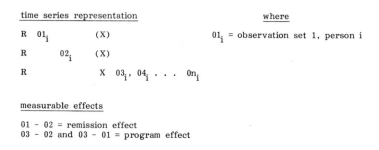

time series representation

R 01_i (X)

R 02_i (X)

R   X 03_i, 04_i . . . $0n_i$

where

01_i = observation set 1, person i

measurable effects

01 - 02 = remission effect
03 - 02 and 03 - 01 = program effect

Analysis and Statistical Tests

01–02 provides a measure of the remission effect. 03–02 and 03–01 can be used to assess the value of the intervention. On–02 detects long-run effects of the intervention. If the remission effect is larger or about the same as the effects of the intervention, the psychological impact of treatment may be masking its therapeutic value. The data can be analyzed by comparing the population of remission effects (01–02) with the population of program effects (03–02) using an independent t test.

Opinion Polls and Surveys

When seeking opinions about the impact of a variety of inadvertent interventions, evaluators often poll stratified samples of people. Even in stratified groups, people have views that are cluttered or even biased by information beyond the control of the evaluator. For instance, surveys of "investor's confidence" have little validity when taken in the wake of assassinations or other national trauma. At a more pedestrian level, hospitals seeking to determine the attitude of employees toward unionization will learn little about employee attitudes after a unionization drive has been initiated. The same applies for organizations attempting job, morale, or attitude surveys. These surveys have little use if taken in the wake of a real or imagined organizational conflict. Major controversies surrounding wages, working conditions, patient care practices, and the like will serve to depress workers and distort estimates of the overall morale in a work group.

Data Collection

The opinion poll design shown in Table 5-9 can be used to sort out the effects of information beyond the control of the evaluation. Two groups are tracked using periodic assessment of important performance indicators.

Table 5-9.   Opinion Polls And Surveys

Purpose: eliminate exogeneous biases

Time Series Representation:

N . . . OB_1 (X) OA_1 where: OB_1 = observations taken in hospital i before the event

N . . . OB_2 X OA_2 OA_1 = observations taken in hospital i after the event

Measurable Effects

$OA_1 - OA_2$ = the effect of X
$OA_2 - OB_2$ = the effect of X and various biases
$OA_1 - OB_1$ = test for (X), the stability of comparison group

Morale surveys using standard instruments like the job description inventory (JDI) could be taken for work groups within an organization over several time periods.[8] When an important event (designated as X in the design) occurs, observations following the event are compared to the observations prior to the event to determine if a change in attitudes can be associated with this unplanned intervention. A sister organization sharing data collected from the morale survey provides a baseline to judge the impact of the unplanned events. For example, this design could be used to assess the impact of a major malpractice claim on the morale of the nursing staff or others in a hospital. The effect of malpractice litigation can be determined by comparing an index of morale with a sister hospital, a naturally occurring group.

Analysis and Statistical Tests

Observations $0B_1$ and $0B_2$ are monitored to insure that organizations 1 and 2 have a history of similar morale. $0A_1$ and $0A_2$ are compared to isolate the effect of X, the intervention. An independent t test can be used to test the equivalency of the groups ($0B_1$ and $0B_2$) and the impact of the unplanned event ($0A_1$ and $0A_2$).

Dropout Controls

Participants in an evaluation study often drop out before the study is completed. For instance, a recent evaluation of the implications of national health insurance was initiated by HEW.[9] The study sought to determine the general health and health–seeking behavior of those in prepaid health care practices, compared with a matched group receiving conventional care through private–practice fee–for–service physicians. Comparison groups must be very carefully matched so that the characteristics like age, current health status, and the like were controlled. When some study participants drop out, the matching precision begins to break down. Differences in the groups may develop which can account for the evaluation conclusions. When these circumstances are likely, a dropout control should be used.

Data Collection

To control for the effects of losing evaluation participants, the experimental group is randomly divided into two more groups prior to the study, as shown

Table 5-10.   Dropout Controls

Purpose:	check effects of mortality on evaluation data

Time Series Representation

R 0_1 X 0_2 X% drop out
R 0_3 X 0_4 Y% drop out

Measurable Effects

$04 - 03$ VS $0_2 - 01$ = effect of different dropout rates
$04 - 03$ and $02 - 01$ = program effect
(check $0_2 - 0_3 = 0_4 - 0_1$)

in Table 5-10. In each group, measurements are taken to represent their initial status. Both groups are measured following the intervention.

Analysis Statistical Tests

The effect of participants that drop out of a study can be tested by comparing 02–01 and 04–03, using an independent t test. If this difference is zero, the evaluator can merge the data 02–01 with 04–03, and compare them to the control group.

CREATING QUASI-EXPERIMENTAL DESIGNS

The elemental designs discussed thus far can be combined in various ways to create data collection devices with application in a wide variety of evaluation studies. For instance, naturally occurring groups provide several independent observations for an evaluation project. An intervention in one setting will be unnoticed in the other environments. If these environments are carefully matched so their characteristics are similar, a control for both differences among the environments and independence in the observations can be provided. Similarly, randomization within a naturally occurring or a matched group is often possible, even if the groups themselves were not selected by a random process. Randomization typically enhances the validity of evaluation findings.

Selection of a data collection device (or design) should be based on the special needs of the evaluation study as well as the opportunities inherent in the evaluation environment. For instance, naturally occurring groups provide an inexpensive and useful way of making performance comparisons. When uncontrollable processes such as learning or maturation take place during an evaluation study, time–series or time–ordered data often can be useful. Finally, the concepts of matching can be used to check on the comparability of naturally occurring environments, or to construct an environment for an evaluation study.

Naturally–Occurring Groups As Controls

In Table 5–11, two designs are shown that use naturally occurring entities to form the comparison groups. In Design A, an intervention program is initiated in an experimental group, randomly selected from several naturally occurring environments. Another naturally occurring environment is selected to be used as a control. (The design can also be used when the naturally occurring groups were not randomly selected.) When several evaluation environments are randomly drawn from a population, these designs become true experimental designs. For example, neighborhood health centers could be

Table 5-11.   Naturally Occurring Groups As a Control

DESIGN A: External Controls

   Design Purpose: determine remission effects in naturally occurring
                     groups and the effects of base line measurement
                     to isolate the generalizability of the program's
                     effects.

   Time Series Representation

        R   01   (X)
   RN
        R   X   02

        R   03
   RN
        R   04

   Measurable Effects

        02 - 03 = 0, groups were similar
        02 - 01 = program effect
        02 - 04 = remission effects

DESIGN B: Program Strategy

   Design Purpose: compare several program intervention strategies

   Time Series Representation

        R   01   (X)   03
   RN
        R   02   X1   04

        R   05   (X)   07
   RN
        R   06   X2   08

   Measurable Effects

        04 - 03 = effect of intervention X1
        08 - 07 = effect of intervention X2
        08 & 04 = cpmpare X1 & X2 program effects
        01 + 02 less 05 + 06 = 0 when groups equivalent
        03 - 01 and 07 - 05 = maturation effects that occurs in each setting
        07 - 03 = differential maturation effects that occurs across groups

randomly selected by HEW officials for evaluation studies.[10] In other situations, a near 100 percent sample of the population may be obtained, and randomization is superfluous. For example, randomization is unnecessary, except as a means to reduce evaluation cost, when all hospitals that have a contract relationship with a particular multihospital system participate in an evaluation project.

In Design A, each naturally occurring group is further subdivided into two groups by some random process. One of the comparison groups in each naturally occurring environment is measured before the intervention and the other group is observed after the intervention. The comparison group serving as the control has no intervention or receives a placebo. The experimental group, further divided into local experimental and control groups, is exposed to a placebo and to the intervention program (see Table 5–11, Design A).

Design A: External Controls

Data Collection

NIH "panel studies" often use the concept of naturally occurring groups (see Design A, Table 5–11). To test the benefits of a new drug, surgical procedure, or the like, a carefully formulated protocol is distributed to competent investigators in a wide variety of clinical settings (naturally occurring environments). In some of these settings, consenting patients are randomly selected to be exposed to either the treatment process or a placebo. Other settings participate as a control. Patients suffering from similar problems are put into two control groups with measurements taken at different periods of time.

Analysis and Statistical Tests

Design A permits the evaluator to determine if groups were similar (01 – 03). The program effect is determined by 02 – 01. "Remission" effects are determined by 02 – 04.

Typically, several hospitals would participate in such a study. The program effect (02 – 01) would be determined in several environments. Similarly, the placebo effects (04 – 03) would be determined in several hospitals. The analysis could consider the significance of the program's effect (04 – 02), the measurement effect (04 – 03), and the group equality (03 – 01) for each hospital using a paired t on each data set. To illustrate, analysis for the program effect is shown below, assuming that hospitals 1 and A, 1 and B, 3 and C, etc., are matched.

Intervention	Placebo	d
02_1	04_A	$d_1 = (02 - 04)$
02_2	04_B	:
02_3	04_C	:
:	:	:

where: 02_1 is the observation after treatment in hospital 1

04_A is the observation after a placebo treatment in hospital A

If the matching process is unfeasible, the data would be analyzed by an independent t.

An ANOVA procedure could be used to study interaction terms as shown below:

		Program Effects	
		Intervention	Placebo
Experimental Group	Site #1	02 – 01	04 – 03
	Site #2	02 – 01	04 – 01
Group Effects	:	:	:
Control Group	Site #1	02	04
	Site #2	02	04
	:	:	:

Using this design, sites, nested in groups, can be tested along with the intervention and the intervention–site interaction. This permits an assessment of the impact of an intervention program across several dissimilar environments. Conclusions drawn from these types of evaluation data can be highly persuasive.

Design B: Program Strategy

Data Collection and Representation

Design B is similar to Design A, except that the naturally occurring environments are used to test program strategies. A slightly different interaction is carried out in the two environments. As shown in Table 5-11, intervention X1 is attempted in the first naturally occurring group, and intervention X2 in the second. (As in Design A, the naturally occurring groups can be selected from those available by some random, or random–stratified, process.)

To illustrate, HEW could use Design B to assess the merits of different teaching programs in independently operated Head Start Program sites. In the first site, Head Start participants would be randomly divided into two groups, with the first group receiving organized play, (X), and the second exposed to a teaching program with specific characteristics, designated X1. This teaching program could rely on certified teachers who use a specific type of curriculum, or have still other differences. In another Head Start site, the same process takes place except that the teaching program X2 is used. This program would be different from program X1 in terms of teacher qualification, the program of instruction, or other factors. Several sites would carry program X1 and several others would carry out program X2. This type of design can assess not only the merit of the basic program, but program variations, to determine how to best carry out an intervention program. The information collected through a single evaluation effort, using Design B, can be highly diagnostic.

Analysis Statistical Tests

04—03 and 08—07 can be used to test the effects of interventions X1 and X2 respectively. Comparing 08 against 04 indicates which intervention is best. Comparing 01 and 02 as well as 05 and 06 permits the evaluator to determine if the randomization procedure produced similar comparison groups at each site. Comparing 01 and 02 with 05 and 06 lets the evaluator assess the similarities of the naturally occurring groups. 03—01 less 07—05 measures the maturation effects that may occur in each setting. 07—03 is a measure of the differential maturation rates that occur across the naturally occurring groups. The data can be analyzed as shown below:

| | | | Program Effects | |
			Intervention	Placebo
	Strategy	Site #1	04 – 02	03 – 01
Program	X1	Site #2	04 – 02	03 – 01
Strategy				
Effects		⋮	⋮	⋮
	Strategy	Site #1	08 – 06	07 – 05
	X2	Site #2	08 – 06	07 – 05
		⋮	⋮	⋮

Study site is nested in program strategy: the analysis detects the performance of each strategy across distinct sites, using an analysis of variance procedure. Conclusions drawn include the impact of the intervention, the relative merits of program X1 and X2, and the program– strategy interaction. On occasion, much of this information is not needed and the analysis can be simplified as follows:

Strategy X1	Strategy X2
04 – 03	08 – 07
04 – 03	08 – 07
⋮	⋮

An independent t is used to compare the strategies, where each datum blocks for the placebo effects. (A paired t cannot be used unless the sites are matched.)
Maturation effects can be detected by arranging the data as shown below:

Maturation Effects

		Before	After
	Site #1	01	03
Site	Site #2	05	07
Effects	⋮	⋮	⋮

The analysis isolates the maturation effects, the site effects, and the site–maturation interaction effects. Again, the analysis of variance procedures are used.

Group equivalency can be detected using the format shown below:

Group Effects

		Control	Experimental
Site	Site #1	03 – 01	04 – 02
Effects	Site #2	07 – 05	08 – 06
	⋮	⋮	⋮

This analysis also applies an ANOVA procedure which determines the group, site, and group–site interaction effects.

Maturation, changes in participants during the study, in each study site can be detected using a paired t test to block for sites, as follows:

Maturation
Effects

X_1 Sites $\qquad$ $d = 03 - 01$

$\vdots$

X_2 Sites $\qquad$ $d = 07 + 05$

$\vdots$

These effects should be nonsignificant, or maturation would be confounded with program effects.

Designs With Matched Naturally Occurring Groups

Many naturally occurring groups lack comparability. For instance, multi-hospital systems offering hospital management contract services may seek to compare hospital performance indicators like cost per patient day or revenue per bed in contract–managed hospitals and noncontract–managed hospitals. The validity of this study can be enhanced by comparing performance indicators in contract–managed and noncontract–managed hospitals with *similar* characteristics. The hospitals can be matched according to the number of services they offer, the size and activity of their medical staff, competition within the community, and similar factors.

Data Collection and Representation

An example calling for an evaluation of a new "management appraisal" approach in contract managed hospitals, is illustrated in Table 5–12. Hospitals 1, 2, 3, 4, 5, and 6 are selected because they have comparable services and revenues. Observations are taken at each hospital before and after the appraisal approach has been initiated. In odd–numbered hospitals, the new management appraisal program is attempted, and in even–numbered hospitals the current appraisal approach is maintained. Effectiveness measures for the appraisal approaches are obtained for each set of hospitals. The effects of the appraisal approaches are determined over the same time intervals for all hospitals. Again, each of the six hospitals shown in Table 5–12 are carefully matched so they have such similar characteristics as service intensity or number of beds.

Statistical Tests and Analysis

The significance of the policy variable, the appraisal approach, can be determined using an independent t test. The net effect of the appraisal

Table 5-12: Designs Using Matched Comparison Groups

Purpose: To insure the comparability of comparison groups selected from a set of naturally occurring groups.

Representation A

Hospital[a]	Program Observation	Time Period
1	O1 X O2	t1 to t2
2	O3 (X) O4	t1 to t2
3	O5 X O6	t1 to t2
4	O7 (X) O8	t1 to t2
5	O9 X O10	t1 to t2
6	O11 (X) O12	t1 to t2

X = new management appraisal approach

(X) = current management appraisal approach

Representation B

		Intervention	
		X	(X)
Time	t1	O1,O5,O9	O3,O7,O11
	t2	O2,O6,O10	O4,O8,O12

[a]Matched naturally occurring groups (e.g., contract-managed hospitals with comparable services and revenues)

processes can be determined by the before–and–after indicators measured in each hospital. The data arrangement is shown below:

"Independent t"

New Appraisal Approach, X	Current Appraisal Approach, (X)
02 − 01	04 − 03
06 − 05	08 − 07
010 − 09	012 − 011
⋮	⋮

This analysis uses the baseline to assess the amount of performance improvement associated with the new appraisal approach. The control hospitals, those continuing to use the current appraisal approach, are used to measure improvement which occurred, independent of the new appraisal scheme.

Matching hospitals in the experimental and control groups permits the evaluator to compare the performance of the appraisal scheme, blocking for the effect of nonequivalent hospitals. The data can be paired as shown below:

"Paired t"

Pairings	d = X − (X)
Hospital 1 & 2	(02 − 01) − (04 − 03)
Hospital 3 & 4	(06 − 05) − (08 − 07)
Hospital 5 & 6	(010 − 09) − (012 − 011)
⋮	⋮

The paired t would test the differences in performance against zero. If differences are observed (the appraisal scheme enhanced performance across the hospitals), the difference must be large compared to the measurement error. The independent t would provide the same level of analytic validity if all six hospitals in the sample could be matched. As this is often impractical, the more restrictive situation has been described.

Matched Naturally Occurring Groups With Internal and External Controls

Naturally occurring groups, like neighborhood health centers and hospitals participating in NIH panel studies, have been shown to be a powerful aid in evaluation studies. The independent origin and behavior of these environments permit evaluators to use them as either control or experimental groups. Matching the naturally occurring groups can reduce the chance that group differences will influence the evaluation conclusions. The design illustrated in Table 5-13 is a refinement of design 12, using matched naturally occurring

Table 5-13.   Matched Naturally Occurring Groups Used To Provide Internal and External Controls

Purpose: To test the effects of environmental influences on the intervention program.

Representation A

Intervention - Observation			Center	Time
*MN M	01	(X)	1	t1
M	X	02	1	t2
MN M	03	(X)	2	t1
M	X	04	2	t2
MN M	05	(X)	3	t1
M	X	06	3	t2
MN M	07	(X)	4	t1
M	X	08	4	t2

X = a new medical record

Representation B

Time		Old Record	New Record
	t1	01, 02, 05, 07	
	t2	04, 08	02, 06

groups matched for internal and external controls to insure the equivalency of settings.

Data Collection and Representation

Assume that a new medical record system has been initiated in several neighborhood health centers and that a federal agency hopes to determine its acceptance in the field. In the example, shown in Table 5-13, four neighborhood health centers participate in an evaluation study to determine the acceptance of a new medical record. Centers 1, 2, 3, and 4 are matched according to characteristics that may influence the record's acceptance. Physician compliance rates, measured by the number of completed records over a certain time period, can be used as a proxy measure of acceptance. Compliance is determined by assigning a matched group of physicians to experimental groups, those that use the new medical record, and control groups, those that continue to use the old record in centers 1 and 3. (Alternatively, the physician groups could be matched according to their a priori views of the current record.) In neighborhood health centers 2 and 4, physician compliance could be measured without changes in the system, again matching physicians according to their views.

Statistical Tests and Analysis

The measurement effect can be determined using a paired t test comparing differences in $04 - 03$ and $08 - 07$. If these differences prove to be greater than zero, the measurement process had an effect on the behavior of the physicians. The data are formatted below.

(Block Variable)
Measurement Effects

$$d1 = 04 - 03$$
$$d2 = 08 - 07$$
$$\vdots$$

This design can also verify the comparability of the evaluation environments when $01 = 03 = 05 = 07$. The similarity of the evaluation environments is determined by comparing the internal and external control groups using a paired t test. This analysis is shown below.

Centers	Internal Control Groups	External Control Groups	d
1 & 2	01	03	$d1 = 01 - 03$
3 & 4	05	07	$d2 = 05 - 07$
	$\vdots$	$\vdots$	$\vdots$

The policy variable assesses the impact of the medical record in terms of physician compliance rates. Compliance rates 02 and 06 (stemming from the new medical records) can be compared with the internal control groups 01 and 05, and with the external control groups 04 and 08. A paired t can be used as illustrated below.

(Policy Variable)
Medical Record Compliance Rates

$d1 = 02 - 01$
$d2 = 06 - 05$
$\vdots$

Assuming centers 1 and 2 and centers 3 and 4 are comparble, the analysis can extract trends by folding in the external control group.

(Policy Variable)
Impact of Medical Record

$d1 = (02 - 01) - (04 - 03)$
$d2 = (06 - 05) - (08 - 07)$
$\vdots$

Cycle Designs with Partial Randomization

In Table 5–14, a cycle design with partial randomization is illustrated. This data collection device exposes naturally *recurring* groups to an intervention program. For instance, all patients admitted to a hospital on Monday with a given diagnosis can be compared to determine how a public relations program influences patients' perceptions of the hospital.

Data Collection and Representation

Cycle designs with randomization take the naturally occurring groups and randomly subdivide them into two additional groups. One segment of the naturally occurring group receives an intervention, and the other a placebo or no treatment. The data collection protocol can be applied over long periods of time to damp fluctuations due to individual differences. These designs can be effectively used when the attributes of participants in an evaluation program are not understood or cannot be anticipated through a forecast. Cycle designs

Table 5-14.   Cycle Designs with Partial Randomization

Purpose: to study the effects of an intervention program in an institution
when determining performance in several settings is impractical,
or when comparable settings cannot be found.

Conventional Representation:

	Intervention Program	Group	Block	Time	Observation
Naturally Occurring Groups	R (X) N	1A	Pre Test	t1	01
	R X	1B	Post Test	t2	02
(e.g., patients admitted to hospital with given diagnosis on Monday)	R (X) N	2A	Pre Test	t2	03
	R X	2B	Post Test	t3	04
X = new patient care practive	R (X) N	3A	Pre Test	t3	05
	R X	3B	Post Test	t4	06
	R (X) N	4A	Pre Test	t4	07
	R X	4B	Post Test	t5	08

etc.

Time-Series Representation:

N 01 (X)						group 1-A
X 02						group 1-B
N 03 (X)						group 2-A
X 04						group 2-B
N 05 (X)						group 3-A
X 06						group 3-B
N 07 (X)						group 4-A
X 08						group 4-B
N 09 (X)						group 5-A
X 010						group 5-B
t1 t2 t3 t4 t5 t6						

Split into two naturally occurring groups

also find applications in situations where extrainstitutional comparison groups are prohibited. Examples include evaluations that collect confidential financial data, assessments of medical staff views of supercharged incidents, and evaluations of institutional contingency plans. Cycle designs are similar to the designs that use naturally occurring groups as a control (Tables 5–11 and 5–12). Cycle designs define naturally occurring groups within a single environment, whereas the designs in Tables 5–11 and 5–12 use comparison groups from several environments (organizations). Both a conventional and a time series representation of the cycle design, with randomization, are shown in Table 5–14.

Analysis and Statistical Tests

The first step in the analysis is to remove trend effects from the data to keep these effects from cluttering up the analysis. To isolate the trend effect, all premeasurements (01, 03, 05, 07, 09) are plotted, as are all postmeasurements (02, 04, 06, 08). If a trend is apparent in these plots, the covariant is identified and removed. As described previously, this procedure may reduce the data's inherent variability, which removes some of the conservatism built into statistical tests.

To assess the impact of the policy variable, observations taken after the intervention program are compared to the initial observations taken before the placebo, for each naturally occurring group (see Table 5–14). Either an independent or a paired t test can be used, as the following shows:

	Independent t			Paired t
	X	(X)		$d = X - (X)$
Group 1	02	01	Group 1	02 − 01
Group 2	04	03	Group 2	04 − 03
Group 3	06	05	Group 3	06 − 05
Group 4	08	07	Group 4	08 − 07
⋮	⋮	⋮	⋮	⋮

A paired t test is generally preferable because it blocks for differences among participants in *each* of the naturally occurring groups. Most block variables cannot be assessed. In this case, the block variable, measurement bias, is mixed in with the cycle or trend effects. If a measurement bias exists, it will tend to deflate the trend effect which may be present in the data. Nevertheless, cycle designs with partial randomization provide an excellent method to block for individual differences while assessing the impact of the policy variable or an intervention program.

Cycle Designs without Randomization

On many occasions, randomization within a naturally occurring group is infeasible or impractical. For instance, to assess a new method of debt collection, a hospital may find it impractical to randomly assign, each week, admitted patients into two groups so that current debt collection practices can be used with one group and a new practice applied to the other. However, patients with more than a 90–day nonpayment history can be determined quarterly. Exposing those who turn up in odd–numbered months to current

Table 5-15. CYCLE DESIGNS WITHOUT RANDOMIZATION

Purpose: The design permits a study of programs using naturally occurring groups, within a particular setting, when partioning each naturally occurring group, using randomization is impossible or impractial

Conventional Representation

	Intervention Program	Group	Time	(Compliance) Observation
Naturally occurring	N (X)	1	t1, t2	01, 02
groups (e.g., patients	N X	2	t2, t3	03, 04
with more than a 90	N (X)	3	t3, t4	05, 06
day non-payment history	N X	4	t4, t5	07, 08
in any quarter of the	N (X)	5	t5, t6	09, 010
year.	N X	6	t6, t7	011, 012
	N (X)	7	t7, t8	013, 014
X=New Collection	N X	8	t8, t9	015, 016
Approach	etc.		etc.	etc.

Time Series Representation

group 1   01 (X) 02

group 2   03 (X) 04

group 3   05 (X) 06

group 4   07 (X) 08

group 5   09 (X) 010

group 6   011 (X) 012

group 7   013 (X) 014

group 8   015 . . .

time   t1   t2   t3   t4   t5   t6   t7   t8

bad debt collection practices and those in even–numbered months to a new procedure, can be used in place of randomization.

Data Collection

Cycle designs without randomization are shown in Table 5–15. Compliance rates can be used as the measure of effectiveness. In every month, the initial percent of bills paid can be compared to the percent paid following the current or proposed collection program.

Statistical Tests and Analysis

The trend effect is determined the same way described for cycle designs with randomization. The before measures and after measures are plotted to reveal patterns in the data. In the analysis a baseline, which is used to measure improvements over the current collection rate, is used to control for changes in rates of payment related to factors beyond the control of the study, like the receipt of a welfare check. An independent t test can be used to compare the rates of payment for the debt collection approaches, as shown below.

Independent t Test

New Collection Method X	Current Collection Method (X)
04 − 03	02 − 01
08 − 07	06 − 05
012 − 011	010 − 09
016 − 015	014 − 013
⋮	⋮

The policy variable (debt collection method) can also be assessed by eliminating (blocking) for time–related effects in the data. A paired t test would be used as shown below:

Paired t

Time Period	$d = X - (X)$
t_1 to t_2	(04 − 03) − (02 − 01)
t_3 to t_4	(08 − 07) − (06 − 05)
t_5 to t_6	(012 − 011) − (019 − 09)
t_7 to t_8	(016 − 015) − (014 − 013)
⋮	⋮

In this case, observations taken at adjacent time periods for nonintervention and intervention groups are paired. This procedure blocks for changes that occur over time.

NONEVALUATIVE METHODS

Through ignorance and misguided pragmatism, "nonevaluative" methods such as case studies, before–and–after comparisons, and/or single–comparison groups, are often used to answer important evaluation questions. These methods have few diagnostic abilities. Nonevaluative approaches can seldom yield information of sufficient quality to justify the cost of data acquisition and analysis.

Nonevaluative approaches have several common problems. Causal inferences drawn from these approaches can be easily challenged and argued away, because it is impossible to relate the observed performance with a particular intervention. A variety of other factors can provide equally plausible explanations of the change in performance which follows the initiation of an intervention program. A decline in costs, increase in satisfaction, and the like, may be due to the intervention and/or an inadequate or a biased sample of cases. The natural variability of the responses to most interventions makes it essential to make several independent estimates of performance and to carefully construct a baseline of performance to measure these effects against. Without such precautions, what appears to be a good outcome may prove to be illusory. Finally, nonevaluative methods often use nonequivalent comparison groups. The control group may differ substantially from the experimental group, making comparisons totally invalid. To dramatize these problems, three common nonevaluative approaches are discussed.

Table 5-16. Nonevaluative Data Collection Methods

Case Study
    time series representation:
        X0
    test: compare 0 to expectations

Before-and-After Study
    time series representation:
        01 X 02
    test: 02 − 01 = program effect

AD Hoc Comparison Groups
    time series representation:
        X 01
        02
    test: 01   02 = program effect

Case Studies

Table 5-16 illustrates a time series representation of a case study. A case study is similar to a "narrative history."[11] A retrospective analysis of past events or a reconstruction of these events is used to isolate cause-and-effect relationships. These observations can serve as little more than a tentative basis to draw inferences about a program's success. Even when the effects of the program have been carefully observed, they have limited value until they are compared to a before measure collected with equal care and precision.

Case studies rely on nonsystematic observations after an intervention takes place. For instance, a case study is used when an administrator installs a materials handling system for ward supplies in a hospital and evaluates its effectiveness using personal observations or testimonials. Case studies are often indistinguishable from an authoritative, or even nonauthoritative, opinion. Evaluation in many organizations relies on the views of experienced, if not knowledgeable, practitioners. As Mintzberg points out, imitation and tradition form the basis for many strategic organizational choices.[12]

Case studies provide little in the way of policy guidance to administrators. At best they can be used to suggest some of the intertwined factors which may be influencing the performance of an intervention program. Case studies can be helpful in defining evaluation issues by providing a historical view of events that may have caused success (or failure). A careful listing of block variables, performance measures, and protocols for the implementation of the intervention program may result.

The Before-and-After Study

A time-series representation of the before-and-after study is shown in Table 5-16. This evaluation approach is superior to the case study but still lacks the precision of quasi-experimental approaches. Long time periods between the measurements increases the chance that factors other than the intervention program cause the observed changes in 02. For example, a survey to determine patient attitudes, stemming from new patient care practice in the hospital, may be influenced by spurious contact with physicians and nurses as well as the intervention program. This design is unable to separate increases in performance as a natural outgrowth of repetition or learning, from the effects of the intervention program. Inflation and other exogenous factors cause a growth in the value of certain performance indicators. If these effects are not extracted from the evaluation data, the effects of these processes and the effects of the intervention program will be confounded. The inability of this design to control for block variables is a major limitation. The before-and-after study cannot sort out the impact of block variables including the accuracy of measurement process, changes in the observers or recording process, and the participants themselves. In most circumstances, these factors are likely to be present, and must be controlled, so before–and–after studies cannot be used.

Ad Hoc Comparison Groups

The ad hoc comparison groups is another common evaluation approach. Essentially the evaluator/sponsor recognizes the need for a control group but is unwilling or unable to establish one. Another conveniently available group not a part of the study (shown as 02 in Table 5-16) is assessed along with the group that receives an intervention. If the intervention group performs better than the comparison group, the intervention is termed a "success."

When comparison groups are carefully selected, or when they occur naturally, these comparisons can provide the evaluator with useful information. However, selecting a reference group without careful consideration of the similarities between the environments or participants typically yields highly inaccurate evaluation conclusions. For example, hospitals assessing their financial management activities may compare their bad–debt rate with rates in other community hospitals. The differences between the hospitals may be dramatic. Some hospitals in the community have a very high proportion of low–income patients. If so, it is likely their bad–debt rates are high, regardless of the quality of the financial management program. These differences are likely to be the primary cause of a particular bad rate. To make meaningful comparisons, these hospitals must be compared to meaningful reference groups, those with similar clientele.

Comparisons of performance between nonmatched groups are pervasive in the health care industry. For instance, if an 80 percent occupancy rate is the highest rate achieved by hospitals in the community, it is often used as a benchmark. In other cases, administrators employ social tests, mimicking the activities and programs or other organizations because their cost–per–patient day is low or because the organization's medical/staff relations are believed to be "good." Organizational differences as well as exogenous factors make such comparisons misleading and not worth the effort.

SUMMARY

A variety of quasi–experimental data collection devices have been presented. Several of these approaches can be applied to most evaluation problems. The evaluator should always select the most powerful evaluation approach that is feasible for the evaluation task. The following chapter provides some guidelines for this selection process. Experimental approaches are compared with nonevaluative methods and quasi–experimental approaches. The framework is provided to aid the evaluator in assessing the strengths and weaknesses of these methods.

NOTES

1. Kershaw, P.N., "Issues in Income Maintenance," in P. Rossi, et al. (eds.) *Evaluating Social Programs.* New York: Seminar Press, 1972.
2. Campbell, D.T. and J.C. Stanley, *Experimental and Quasi–Experimental Designs for Research.* Chicago: Rand–McNally, 1963.
3. Rosenthal conducted several experiments in which the experimenter could select between data that confirmed or discredited the experimenter's hypothesis. His experiments revealed that experimenters will actively seek out information that confirms their hypothesis. This bias is subtle and often unconscious. Often experimenters structure data collection and search out cases which help them substantiate their views. Evaluation projects can be subject to the same kind of biases. The evaluator may feel pressure to confirm the views of important, powerful figures who favor either a new or the current approach. Rosenthal, R., "On The Social Psychology of the Psychological Experiment: The Experiments Hypothesis As An Unintended Determinant of Experimental Results," *American Psychologist,* Vol. 51, No. 2, June 1963, pp. 268–283.
4. Likert Scales are described in Likert, *New Patterns of Management.* New York: McGraw–Hill, 1961. For an illustration of Hackman Items see Hackman, J.R. and E.E. Lawler III, "Employee Reactions to Job Characteristics," *Journal of Applied Psychology Monographs,* Vol. 55, No. 3, June, 1971, pp. 259–286. Anchored rating scales are discussed in Nutt, P.C., "Comparing Internal & External Criteria Weighting Techniques," *The Midwest Institute of Decision Sciences Proceedings,* Vol. 9, May 1978.
5. Webb. E.J., D.T. Campbell, R.D. Schwartz, J. Sechrest, *Unobtrusive Measures: Nonreactive Research in the Social Sciences.* Chicago: Rand–McNally, 1972.
6. Suchman, E.A., *Evaluative Research: Principles and Practice in Public Service and Social Action Programs.* New York: Russell Sage Foundation, 1967.
7. Williams W. and J.W. Evans, "The Politics of Evaluation: The Case of Head Start," in P. Rossi et al. (eds.) *Evaluating Social Programs.* New York: Seminar Press, 1972.
8. The *job description inventory* is a questionnaire that measures job status factors keyed to standard job descriptions and perceived opportunities for promotion, pay increases, supervision, and the like. The baseline provided through a comparison of job satisfaction across organizations and industries for comparable jobs can be quite useful. Without such a baseline, morale surveys have little value.
9. Newhouse, J.P., "A Design for a National Health Insurance Experiment," *Inquiry,* Vol. 11, March 1974, pp. 5–27.
10. Table 5–13 describes data collection when randomization (or population based estimation) is infeasible.
11. Filley, A., R. House, and S. Kerr, *Managerial Process and Organizational Behavior.* Glenview, Ill.: Scott, Foresman, 1976 (Revised Edition).
12. Mintzberg, H., D. Raisinghani, and A. Theoret, "The Structure of 'Unstructured' Decision Process," *Administrative Science Quarterly,* Vol. 26, No. 2, 1976 pp. 246–275.

Contrasting Evaluative Methods

> ...the love of wisdom...returns to the Socratic principle equipped with a
> multitude of special methods of inquiry and tests.
>
> John Dewey

This chapter compares results that stem from experiments, quasi–experiments, and nonevaluative methods. The strengths and weaknesses and range of application of these data–collecting arrangements are presented.

JUDGING VALIDITY

To provide convincing evaluation results, Campbell and Stanley contend that evaluation findings must have both internal and external validity.[1] *Internal validity* describes the ability of an evaluation method to relate the observed performance measures (effects) to a specific cause or set of causes. The "cause–and–effect relationship," or model, contains one or more performance measures or dependent variables as well as two classes of causal or independent variables: policy variables and block variables.[2] An internally valid evaluation project can relate particular outcomes to specific levels of the policy and block variables. Internal validity is the sine qua non of an evaluation project.

An *externally valid* evaluation finding can be extrapolated or generalized to a wide range of situations or circumstances. Many evaluation projects seek to generalize their findings beyond the data collected. When an evaluation suggests policy actions that are useful in a variety of settings, or environments, its findings are termed externally valid.

Internal validity is concerned with controlling bias. Bias occurs when factors not controlled in the data collection become confounded with the intervention and inflate (or deflate) performance measures. External validity is inductive. For example, evaluation data can be collected for several socioeconomic strata. Inferences can be drawn for strata, such as levels of income, not represented in the evaluation study. Economy dictates that some strata must be deleted. Others simply escape the attention of the evaluator. As a result, the external validity of an evaluation has practical limits. External validity declines as conclusions are extended to more and more strata not considered in the project. The findings of any evaluation effort must be carefully qualified to indicate circumstances in which the evaluation findings are likely to hold.

Internal Validity

The credibility of evaluation findings increases as other plausible explanations for the findings can be discredited. Evaluation data are collected so these factors will be implausible as explanations of the evaluation findings. For example, repetition invariably improves skill, often making controls for practice or learning effects mandatory. Elton Mayo's famous experiments failed to control for motivation during a study of how productivity was affected by work environment, lighting, music, and the like. Ultimately motivation, not the environmental factors, explained *all* of the observed increases in productivity.[3] Learning, performance enhancement through participation, and the like, have taken on the status of empirical laws. Unless they are carefully controlled in the evaluation project they can provide compelling reasons to discount, or even dismiss, an observed performance improvement that follows a managerial intervention. In statistical terms, these factors become confounded with the policy variable. The credibility of the evaluation findings always improves when the influences of factors like skill are either controlled or distributed equally across comparison groups.

Campbell and Stanley identified eight factors that influence internal validity.[4] If not controlled, history, maturation, regression, testing, instrumentation, selection, mortality, and various selection interaction effects may provide plausible explanations of evaluation findings. Performance measures in most evaluation projects can be inflated or deflated by one or more of these factors unless they are carefully controlled during data collection.

History depicts unplanned events which occur as the intervention program is initiated. These events often influence measurements of the intervention program's success. For instance, opinion surveys that follow a new management practice carried out while employees are agitating for a union, measure both the effects of unionization and the effects of the intervention. Generally, the longer the time interval between the pre– and postintervention measures, the higher the likelihood that events will occur that will inflate or deflate (bias) the measures taken.

Maturation describes various processes or natural changes that occur with the passage of time. For example, the aging process produces both mental and physical changes in human beings. In comparatively short time intervals, people grow hungrier, become tired or fatigued, engage in vicarious learning, and acquire information from a variety of sources not documented in the evaluation data. This acquisition of insights and information as well as changes in the physical status of people during the evaluation can bias evaluation findings. For instance, the age–specific learning rates of children must be considered when assessing the impact of new instructional methods. Whenever people or even organizations perform certain tasks, performance will improve through repetition. If an evaluation process is initiated soon after an intervention program is installed, a learning effect may be mixed with the effect of the program.

Test reactions may occur as a consequence of any measurement process. By merely asking questions or by making observations, people, and even organizations, become sensitive to the kinds of results preferred. As a result, people either conform (or refuse to conform) to the implied expectations. The data reflect this capriciousness, making the evaluation findings suspect. Surveys and questionnaires that explore the attitudes or preferences of people can be rendered invalid by testing effects if the initial measurement process was reactive. For instance, pretests are often used to determine a person's initial state of knowledge. However, pretests suggest a course of study which will optimize the performance on a post test, a process quickly adopted by students seeking to optimize their grade. Thus, the act of measurement interacts with the educational program. When an initial measurement process sensitizes participants to the program's objectives, the merits of the intervention program are often overstated. In other instances, people, work groups, or even entire organizations participating in an evaluation project may believe they were selected because they are outstanding in some way, when in fact selection was the result of a random process. The benefits of participation can stimulate a greater than normal effort during the period the evaluation project is being conducted, making performance levels atypical.

Instrumentation refers to changes in the calibration of the instruments used to measure the results of the intervention program. Survey respondents may interpret the questions on a survey differently. A tired or careless surveyor may irritate some respondents, thus altering their responses. Interviewers and observers tend to be more skillful and perceptive as they gain exposure to the evaluation topic, and their questions are phrased more succinctly and with less ambiguity. For example, a careful set of instructions must accompany a hospital closed–claims malpractice survey, or the responding hospitals may selectively define variables such as mode of settlement, amount of settlement, misadventures in diagnosis and treatment, and the like. Physical measurement processes also require calibration. Accounting systems often measure particular costs with varying error rates and may *not* permit segregation of costs into categories meaningful for evaluation. The number of retakes in an x–ray department may be recorded haphazardly and/or not segregated into poor procedure and verification categories. As a result, changes in the calibration of evaluation instruments can be an important source of bias in evaluation results.

Regression effects may occur when individuals are selected because they have extreme scores or unique characteristics. For instance, the mean performance of individuals often improves with retesting. As a result, evaluating the effects of a reading program by using slow readers as a test group will overstate the benefits of the program. To determine the effects of satellite clinics, an evaluation project may select groups of users and nonusers, matching the two groups across characteristics such as income. Characteristics like income are likely to change as people are laid off from their jobs, gain employability through training, and so on. Thus, regression effects often result when extreme cases are selected. Looking at each characteristic, (such as individual income) as a distribution, the likelihood that people will fall on the tails of the distribution is very low. On retesting or remeasurement, regression to the mean often occurs. The differences between groups become less distinct.

Selection procedures identify evaluation participants. These procedures are used to select a target group for the evaluation and to divide the target group into experimental and control comparison groups. Inconsistent selection procedures produce nonequivalent comparison groups. Differences in the comparison groups may account for differences in performance and satisfaction which are observed when comparing the experimental and control groups. For example, evaluation projects to determine the effectiveness of drug abuse programs or antismoking clinics can overstate (or understate) the program's effectiveness unless they carefully account for the nature of the program's clientele.

Mortality occurs when some comparison groups or members of a comparison group drop out of the evaluation project. For instance, a multihospital system administering several community hospitals under a contract may attempt a job–enrichment program in several of their contract–managed hospitals. Sample mortality occurs when some of the hospitals serving as controls drop the contract during the evaluation of the job–enrichment program. The hospitals that dropped out of the study may have experienced a highly successful or quite unsuccessful job–enrichment program, biasing the overall estimates of program effectiveness. Mortality in either the experiment or control group may make comparisons invalid.

Selection biases can also produce interactions with several other factors. A *selection–maturation interaction* may occur when those selected for *one* of the comparison groups exhibit different rates of compliance, performance, learning, etc. Performance measures would detect changes in the selective maturation of people as well as the program effects. A confounding or mixing of program and selection–maturation effects results. For example, hospital administrators may send employees who lack ability or interest to continuing education programs and conclude that educational programs have little value. *Selection-measurement* or *selection-instrumentation* interactions may occur when selection procedures for the comparison groups differ. Selection interactions can be controlled by including various measurement approaches as block variables. For example, using distinct measurement processes (such as parallel measurement) can detect the selective effects of reactive pretests, which provides a control for selection–measurement interactions.

External Validity

Externally valid evaluation findings can be extended to other settings or target groups. Huston identifies several factors that restrict the generalizability of evaluation findings.[5] They include units, block variables, measures, interactive testing, selection-program interference, reactive arrangements, treatment interference, and naturally correlated variables. Dealing with each of these factors can often improve the generalizability of the findings.

The *units* studied in the evaluation project stem from samples drawn from the program's clientele or beneficiaries. To provide compelling evidence linking the program to observed effects in its intended *target group,* this sampling process must be carefully carried out. For instance, random samples that draw age, sex, and health status strata from the target group are preferred. When the participants (units) in an evaluation are not representative of the target group, the external validity of the study can be poor. For example, the negative income tax experiments were criticized for selecting low–income people in a particular community in New Jersey as participants in an evaluation because unemployment in that region had been particularly volatile due to periodic layoffs by local firms.[6] Participants in the comparison groups hardly characterized the hard–core unemployed—those without any income for several years. Sample adequacy was also a problem in the Job Corps program. The Job Corps was initiated to seek out young people from low–income families, who failed to finish high school. The program administrators, hoping to operate a successful program, made a special effort to find and enroll students with good high school performance. The program administrators found that the effectiveness of the Job Corps declined dramatically when applied on a large scale.

Block variables can be used to control for environmental factors and other variables that provide important qualifications to the evaluation findings. For example, when investigating the effectiveness of a highway safety program, an evaluation should consider holidays, bad weather conditions, and the time of day when accidents occur. If highway accidents and/or fatalities decline in the wake of a highway safety initiative, these block variables offer important qualifications to the program's effects for policy makers.

The *measures* of the intervention program effectiveness may or may not capture the intent of the program's objectives. Evaluation projects often measure convenient effects which have little or no relationship to the objectives of the program. For example, the program administrators of HEW's contact centers have used the number of contacts to assess the center's effectiveness. Disposition of referrals would have been a better measure for these programs because it is tied to the (implicit) objective of contact centers: improved entry into the health care system.

Interactive testing occurs when a measurement procedure implies or suggests the kind of behavior an evaluator and/or sponsor prefers or endorses. These implicit suggestions may cause participants to react favorably (or unfavorably) to the intervention, making satisfaction measures unrepresentative of the program's effects when applied on a large scale to its intended clientele. For instance, hospitals may use "T–groups" to dramatize to their employees the need for tact when dealing with patients. To evaluate the merits of the T–groups, a pretest may be used to determine their employee's approach to the uneasy or frightened patient. The pretest may sensitize employees, making the T–groups superfluous. (In this case, the pretest should be included as an evaluation variable to measure its effects.)

Suchman points out that the apparent effectiveness of many treatments stemmed from the symbolic power of the physician, the social pressure on the patient to respond, and the belief of both patient and physician in the effectiveness of therapy, not from the treatment itself.[7] This placebo effect stems from the intense hope, by both patient and physician, for a cure. Frank points out that until the past few decades, most medications prescribed by physicians were pharmacologically inert.[8] Physicians were getting positive results by prescribing placebos. Suchman extends this idea to social action programs, contending that the programs may appear to work largely because both consumers and practitioners have faith in them.[9] As a result, dummy programs (placebos) are used to detect responses which stem from the hope or expectation of benefits implicit in most interventions.

A *selection–program interaction* occurs when participants particularly amenable to an intervention program are placed in one of the comparison groups. This, for example, occurred in the Job Corps program when its administrators sought candidates with good high school achievement records. Evaluation data drawn from these participants lacked external validity: the findings failed to suggest how the typical high school dropout might respond to the program.

Reactive evaluation arrangements are elements in the evaluation setting which carry special and unintended significance to participants. For instance, when assessing the merits of a new personnel appraisal program, the interview should not be carried out in the boss's office, but on neutral turf. The boss, sitting behind a desk cluttered with symbols of his supervisory power, is unlikely to elicit candid responses from the person being appraised. To reduce the reactiveness of an appraisal, the meeting could take place in an informal setting like a cafeteria. Some administrators provide couches in their office to help reduce the social distance between them and their subordinates.

Treatment interference occurs when an intervention program influences participants in a way that cannot be nullified or erased. For example, when evaluating educational achievements, prior skills cannot be erased. In the treatment of Hodgkin's Disease, patients may have been inappropriately treated with a low KV cobalt. When this occurs, patients cannot receive optimal treatment with a high–voltage linear accelerator, because the body can only receive certain amounts of radiation without highly undesirable side effects. Thus, an inappropriate initial treatment limits the effectiveness of subsequent treatments. An evaluation of the benefits of radiation therapy should carefully exclude patients with exposure to low KV cobalt, or the evaluation studies will understate the benefits of radiotherapy.

Finally, *naturally correlated variables* may be confounded or mixed with the intervention program. For instance, an evaluation program seeking to control for race and religion may be unable to locate sufficient numbers of Oriental Muslims or white Buddhists to permit analysis.

The intrusion of uncontrolled factors into an evaluation project is often subtle and difficult to detect. Antagonists and critics of evaluation results, in particular those who can benefit from a certain evaluation finding, are quick to point out plausible (if not probable) weaknesses in an evaluation study. Further, the factors that influence external validity may be latent. A careful study of these factors before the project begins, with the help of those familiar with the evaluation topic, can suggest factors that merit control. Many threats to external validity can be controlled by selecting an appropriate data–collection device (or design).

COMPARING EVALUATION APPROACHES

The advantages and disadvantages of the data collection devices (designs) discussed in Chapter 5 will be described by their internal and external validity. Each design is ranked by the extent that factors influencing internal and external validity are likely to cause difficulty in interpreting evaluation findings. For simplicity, Campbell and Stanley's scale is used.[10] A minus sign signifies that the design is likely to be affected by the factor, whereas a plus indicates that the data collection device seems immune. A blank indicates factors that are not relevant. A question mark depicts a weak causal connection: the factor may cause problems if not controlled in certain types of evaluation projects.

The scoring of the data collection approaches (or designs) in Tables 6–1, 6–2, 6–3, and 6–4 differs dramatically from those suggested by Campbell and Stanley.[11] The limitations of data collection devices seem situational. The merits of these approaches in particular application areas are unlikely to extend to others.

The designs summarized in Tables 6–1, 6–2, 6–3, and 6–4 have been assessed to isolate their *overall* merits when applied to the evaluating intervention programs in human service industries. These conclusions must be interpreted with care. The merits of a given design are less dependent on the application area (like health or education) than the specifics of each evaluation project. This suggests that evaluators should carefully compare the merits of feasible data collection devices *for each evaluation project* by following the rationale outlined in this chapter. Index numbers can be developed to score designs, based on their application to particular evaluation topics. For example, a five–point scale could be used. Five could signify that a particular evaluation approach seems immune from the influences of a factor, and 1 used to identify factors that seem uncontrolled and likely to distort the measures of program effectiveness in the project. Scoring the designs in this way helps the evaluator to systematically consider factors that may bias or limit the scope of application of the evaluation findings. A data collection device is selected, for a particular project, to control for factors likely to influence the project's findings.

NONEVALUATIVE APPROACHES

Much evaluation carried out in the health and human services industries follows the dicta of designs 1, 2 and 3 as shown in Table 6–1. Evaluation consists of a follow–up measurement after the intervention. This evaluation approach is called a case study. Represented as a time series,[12] the design is shown diagramatically below:

$$X \ O$$

When an intervention program is evaluated in the absence of careful baseline measurements, the equivalent of a case study results. Case studies compare the measure O to some set of expectations. When results seem good because the measurement process confirms the sponsor's expectations, the program is adopted. For instance, a nursing supervisor may free staff nurses from clerical duties to increase their patient contact, hoping to alter patients' behavior or perceptions. The merits of this intervention program would be based on the

Table 6-1. Factors Influencing The Internal and External Validity of Non-Evaluative and Experimental Designs

	INTERNAL								EXTERNAL							
	History	Maturation	Measurement	Instrument	Regression	Selection	Mortality	Selection Interactions	Target Group	Selection	Block Variables	Testing	Outcome Measures	Correlated Variables	Reactive Setting	Multiple Treatments
NON-EVALUATIVE DESIGNS																
1. Case Study X O	−	−	−	−		−			−	−	−	?	−	?	?	?
2. Before-After Study 01 X 02	−	−	−	−		−			−	−	+	+	−	?	?	?
3. Adhoc Comparisons X 01 / 02	+	+			?	−	?	−	−	+	−	−	−	?	?	?
EXPERIMENTAL DESIGNS																
4. Factorials with (pre-test block variable) R 01 X 02 / R 02 04 / R X 05 / R 06	+	+	+	−		+	?	+	+	+	+	+	−	+	?	?
5. Factorials (with instrument as block variable) R XA 01 / R (X)A 02 / R XB 03 / R (X)B 04 A & B distinct measurement instruments	+	+	?	+		+	?	+	+	+	+	−	−	+	?	?
6. Factorial (with parallel measures as a block variable) R X 01 / R 01 / R X 02 / R 02 0 & 0 distinct measures	+	+	?	+		+	?	+	+	+	+	+	+	+	?	?

Where:
?: factor may be uncontrolled in certain applications
−: factor not controlled in design
blank: factor not relevant
+: factor is controlled in design

supervisors' expectations of what is an adequate level of satisfaction or appropriate behavior in patients.

As shown in Table 6–1, a wide array of factors could explain away the evaluation findings stemming from a case study. For instance, if learning can occur, learning effects would be mixed with the program effects, "X." The measurement "O" will detect the program effect *and* the effects associated with each of the uncontrolled factors. As shown in Table 6–1, none of the relevant factors that influence internal and external validity can be controlled in a case study. As a result, case studies have little value in isolating the effects of intervention programs and seldom provide evaluation information with policy significance.

The Before–and–After Study

Before–and–after studies are also commonly used to assess the impact of managerial interventions. These are essentially case studies with the addition of a baseline measurement. A measurement is taken before and following an intervention. If the differences between the before and after measures are large, the program is assumed to be good and thus is implemented.

This evaluation approach is shown diagramatically below:

$$O1 \quad X \quad O2$$

As shown in Table 6–1, the before–and–after study permits an evaluator to gauge the magnitude of the O2–O1 difference, which the before–and–after study assumes was caused by the program X.

Linking this difference to the program, X, can be challenged then on several grounds. A key factor influencing internal validity is history. During the time which elapses between the measurements O1 and O2, events may have occurred that influence these measures. For example, when effectiveness measure was taken from a survey, history effects can be particularly troublesome. The effect measured by the survey is likely to be small in comparison to external events which stimulate hostility, warmth, or other responses in the respondent. Similarly, surveys to determine a hospital's views of various prospective reimbursement schemes may be biased if HEW proposes a cap on all hospitals costs during the survey period.

Systematic changes which occur with the passage of time cannot be controlled in a before–after study. Between measurements O1 and O2, participants may have grown older, become bored, or experienced fatigue which may serve to depress their performance. O2 would be abnormally low. In other cases, O2 is inflated by the passage of time. Illustrations include learning, which often occurs within the context of any new program.

Often measurement processes are obtrusive: the process of taking the measurement changes the object being measured. For instance, students taking graduate placement exams often do better when taking the test for a second time. Personality tests often show better adjustment when the test is repeated. Measures of attitudes, perceptions, and beliefs are particularly susceptible to obtrusive measurement processes. For example, naive subjects are more likely to be candid in their responses but subsequently begin to understand some of the ramifications of being candid. The second set of responses may be tailored to meet what is in the respondent's best interests. Reactive measurement often stimulates reactions that are mixed with the effects of the intervention program. The value of O2 may be caused by the intervention program, or a stimulus implicit in a reactive process of measurement. For example, Elaine Powers Weight Control Programs require a public weigh–in before the program begins. The weigh–in itself may provide a sufficient impetus for many people to attempt to reduce their weight.

Survey instruments like Hackman items are likely to be influenced by history. A Hackman item offers respondents an opportunity to provide open–ended responses to general questions. This type of instrument can be dramatically affected by changes in mood, interaction with peers, and other factors.

Differences in calibration of the measurement instrument may account for the O2–O1 differences observed in before–after designs. For example, human observers may experience learning, fatigue, and the like, which influence the accuracy of their observations. Survey interviewers may get on with one set of respondents, creating favorable responses, and create hostility in another group, creating unfavorable responses. In other instances, the calibration used in the measurement process may be subject to change with the passage of time. If survey instruments are long, respondents may become exasperated, giving later questions only superficial attention.

In short, before–and–after studies have very little ability to link cause and effect (a performance measure with an intervention program). History, maturation, reactive measurement, changes in instrument calibration, and still other factors can explain the observed evaluation findings. Discussions of the generality (external validity) of effects which are highly uncertain are pointless.

Ad Hoc Comparisons

An ad hoc comparison takes two types of observations following intervention programs. Hospitals seeking to evaluate their bad–debt collection procedures may compare their experiences to others in the community or to rates reported by data services for a region.[13] Administrators often initiate evaluation studies of this type, hoping for quick answers. For instance, to determine if the new outpatient clinic has stimulated hospital admissions, the hospital may compare its admissions rate with others in the community. These ad hoc comparisons are nonevaluative because the differences among the hospitals are likely to render the comparisons meaningless.

As shown in Table 6-1, ad hoc comparisons can control for history and maturation effects, but additional problems arise. The most serious problem is selection. Comparing hospitals in terms of their bad–debt experience has little diagnostic value unless the hospitals are similar. A particular hospital's clientele may have a high proportion of low–income (no–pay) patients, which is bound to drive up its bad–debt rate. Comparisons stemming from dissimilar hospitals provide little diagnostic information. Clever administrators often make invalid comparisons of this type to deflect legitimate criticisms.

Evaluation carried out in the health care industry is often based on ad hoc comparisons. For instance, HAS data compare hospitals on a regional basis, but disregard factors such as hospital size, number of services, composition of the medical staff, and the like in these comparisons. Standard reporting forms in hospitals often accumulate performance and other data with only minimal attention to how wards in a hospital differ in terms of case mix and other factors.[14] This has led organizations to collect enormous amounts of data that have only marginal diagnostic value.

Mortality may bias evaluation data based on ad hoc comparison groups. For instance, a multihospital system may have initiated new management practices in some of their hospitals to compare these hospitals' performances to those in a control group. Mortality occurs when the proportion of hospitals that fail to participate varies in the experimental and comparison groups. If the mortality rate is higher in one group than the other, mortality effects may explain away the evaluation findings. Similarly, if a large hospital seeks to investigate the effects of a new management control procedure and it involves all departments in the evaluation, the transfer or resignation of the department head may limit participation of some departments, causing them to drop out of the study.

Ad hoc comparison groups also may induce a selection–maturation interaction. Different learning rates and other changes in comparison groups may accentuate or damp out performance comparisons.

The inability of ad hoc comparison groups to control for factors that influence internal validity makes unnecessary a full discussion of their limitations in extrapolating their findings.

The discussion of nonevaluative methods serves to discourage the use of these data collection devices for most serious evaluation efforts. Nonevaluative approaches are unlikely to provide diagnostic evaluation information, no matter how carefully they are carried out.

EXPERIMENTAL DESIGNS

The essential ingredient in experimental designs is randomization. The assignment of people, organizations, departments, etc., to treatment and nontreatment categories is dictated by a random process in a true experimental design. These designs can also estimate the importance of extraneous variables and their interaction with the program effects. In Table 6–1, a factorial design is shown which attempts to control for three distinct types of extraneous variables. In Design 4, test effects are measured. Design 5 manipulates the data collection instrument, and parallel measures are used in Design 6.

Controls for Internal Validity

Table 6–1 illustrates the power of Designs 4, 5, and 6 to isolate the effects of an intervention program. For example, history effect is equally distributed across the measurements taken. As a result, comparisons among these measurements can be made independent of the history effect. A blocking strategy can be used to control for history, maturation, selection, and selection–maturation interactions in these designs. Further, these designs can control the impact of reactive measures by taking baseline measures and extracting their effects in the analysis. Instrumentation effects (changes in the way measures are taken) can be controlled in Designs 5 and 6. The randomization process provides a control for selection. It is unlikely that organizations or individuals in comparison groups will differ systematically when randomization principles have been followed. To detect impact of mortality, a special type of design can be used (see Design 14 in Table 6–2).

Controls for External Validity

Experimental designs, like Designs 4, 5, and 6, have considerable internal validity. Measure of effectiveness can be linked to the intervention program, controlling for factors that lower internal validity. Once a cause–and–effect relationship has been established, the evaluator tests the relationship to determine whether it generalizes to other populations. External validity determines whether evaluation findings extend to a range of settings. For example, when a hospital administrator reviews an article describing the influence of patient case review on physician behavior, the dominant concern is the study's external validity, its application in the administrator's setting.

Unlike internal validity, external validity is seldom demonstrable. Typically the evaluation findings are *not* likely to hold for some circumstances that may arise in the field. The ability to extrapolate evaluation findings to circumstances not represented in the study is always tenuous. If study participants fall into specific age, and socioeconomic categories, the results cannot be extrapolated to groups with radically different ages and socioeconomic status. Generalizing the evaluation findings to a population not represented in the study hinges on logic. If the intervention is unlikely to interact with sex, the evaluator can disregard the sex variable. For instance, the effects of a collection procedure are unlikely to be influenced by the sex of people with bad debts. The evaluation can extrapolate the findings to both sexes. In contrast, socioeconomic status seems tightly correlated with bad debts, so the evaluation findings would be restricted to socioeconomic strata similar to those considered in the study.

External validity is enhanced when data collected are similar to the conditions expected in the field. When evaluation environments do not or cannot duplicate conditions expected in the field, the entire experiment should be repeated. The repeatability of evaluation findings upon successive trials, is the hallmark of a quality evaluation project. When evaluation findings have considerable policy significance, considerable rigor is justified. Indeed, a strong case can be made that evaluation rigor is far below that justified by the types of policy guidance sought from the typical evaluation projects. The negative income tax experiments and the HEW–Rand evaluation of prepaid medical care are examples.[15]

Factors Influencing Generalizability In Experimental Designs

A careful definition and selection of the *target group* of an intervention program or service dramatically improves the external validity of an evaluation. When the target group (clients or beneficiaries) of the intervention program is carefully defined and comparison groups are drawn from the target group following the principles of randomization, the evaluation findings are likely to generalize. For example, if the Job Corps had initially selected high school dropouts from the population of dropouts, using a random process, the success of the program would have been far below that initially reported. Carefully identifying and sampling the program's target group can dramatically enhance the generalizability of the evaluation findings.

Experimental designs incorporate block variables to enhance their external validity. Evaluation findings have relative higher credibility when they can be related to important processes known to be operating at the time of the study. For instance, when test effects are controlled with a block variable, the interaction of testing and the policy variable can be assessed. Reactive testing can be discounted if this interaction is not significant.

Outcome measures must be carefully related to the objectives of the intervention program if the findings are to generalize. When objectives are multiple, or difficult to measure, agreement among several similar (or parallel) measures can improve the external validity of an evaluation effort (see Design 6, Table 6–1). For example, a management contract is thought to lower costs but have unfavorable effects on the quality of patient care contracting hospitals. Measuring the "cost per patient day" and "nursing hours per patient day" provides a basis to counter critics who contend that these factors trade off.

Naturally correlated variables occur when populations of unequal size must be included in an evaluation project. For instance, cervical cancer screening programs appear to stimulate repeated participation of Jewish women and the very little participation of black women. The availability of preventive care may cause excessive consumption by one group, and little consumption by the other. If few blacks participate and if blacks have the greatest need for the services, the cost effectiveness of screening based on these participants will not generalize.

In other instances, specific combinations of experimental variables are impossible to realize. Consider an evaluation project to determine the effect of a new treatment procedure in a neonatology ward. Severity indicators like weight and diagnosis are naturally correlated. For instance, high body weight infants are unlikely to have hylaine membrane disease, and those with low body weight are unlikely to be diagnosed as muconium aspirations. Factorial designs can sort out these factors and fractional factorial designs may be able to skip diagnosis–weight combinations that never occur.

Testing–program interactions can be controlled by unobtrusive measures or by Design 4 in Table 6–1. The block variable in Design 4 controls for the reactive effects of testing. The use of random processes to assign participants drawn from a target group to experimental and control groups controls for selection–program interactions. In the same way, randomization controls for other interactions with the intervention program and renders these rival explanations of the evaluation findings implausible.

Reactive arrangements can bias evaluation results. Intervention programs implemented in laboratories and other artificial environments are often distracting, altering the behavior of participants. Field conditions or following normal organizational practices is encouraged when evaluating intervention programs. For example, a controller in a multihospital system may initiate a new budgeting procedure and compare its effectiveness with hospitals employing traditional procedures. If the financial managers in the experimental group carry out the budgeting procedure, in addition to their normal budgeting activities, the new procedure would be implemented in a somewhat artificial manner. This encourages department heads in the experimental group to try to outguess or even mislead the evaluator. As a result, the information gathered may not be representative. Blind and double–blind measurement overcomes some of the problems that stem from a reactive arrangement. When the hospital financial managers are unaware that they are being observed, observations cannot be reactive. Unobtrusive measures also minimize reactivity.[16] Designs 4, 5, and 6 in Table 6–1 were judged questionable in their ability to deal with reactive arrangements unless field performance data or unobtrusive measures can be used.

Multiple treatment interference, like reactive arrangements, is strongly related to the phenomenon under study. For instance, when assessing individual performance, skill improves as the task is repeated. Thus, employing these same individuals in a subsequent evaluation confounds the effect of skill with the intervention. As pointed out in Table 6–1, multiple treatment interference can be a problem in experimental designs.

QUASI-EXPERIMENTAL DESIGNS

Evaluation is often carried out in environments where randomization is impossible or only partially feasible. When the evaluator lacks full control over when measurements can be taken and/or who will be exposed to an intervention program, a quasi–experimental design can be used to collect evaluation data.

As pointed out in Chapter 5, quasi–experimental designs overcome many of the limitations of nonevaluative designs. The purpose of this section is to point out the strengths and weaknesses of several quasi–experimental designs and to indicate appropriate applications for each data–collection device. To illustrate these points, the quasi–experimental designs described in Tables 6–2, 6–3, and 6–4 are systematically assessed considering the factors that influence their internal and external validity. It should be stressed however, that true experimental designs should be applied wherever conditions permit.

Alternative Comparison Groups

Design 7, shown in Table 6–2, illustrates the use of a matched group as a substitute for randomization. The comparison groups are not formed by a random sampling of program beneficiaries. Rather, the members of the experimental and control groups are matched according to important characteristics. This design is shown below:

M O X O

M O   O

Matched group designs can control for history, maturation, and measurement effects (Table 6–2). However, statistical regression often creates problems when matched groups are used. Regression may occur because the members of matched groups have unstable characteristics. For example, to account for the effect of income, a questionnaire might be administered to high– and low–income service users of a neighborhood health center. The average income of each group is likely to shift from time period to time period, perhaps dramatically. Thus, matching groups according to income may be illusory. Similarly, a children's hospital association used a matching strategy

Table 6-2. Factors Influencing Internal & External Validity of Quasi-Experimental Designs

	INTERNAL								EXTERNAL							
	History	Maturation	Measurement	Instrument	Regression	Selection	Mortality	Selection Interactions	Target Group	Selection	Block Variables	Testing	Outcome Measures	Correlated Variables	Reactive Setting	Multiple Treatments
ALTERNATIVE COMPARISON GROUPS																
7. Matched Group Designs M 01 X 01 M 03 04	+	+	+	?	-	-	+	?	?	-	+	+	?	+	?	?
8. Naturally Occuring Groups N 01 X 02 N 03 04	+	+	+	?		?	+	?	?	+	+	+	?	+	?	?
TIME ORDERED DATA																
9. Time Series Designs . . . 0 0 0 X 0 0 0 . . .	-	+	+	?			-		?	-	-	-	+	-	?	-
10. Multiple Time Series . . . 0 0 0 X 0 0 0 . . . . . . 0 0 0 0 0 0 . . .	+	+	+	?	?	-	-	-	?	-	+	-	+	-	?	-
SPECIAL PURPOSE DESIGNS																
11. Switch Back (longitudinal) designs 01X 02(X) 03X 04 . . .	+	+	+	?		-	-	-	?	?	+	+	?	-	?	-
12. Remission Designs R 01i (X) R 02i (X) R X 03i	-	+	+	?	+	-	+		+	+	?	+	?	?	?	+
13. Opinion Polls N . . . OA,1 (X) OA,2 . . .	+	+	-	?	+	-	+		+	+	?	-	-	?	+	-
14. Dropout Designs R 01 X 02 (X%) R 03 X 04 (Y%)	-	-	+	?	+	+	?		+	+	?	+	+	?	+	

to compare its care costs with costs in similar hospitals.[17] Each children's hospital participating in the study were matched with a community hospital that has comparable admission rates, occupancy, services, and the like. As many of these factors change from time to time, particularly those dealing with utilization and admission, the precision of the matching process will tend to degenerate during the study.

Regression to the mean occurs when groups are selected because they have extreme properties. For these reasons, *selection* becomes a possible source of bias when matched groups are used. If the selection process is biased, those participating in comparison groups may differ and selection may interact with maturation and similar factors to bias performance measures.

The discussion reveals that substituting matching for randomization has several important drawbacks. Similarly, generalizing findings based on matched–group evaluation data can be suspect on several counts. First, the matched groups may not be descriptive of the target group's population because the characteristics used to select comparison groups tend to be unstable. As a result, matched group data may fail to characterize the behavior of a target group. For these same reasons, an interaction between the selection process and the intervention program may occur. Some matched groups may be particularly susceptible to the intervention process while others are not. However, matched–group designs can control for block variables, testing–program interactions, and naturally occurring variables which make these designs superior to nonevaluative approaches cited in Table 6–1.

Naturally Occurring Groups

Naturally occurring groups (Design 8 in Table 6–2) are experimental sites where intervention programs can be tried in relative isolation. For example, the hospitals in a multihospital system are often geographically dispersed in such a way that intervention programs tried at one setting will not influence the other hospitals. This design is illustrated below:

$$N \; O \; X \; O$$
$$N \; O \quad O$$

Naturally occurring groups are superior to matched groups because they avoid regression effects. However, selection of the naturally occurring group can be a significant problem unless a large proportion of the target group participates or stratified samples are used to control for selection effects.[18] For instance, management in a multihospital system, seeking to evaluate the merits of a statistical package to improve Medicare reimbursement in contract-managed hospitals, has several hospitals that may vary in terms of their quality of financial management, size, or the number of services. A stratified sample of the contract–managed hospitals can be selected to represent a profile of the financial management skills that exist in the hospitals. By involving management skills in the evaluation proportional to that found in the field (the multihospital system), selection-maturation effects can be controlled. The merits of the statistical package would be overstated if only hospitals with well–trained financial managers participate in the study.

To generalize the findings from naturally occurring groups, the comparison groups must be representative. For example, the merits of the intervention can be extrapolated to all hospitals in the multihospital system if a stratified sample of hospitals in the system participated in the study.

Time–Ordered Data

Time–series designs make periodic measurements prior to and following an intervention program. The time series design is shown below:

OOO X OOO

This mode of data collection was developed for the physical sciences. The design permits the evaluator to check the reliability of instruments and the measurements they provide. A series of measurements are taken to learn as much as possible about the inherent variations in the measures. The intervention or other phenomonon study is assumed to be unlikely to change and relatively easy to control. For example, students in a freshman physics class drop steel balls and corks from varying heights to verify Newton's law of gravity. The same steel ball and cork can be used on repeated occasions, but the measurements are likely to vary.

As shown in Table 6–2, the inability to control for history is the most serious drawback in a time series (Design 9). The biasing effects of external events which occur as the measurements are taken can never be completely ruled out. A variety of exogenous variables are associated with history effects. For example, trend effects and seasonal fluctuations can be confounded with the measurements taken in the time–series design. It may be possible to control for history in a time series by a process called experimental isolation. If the intervention program and subsequent measurement process takes place during a relatively short period of time, the likelihood of history effects can be discounted.

Because time–series designs tend to be "population specific," they have limited ability to generalize their findings. The participants may be particularly amenable (or not amenable) to the intervention program. Further, time–series designs cannot control for test effects. Repeated measurements taken before an intervention program are likely to be reactive. For example, establishing a firm baseline which measures attitudes before the intervention may suggest the behavior management expects. Block variables are not explicitly controlled in a time–series design. Rather, each observation, "O," represents a composite of the performance for the organizational participants. Finally, time–series designs cannot isolate and control the effects of naturally correlative variables or multiple treatments.

A multiple time–series (Design 10 in Table 6–2) can overcome some of these problems. This design is shown below:

$$...OOO \ X \ OOO...$$
$$...OOO \quad OOO...$$

A multiple time series helps to overcome a major limitation of the single sample time–series design: history. Another group is measured along with the group that will receive the intervention program. Trends and cycles, caused by exogenous events, can be extracted by plotting measures in the experimental and control groups. The validity of multiple–time–series evaluation data can be quite good when the control is a matched naturally occurring group. But, when matched naturally occurring groups are used, the same problems cited for Designs 7 and 8 in Table 6–2 crop up.

Multiple–time–series designs have somewhat better external validity than a single time series. By using two groups, the generalizability of the findings can be increased. Some degree of control over block variables is also possible. For example, trends and other factors can be removed by comparing the after indicators in the experimental and control groups. While this approach does not permit the evaluator to account for the effects of the specific block factor, it does permit the evaluator to study the pattern of these external events.

This design has been used for evaluations carried out in school systems. Grades in a school system are assumed to be homogeneous. An intervention can be attempted in one grade and compared with student performance in other grades. Campbell and Stanley somewhat overstate the value of time–series designs.[19] The merits of multiple time–series designs are quite dependent on the availability of homogeneous test sites.

SPECIAL PURPOSE QUASI–DESIGNS

Switchback and Longitudinal Designs

Switchback designs are used to detect the permanency of intervention program effects (Design 11, Table 6–2). They are particularly useful when the evaluator *can* stop and start an intervention and track changes in performance indicators. For example, the administration in a hospital may believe that closer supervision will increase productivity in certain departments. To determine the effects of current supervisory practices, productivity measures could be tracked to provide a baseline. Next, closer supervision will be initiated by, for example, carefully monitoring when employees arrive, working hours, checking the accuracy of reports or forms, or by pointing out to employees their contentious encounters with others. After a certain period of time, these practices are abandoned, but arrival time, hours worked, report accuracy, and critical incidents continue to be recorded. Depending upon the subtlety of the intervention program, such designs may wish to switch back and forth several times to verify the permanency of the effects sought by an intervention program.

This design is shown below:

$$...OOOXOOO(X)OOOXOOO...$$

A simple form of the switchback design is called a longitudinal design. This design detects decay in the measures of effectiveness after an intervention program has been initiated. Returning to the example cited above, the measurement process may be continued concurrently with the practice of closer supervision to insure that performance measures are maintained at a high level. This design is shown diagramatically below:

$$O XOOOO...$$

Switchback or longitudinal designs are particularly useful in detecting transient changes in performance indicators that often occur through time. These designs can control for history, maturation, and measurement. But participants must be carefully selected to avoid selection bias similar to these found in time series designs. Selection and selection–maturation interactions may increase (or decrease) performance indicators collected using a switchback design.

If the measurement process is unobtrusive, it is unlikely that testing–program interactions will limit the generalizability of the findings from switchback or longitudinal designs. Block variables are controlled in this design by repeatedly measuring performance.

Selection is the dominant problem in generalizing the results from a switchback study. If the participants in the study were selected from the target group following randomization principles, the results can have considerable external validity. The results from switchback design have excellent generalizability.

The basic limitation to switchback designs is multiple–treatment interference. For instance, the administrator blatantly switching his tactics of supervision back and forth may confuse subordinates. It may not be possible to erase the spectre of capricious supervision.[20] While these effects decay with the passage of time, residual hostility may remain. To illustrate, in the supercharged environment of first appraisal interview, a tactless or flippant remark may be recalled long after favorable observations have been forgotten.[21]

Remission Designs

Design 12 in Table 6–2 illustrates a data–collection device which measures the changes in people, independent of an intervention program. In this design, a pretest is used to characterize a population at an initial point in time and again at some subsequent point in time. The design is shown below:

$$
\begin{array}{lll}
R & O1 & (X) \\
R & O2 & (X) \\
R & & XO3
\end{array}
$$

Changes in the population, i, that occur spontaneously can be detected by the difference between O1 and O2. These designs have several useful applications in health care because people often undergo spontaneous remissions of symptoms, independent of the treatments that are applied. For example, an evaluation of the merits of psychotherapy is difficult to interpret because changes in patients occur independent of the treatment that is used. Remission designs permit the evaluator to extract the effects of spontaneous changes from effects of a treatment.

The internal validity of remission designs is damaged by the history effect. One cannot separate the history effect from the remission effect, particularly if the time period between measurement O1 and O2 is lengthy. A time–series design could be used in conjunction with a remission design to detect history effects.

Instrumentation can also cause problems. Surveyors may become cynical as they are exposed to the hang–ups in those being surveyed and act out their disapproval in ways that influence those being surveyed. Patients may not initially detect or respond to surveyor attitudes (O1), but may in subsequent measurements (O2 and O3). Self–administered surveys or questionnaires may also engender changes in attitude with repeated applications.

Mortality can be a problem because each of the three comparison groups shown in Design 12 (Table 6–2) must be carefully isolated. Differential dropout rates in the three groups or information leakage between the groups may influence the evaluation findings. Nevertheless, remission designs often provide an excellent way to characterize the behavior of a *charter group* or to check for bias in the selection process. Changes in behavior of participants that are independent of the treatment process can also be controlled. Other block variables are less susceptible to controls and may influence evaluation findings. For instance, the transmission of viewpoints between the comparison groups may distort their response to treatment programs or their attitudes.

Reactive arrangements can be caused by remission designs. This is particularly troublesome for medical research carried out in a laboratory. The treatment applied to the experimental group is surrounded by hoopla, and patients received abnormal levels of attention. The patients respond to the attention and their condition improves. When the treatment program becomes routine, the amount of interpersonal contact permitted in a *research* environment declines. Attention declines, as do treatment benefits.

Opinion Polls

Neighborhood health centers, community hospitals, and other organizations have considerable interest in monitoring how their institution or organization is perceived. Surveys and opinion polls are often used to assess these attitudes and to assess the influence of an unplanned event that interrupts a normal relationship between the organization and its clients. For example, a hospital facing a large number of lawsuits may seek to assess the impact of these lawsuits on views of the hospital. Surveys will provide substantially improved information if a naturally occurring group, unaware of the stimulus (e.g., the lawsuit), is surveyed simultaneously. This design is shown diagramatically below:

$$N \ldots OOO(X)O$$
$$N \ldots OOO \ X \ O$$

A professional pollster is aware that attitudes are formed by a variety of factors which the survey cannot control. The attitudes stemming from the advent of lawsuits, the previous example, cannot be separated from people's general views of health and the health care system. The opinion poll design controls for a very important source of invalidity: the effects of history.

This design, however, has several drawbacks. The first concerns measurement. Repeated measurement is costly and may not be feasible. Those filling out repeated surveys will become disenchanted and may refuse to cooperate. To overcome this difficulty, surveyors often use random samples of a reference group they seek to characterize. Also, mortality within any given sample often occurs and will have potentially biasing effects on the evaluation, as shown in Table 6-2.

Opinion polls can nicely characterize the behavior of target groups and minimize the likelihood that selection procedures interact with interventions. However, the potential for interaction between the measurement (survey) and the attitudes the poll seeks to measure, limits the generalizability of the findings. Further, the device (Likert scales and the like) used in a survey may fail to characterize the attitudes of those being surveyed. For example, pollsters seeking to characterize "confidence" in the current administration, often fail to ask questions which permit the respondent to discriminate between equally undesirable responses, such as approve or disapprove. When people's views do not fall into these categories, the measurement process does not represent the views of respondents. Finally, it is difficult to select measures that bring out basic issues which influence the beliefs or viewpoints of respondents.

Repeatedly surveying a group suggests something has occurred that is of interest to the surveyor. The survey implies that an intervention, advertent or inadvertent, has occurred. Respondents may seek to qualify their views according to their perceptions of recent events. As a result, multiple treatment interference may be a major source of invalidity in opinion polls. Members of the naturally occurring group, used as a comparison, may wonder why they are being surveyed and make inappropriate assumptions concerning the motivation behind a questionnaire.

Dropout Controls

Many evaluation projects cannot tolerate sample mortality and must make special arrangements to test for the effects of mortality. For instance, when huge samples are drawn for a population, small changes in response rates may alter performance measures. In many small–scale studies, 100 percent participation may be hard to maintain, even with personal attention by the evaluation staff.

Dropout designs have been devised as a precaution to measure the effect of mortality, discovered after data have been collected, as shown diagramatically below:

$$RO1XO2-X\%$$
$$RO3XO4-Y\%$$

To measure effect of mortality, the experimental group is divided — two additional groups to measure performance and dropout rates in each group. (The control group is also split into two groups to determine the effects of mortality on the baseline measures. Also the measures O1 and O3 can be reconstructed from the initial measures of participants who remained in the study.) By plotting the mortality rates against the performance measures O2 and O4, the impact of dropout rate on the performance measures can be determined, as shown in Figure 6–1.

These designs have limited validity and are seldom applied when trend effects and changes due to maturation are likely to occur. Dropout controls are used to detect selection interactions which occur when the dropout rates are thought to be significant. Qualifying the effects of samples that become

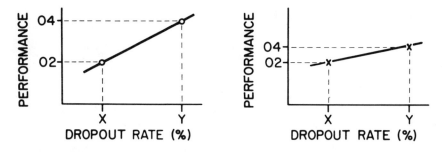

Figure 6.1 THE IMPACT OF DROPOUT RATE ON PERFORMANCE

nonrepresentative improves the external validity of data that has sample mortality.

Dropout controls are often used to qualify the effects sample mortality have on performance data collected for designs like 4, 5, 6, 7, or 8 (see Tables 6–1 and 6–2). Combining the analytical features of these designs improves the internal and the external validity of evaluation data.

OTHER QUASI–EXPERIMENTAL DESIGNS

Many special purpose designs can be constructed by combining the data collection principles described thus far. Each of these special purpose designs uses randomization where possible, and naturally occurring groups, matched groups, or time–series, in various combinations, when randomization is prohibited.

Naturally Occurring Comparison Groups

Design 15a in Table 6–3 uses a naturally occurring group as an external control group. To judge the effects of an intervention program, two naturally occurring groups are randomly divided into two additional comparison groups. This design becomes the equivalent of Design 4, except that the initial environments were not randomly selected. This design follows:

```
              R     01    (X)
        N
              R            X     02
        ----------------------------------
              R     03
        N
              R                  04
```

Table 6-3. Factors Effecting Internal and External Validity
of Quasi-Experimental Designs

	INTERNAL								EXTERNAL							
	History	Maturation	Measurement	Instrument	Regression	Selection	Mortality	Selection Interactions	Target Group	Selection	Block Variables	Testing	Outcome Measures	Correlated Variables	Reactive Setting	Multiple Treatments

15. Naturally occurring comparison groups

a. one program

```
  R   01  (X)
N R        X    02
  R   03
N R             04
```

| | + | + | + | + | ? | + | - | | + | - | + | + | + | - | ? | + |

b. program strategy (X1&X2)

```
  R   01  (X)  03
N R   02  X1   04
  R   05  (X)  07
N R   06  X2   08
```

| | + | + | - | + | ? | + | - | | + | - | - | - | + | + | + | + |

16. Matched Naturally Occurring Group As External Controls

```
   R    (X)   01
MN R     X    02
   R          03
MN R          04
   R    (X)   05
MN R     X    06
   R          07
MN R          08
```

| | + | + | - | + | - | + | + | + | + | + | - | + | ? | - | ? | + |

For example, HEW may try out a new screening program in federally funded contact centers. Each contact center represents a naturally occurring group. X represents the new screening program. Within one naturally occurring group, potential recipients of services are divided into two groups by a random process. In the first, initial observations, O1, are based on a history of patient's health status and the placebo administered. In the second, the new screening program is used and health status, O2, measured by the screening program. In the control group, users of the contact center are also randomly divided into two groups. In each of these groups health status is measured by a history taken at the two different points in time.

As shown in Table 6-3, this design has few defects. However, when the naturally occurring groups differ, internal validity can be a problem. Biases due to selection and selection–interacting with maturation may result. To apply Design 15a (Table 6-3), the evaluator assumes that programs, like contact centers, appeal to a homogeneous type of clientele, suggesting that selection biases are unlikely.

The external validity in naturally occurring comparison groups is limited by selection–program interactions. One group may exhibit dramatically different behavior or performance than another. For instance, the population served by one contact center may differ from another and the health status of its clientele may exhibit considerable differences. Comparing the health status of contact centers (O1 and O2) before the evaluation begins is necessary to test for the selection interaction.

Design 15b (Table 6-3) is used to compare various strategies for carrying out an intervention program.[22] This design is summarized below:

$$
\begin{array}{cccc}
 & R \quad O1 & (X) & O3 \\
N & & & \\
\hline
 & R \quad O2 & X1 & O4 \\
 & R \quad O5 & (X) & O7 \\
N & & & \\
 & R \quad O6 & X2 & O8 \\
\end{array}
$$

The screening program in the previous example can be carried out in both of the naturally occurring groups to compare the discriminating power of two screening approaches. Each naturally occurring group is randomly divided into two comparison groups. In each setting, one of these groups received the placebo and the other group is exposed to a version of the screening program. The screening program can be carried out with two distinct batteries of tests in each setting. Design 15b is used to compare the merits of the two distinct profiles of tests (designated X1 and X2) that could be used as a screening device.

The internal validity of Design 15b is very similar to Design 15a (Table 6-3), with the exception of measurement. As baseline measures are collected for all four comparison groups, the effects of reactive measurement cannot be determined. However, unobtrusive measurement can eliminate the reactive aspects of measurement.[23] For instance, a history and physical exam, which follows the normal practices of the center, is an unobtrusive measure of patient health status. The external validity of program strategy evaluations, using Design 15b, is limited by test effects that occur when unobtrusive measures cannot be used, and by the dissimilarities in the naturally occurring groups (see Table 6–3).

Matched Naturally Occurring Comparison Groups

Design 16 (Table 6–3) selects naturally occurring groups by matching them across several important characteristics. This design follows:

$$NMO1 \quad X \quad O2$$
$$NMO3 \quad (X) \quad O4$$

Because naturally occurring groups may differ on important characteristics, these designs may be an improvement over Designs 15a and b in both internal and external validity. For instance, studies of the cost savings resulting from shared services can match hospitals participating in a shared–service consortium with nonparticipating hospitals, considering characteristics like number of services, service intensity, and size.[24] Hospitals are naturally occurring groups, but may have quite dissimilar characteristics. Matching is essential to create comparable comparison groups.

As shown in Table 6–3, the internal validity of Design 16 is limited by regression effects. The precision of the matching can be questioned when matched groups are used, because little can be done to control or eliminate regression effects. To detect shifts in the parameters used to match the groups, they should be periodically monitored during the study. Unobtrusive measures must be used to eliminate measurement bias, as reactive testing goes undetected in Design 16.

The external validity of matched comparison groups are similar to those in Design 7 (Table 6–2). The findings can be extrapolated if the match proves to be stable. Under these conditions, the intervention program is unlikely to interact with the selection procedure. This design, however, is limited in its ability to measure block variables or to assess the impact of the testing program–interaction.

Designs With Internal and External Controls

Designs can be formulated which use several naturally occurring matched groups as shown below:

```
           R      (X)     O1
    MN
           R       X      O2
    ........................................
           R               O3
    MN
           R               O4
    ........................................
                   ⋮
```

Design 17 (Table 6–4) is similar to Designs 7 or 8 (Table 6–2), with many more replications. Collecting evaluation data for several naturally occurring matched groups overcomes many of the limitations of matched or naturally occurring groups used individually. The regresssion effects that occur in matched groups, and the selection effects associated with both matched and naturally occurring groups can be minimized. Measurement problems, as before, are overcome by unobtrusive measurement procedures.

The inability to consider block variables and to control for naturally occurring variables in the data collection process limits the external validity of Design 17 (Table 6–4). These, however, are not serious limitations. Block variables will be mixed with residual variance and thus reduce the prospect of detecting differences caused by the intervention program, when they exist. This makes the evaluation tests overly conservative, but does not create a source of bias. Few designs can cope with naturally correlated variables.

Cycle Designs

Cycle designs can be applied when only limited randomization can be carried out and groups occur naturally within the evaluation environment. Cycle designs are typically used within an institution. To illustrate, all patients with given diagnosis admitted to a hospital on Mondays represent a naturally occurring group. A hospital administrator interested in assessing the impact of patient care practices could measure the attitudes of each patient cohort. A stratified sample of the patients is made by sorting the patients into treatment categories like minor surgery, dialysis, and the like.

Cycle designs can be applied with or without *internal* randomization. Design 18 (Table 6–4) illustrates a cycle design with randomization. In this design, all patients admitted on Monday are randomly assigned to two groups: one is exposed to current practices and another to the new practices

Table 6-4. Factors Effecting Internal and External Validity of Quasi-Experimental Designs

	INTERNAL								EXTERNAL							
	History	Maturation	Measurement	Instrument	Regression	Selection	Mortality	Selection Interactions	Target Group	Selection	Block Variables	Testing	Outcome Measures	Correlated Variables	Reactive Setting	Multiple Treatments
17. Matched-Naturally Occurring Comparison Groups NM 01 X 02 NM 03 (X) 04	+	+	−	+	−	+	+	?	+	?	−	−	+	−	?	+
18. Cycle Designs (with randomization) N R 01 (X) R X 02 N R 03 (X) R X 04 N R 05 (X) R X 06	+	+	+	?		+	+	+	+	+	+	+	+	−		
19. Cycle Designs (without randomization) N 01 (X) 02 N 03 X 04 N 05 (X) 06 N 07 X 08	+	−	+	−		+	+	+	+	+	?	−	+	−	−	

(intervention). As shown below, each set of patients admitted to the hospital on Monday would be treated in the same way.

```
      R01(X)
    N
      R    X 02
    -----------------------------------------------
      R         03(X)
    N
      R            X 04
    -----------------------------------------------
      R              05(X)
    N
      R                 X 06
    -----------------------------------------------
                     .

                     .

                     .
```

The internal validity of cycle designs with randomization is limited only by instrumentation problems. Instruments create a possible source of bias because they are applied recursively in the evaluation setting. The evaluator must insure that observations O_2, O_4, etc., are collected so the behavior of patients in the experimental group is not influenced by patients in the control group ($O1$, $O3$, etc.). For instance, if patients in the control and experimental groups are assigned to the same room, the survey may be discussed during convalescence. Taking care that each room has either control or experimental group members will enhance the internal validity of responses.

The external validity for cycle designs with randomization is limited by naturally occurring variables. Naturally correlated variables are troublesome for most designs and do not provide any special problems for cycle designs. As pointed out above, only experimental designs based on factorials can efficiently handle these problems. Many block variables can be controlled by stratifying a naturally occurring group into categories such as admitting diagnosis.

When randomization is prohibited, the naturally occurring group is observed before and after the administration of a placebo or the intervention program. Design 19 (Table 6–4) is shown below:

```
      N01X02
    N    03(X) 04
    N         05X06
    N            07(X) 08

                 .

                 .

                 .
```

The internal validity of cycle designs, without randomization, is limited by its inability to control for measurement and maturation effects. Patients, for instance, experience dramatic changes in mood and the like during hospitalization. Continuing with the previous example, attitudes can be determined at admission and discharge for minor–surgery patients exposed to a new patient-care practice. If these patients had no prior exposure to surgery, they may become quite apprehensive. The relief experienced by such patients during recovery may induce favorable attitudes which may dramatically overstate the impact of the patient care practice. Instrumentation problems like those described for Design 18 may also occur.

The principal limitations to the external validity of cycle designs without randomization are associated with testing and observational arrangements. Because extensive testing is required (both pre- and postmeasurements), the testing may become reactive. Further, controlling for block variables in cycle designs can be complex. The complexity, and thus the potential for errors in data collections, mount rapidly as block variables are added.

Designs 18 and 19 (Table 6–4) are used in settings where evaluation findings are likely to be influenced by many external events, because they can control history effects. Trends, cycles, and other factors that occur with the passage of time can be extracted from the evaluation data using a cycle design. For instance, the Economic Stabilization Act in the early 1970s established price controls for hospitals. These controls had a decisive impact on indicators of hospitals' financial effectiveness. Cycle designs could have been used to track key financial effectiveness measures. The hospital can study trends in "revenue less cost–per–patient day" and the like to isolate the exogenous influences such as price freezes, and extract them from the financial indicators. Block variables can be handled by merely stratifying data into the appropriate categories like diagnoses. The data collection problems are strictly mechanical, not conceptual. Finally, when randomization is prohibited, cycle designs provide an excellent way to develop valid comparison groups for evaluative data collection. Cycle designs can be inexpensive, easy to apply, and highly diagnostic.

SUMMARY

To use information derived from evaluation projects, the sponsor must ask two vital questions. First, does the intervention program meet its objectives? And second, are the results justifiable? The latter question tends to be judgmental, whereas the former is related to the methods used to carry out the evaluation. Judgment has less chance of success when based on evaluation information that is suspect. The sponsor should consider the *precision* of the evaluation information before making judgment calls. Precision is tied to the confidence a sponsor can place in conclusions of an evaluation. Sponsors and practitioners should know *how* the quality of evaluation information is influenced by the *method* used to generate or collect this information. This chapter presented a means to make this judgment.

This chapter provided a description of the strengths and weaknesses of nineteen distinct modes of data collection in terms of their internal and external validity. Internal validity determines the likelihood that observed performance can be attributed to an intervention program. Eight factors which influence internal validity were used to critique the designs. External validity determines the extent to which evaluation findings can be extrapolated or generalized. Eight factors which limit extrapolation of evaluation information were also used to critique the nineteen designs.

The nineteen data–collection devices, or designs, fell into three categories: nonevaluative approaches, experimental designs, and quasi–experimental designs. Nonevaluative approaches were found to be inadequate and should not be avoided. Experimental evaluation approaches tend to be the best methods of data collection. However, circumstances may prohibit using randomization to form comparison groups. When these circumstances occur, quasi–experimental designs were recommended. Quasi–experimental designs are formed using, in various combinations, principles of matched comparison groups, naturally occurring comparison groups, and time–ordered data. Quasi–experimental designs were found to have considerable internal and external validity, close to that of experimental approaches.

NOTES

1. Campbell D.T. and J.C. Stanley, *Experimental and Quasi-Experimental Designs for Research,* p. 5. Chicago, Ill.: Rand–McNally, 1963.
2. Recall that policy variables are subject to manipulation by the sponsor. Block variables are constraints or factors known to influence performance. The sponsor cannot manipulate these variables, nor has he reason to do so. For instance, to determine the impact of prepaid health insurance (the policy variable), the sponsor may realize that people with a history of health problems may select prepaid services but have no interest in the history factor, except to control its influence. A constraint might be the disproportionate number of young people who seem to prefer prepaid health care services.
3. Filly A., R. House, and S. Kerr, *Managerial Process and Organizational Behavior,* pp. 10–15. Glenview, Ill: Scott, Foresman, 1976.
4. Campbell and Stanley, p. 6.
5. Huston, T.R., Jr. "The Behavioral Sciences Impact–Effectiveness Model," in P. Rossi, et al. (eds.), *Evaluating Social Programs,* pp. 59–64. New York: Seminar Press, 1972.
6. Kershaw, P.N., "Issues in Income Maintenance Experimentation," in P. Rossi, et al. (eds.), *Evaluating Social Programs,* pp. 221–240. New York: Seminar Press, 1972.
7. Suchman, E.A., *Evaluation Research; Principles and Practice in Public Service and Social Action Programs,* p. 97. New York: Russell Sage Foundation, 1967.
8. Frank, J.D., *Persuasion and Healing,* p. 66. Johns Hopkins, Baltimore: 1961.

9. Suchman, p. 97.
10. Campbell and Stanley, p. 8.
11. *Ibid.*
12. For simplicity, a time–series representation is used to describe each design considered in Chapter 6.
13. HAS, and other data services, are misused when an administrator evaluates the fitness of the programs and services by comparing their performance with norms based on averages for the performances of hospitals in a particular region.
14. Nutt, P.C. R.J. Caswell, and P.K. Findling, "Comparing Historical & Subjective Methods of Forecasting," *American Institute of Decision Sciences Proceedings,* Vol. 11, Nov. 1979, pp. 309–312.
15. Newhouse, J.P., "A Design of a Health Insurance Experiment," *Inquiry,* Vol. 11, March 1974, pp. 5–27.
16. Webb, E.J., D.T. Campbell, R.D. Swartz, and J. Sechrest, *Unobtrusive Measures: Nonreactive Research In The Social Sciences.* Chicago: Rand–McNally, 1972.
17. "Study to Quantify Children's Hospitals Uniqueness," National Association of Childrens Hospitals and Related Institutions, Aug. 1978.
18. In a stratified sample, the proportion of characteristics found in the field are represented in the sample. For instance, if 20 percent of the target hospitals are less than 150 beds, 30 percent 200 to 250 beds, and 50 percent more than 400 beds, the sample would draw 20 percent "small" hospitals, 30 percent "medium sized" hospitals, and 50 percent "large" hospitals for the study.
19. Campbell and Stanley, p. 55.
20. Collins B.E. and H. Guetzkow, *A Social Psychology of Group Process for Decision-Making,* p. 131. New York: Wiley, 1964.
21. Cummings, L.K. and D.P. Schwab, *Performance in Organization: Determinants and Appraisal,* p. 103. Glenview, Ill: Scott, Foresman, 1973.
22. Wholey, J.S., J. Scanlon, H.G. Duffy, J.S. Fukumoto, and L. Vogt, *Federal Evaluation Policy Analyzing The Effects of Public Programs,* p. 25. Washington, D.C.: The Urban Institute, 1971.
23. Webb, et al.
24. R.E. Berry, Jr., "On Grouping Hospitals for Economic Analysis," *Inquiry,* Vol. X, Dec. 1973, pp. 5–12.

PART II

BEHAVIORAL ISSUES

"Wisdom comes by disillusionment"
George Santayana

CHAPTER 7

Measures

[Alice] "Would you tell me, please, which way I ought to go from here?"
"That depends a good deal on where you want to go to," said the cat.
"I don't much care where," said Alice.
"Then it doesn't matter which way you go," said the cat.

Lewis Carroll, *Alice In Wonderland*

MEASURING OUTCOMES

The objective of an intervention program describes the program's mission or aim, suggesting anticipated benefits. Evaluation determines the extent to which these benefits were realized, within resource and time constraints.

Objectives may be stated in terms of performances or goals. Goals specify a program's long–range aims, indicating a desirable but not necessarily attainable state of affairs. For example, a renal disease program may hope for zero mortality from renal disease. Performance states the program's anticipated benefits in terms of the results sought. For example, performance expectations in a renal program could be successful transplantation for 85 percent of all new dialysis patients within a given time period. Thus, objectives for an evaluation can be phrased in terms of long–range aims or anticipated performance levels. Goal–directed evaluation is carried out to isolate progress toward the goal within certain time periods. Performance evaluation is used to detect the extent to which certain of the anticipated benefits are realized.

Objectives may be established prospectively or retrospectively. In a prospective evaluation the objectives of the intervention are selected before the evaluation begins. In a retrospective evaluation the objectives of the intervention program are reconstructed, a process filled with many potential biases.

Table 7–1 summarizes the prospects for bias in goal and performance evaluations, conducted retrospectively and prospectively. *Goal–directed prospective* evaluations produce a "moderate" level of bias. The objectives are set before evaluation begins, which minimizes tampering, where objectives are altered to match perceived achievements. However, projecting the impact of a program into the future requires the evaluation to anticipate future events.

Table 7-1:   Sources of Evaluation Bias

		TYPE OF EVALUATION	
		Retrospective	Prospective
Type of Objective	Goal Directed	high bias	moderate bias
	Performance Directed	moderate bias	low bias

Important features of a future environment can be overlooked, limiting the ability to extrapolate evaluation findings. For example, attempts to detect the long-range benefits of prepaid group practice from a cross-section of people may understate the benefits of prevention. Such an evaluation of populations enrolled in prepaid health plans is limited to studying the health status of population groups that *elected* such care. Klarman points out that people under 30 dominate the membership of these plans, making it difficult to extrapolate effects of prepaid care to the other age groups.[1] Bias may be introduced when the health status of young adults participating in prepaid programs is qualified to reflect how prepaid programs might apply to the elderly, low-income groups, and others. Generalizing a causal relationship is likely to introduce some degree of bias.

Goal-directed retrospective evaluations have a high potential for bias. Sponsors may sort through performance data and reconstruct a statement of goals that seems defensible. Post hoc objectives create considerable bias, making the interpretation of findings from this type of evaluation difficult at best. Further, because the data are gleaned from an archive, data that are missing or difficult to interpret introduce a second source of bias. For example, a large university hospital took twenty years to construct a new hospital facility after state funding had been appropriated. When the project was finally completed, the state dollars purchased only one-fifth of the planned beds. Retrospective assessments, periodically undertaken by the university administration, uncovered a mosaic of plausible explanations for the delays. The evaluation data were selectively interpreted by each group that had a vested interest in the project. The hospital's clinical staff and administration, the university's administration and trustees, and others periodically sorted through the data to find explanations that suited their purposes.

Performance-directed retrospective evaluations provide findings with a moderate level of bias. The intervention program's costs and benefits are reconstructed, not measured. Retrospective evaluations introduce bias because data that failed to substantiate the sponsor's views may have been pruned. For example, "Early And Periodic Screening, Diagnostic And Treatment Programs" (EPSDT) were initiated by state health departments with federal funds.[2] A performance evaluation could compare health status indicators (like incidence and prevalence of particular diseases) in EPSDT program participants and nonparticipants. Knowing this, local EPSDT program administrators have an incentive to retain only performance data that they scored well on.

Whenever possible, *prospective performance-directed* evaluation should be applied. Prospective–performance evaluations minimize bias because performance data are defined before they are collected. This limits the formation of post hoc objectives and makes interpretation of evaluation findings comparatively straightforward.

THE NATURE OF INTERVENTION PROGRAM OBJECTIVES

The objectives stated for an intervention program must be used to guide the selection of program effectiveness measures. Proxy measures are derived from objectives for prospective evaluations and inferred from objectives in retrospective assessments.

Retrospective Evaluations

Retrospective evaluation projects must *reconstruct* the basic intent of the intervention program and get the evaluation sponsor to endorse the objectives that emerge. In federally initiated programs, the enabling legislation should be consulted. Often states are asked to authorize federal programs, and may add qualifications. The state house may tighten eligibility requirements or add co–payment provisions. The guidelines from state or federal implementing agencies further provide insights. For example, The Coal Miner's Health And Safety Act established federal benefits for miners disabled from Black Lung and other respiratory diseases. States were given financial incentives to establish treatment centers. The objectives found in the guidelines of a state implementing agency are listed below:[3]

1. Expansion on a permanent basis of the provision of ambulatory diagnostic and treatment services for respiratory care.
2. Expansion on a permanent basis of counseling services to assist disabled miners in applying for local, state, and federal benefits.
3. Improvement in the health status and the quality of life of miners.
4. Description of the basic parameters of a respiratory disease program.

Like many federal and state intervention programs, the objectives stated for the coal miner's rehabilitation program were multiple and complex. The objectives vary in terms of time, place, specificity, and importance. Some program objectives even imply a preferred type of intervention. This confusion stems from the origin of many federally initiated intervention programs. Job Corps, Aid to Dependent Children, and the coal miner's program arose from the collective interests of these programs' supporters, amended to counter the objections of program detractors. To gain approval, program objectives are modified to reflect the views of supporters and detractors, resulting in a hodgepodge of aims, constraints, and directives, often without any notion of priority.

Interventions in organizations often have a similar history. For instance, the motives behind a new hospital service like a burn center can be quite diverse. The administrator may seek to improve the hospital's image with its medical staff. The board of trustees may hope to expand service to the community, and the medical staff may seek to stimulate applications to the hospital's residency program. As a result, burn service programs can be stated in image, service, or resident application terms. To disguise conflict among the administrator, trustees, and medical staff, objectives are often stated in terms that are acceptable to all parties. The formal statement of objectives becomes complex because it must reconcile these diverse interests. As a result, the objectives of organizational interventions often seem shrouded in confusion.

The complexity of program objectives often causes disagreement and conflict among the evaluator, the evaluation's sponsor, and program administrators. The evaluator must dispel this confusion and conflict and help sponsors and program administrators to settle on an objective that can be used to measure the success of their efforts.

Methods To Reconstruct Program Objectives

Objectives can be classified by their generalizability. Some objectives found in guidelines or in other documents mandating programs are highly specific;

others are quite general. Nadler contends that a hierarchy of these objectives can be formed for most intervention programs.[4] The hierarchy describes a set of possible actions that were open to the program sponsor. Suchman points out that objectives in such a hierarchy often correspond to the steps needed to carry out a comprehensive intervention program.[5] The hierarchy of objectives forms a continuous series of events. Each objective relies on achievement of a preceding objective and creates the preconditions to achieve the next, higher–level objective. Table 7–2 illustrates how objectives for the Coal

Table 7-2. Reconstruction of Objectives for the Coal Miner's Program

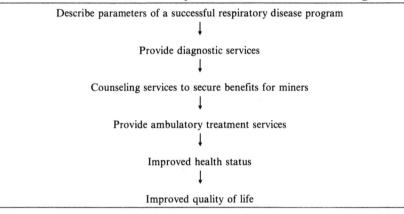

Describe parameters of a successful respiratory disease program

↓

Provide diagnostic services

↓

Counseling services to secure benefits for miners

↓

Provide ambulatory treatment services

↓

Improved health status

↓

Improved quality of life

Miner's Respiratory Disease Program can be reconstructed following these principles. As a final step in this process, the evaluator must present the hierarchy to the sponsor and identify which objective was used to guide the intervention.[6]

Developing Objectives Prospectively

In a prospective evaluation, objectives are selected which best characterize the motives of the intervention program—how the program intends to allocate its resources. For example, objectives for a home health care program are listed in Table 7–3, and objectives for a community health center are provided in Table 7–4. Each objective is linked to an adjacent objective to create a hierarchy, as described above. Lower level objectives must be accomplished before higher level objectives can be achieved. The sponsor selects an objective that seems achievable within a given time period and for a particular level of resources.

Table 7-3. Objectives for a Home Health Program

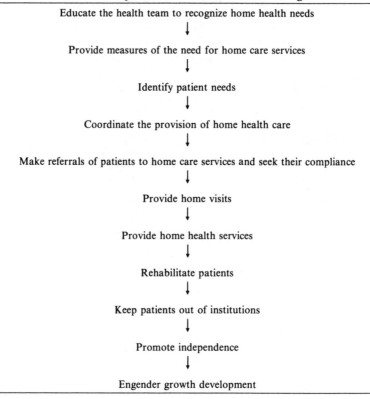

Educate the health team to recognize home health needs
↓
Provide measures of the need for home care services
↓
Identify patient needs
↓
Coordinate the provision of home health care
↓
Make referrals of patients to home care services and seek their compliance
↓
Provide home visits
↓
Provide home health services
↓
Rehabilitate patients
↓
Keep patients out of institutions
↓
Promote independence
↓
Engender growth development

Selecting a program objective is not a trivial task. For example, a medical society may provide funds to develop a pamphlet that depicts the dangers of smoking. Such projects often state that the objective of health education projects like the pamphlet is to reduce mortality and morbidity of lung cancer. To alter health status, a health education program must move through a four–step hierarchy shown in Table 7–5.

Measuring health status as an indicator of the merits of health education materials is misleading at best. It is unreasonable to expect a pamphlet to have any measurable effect on the mortality and morbidity of lung cancer. Meeting the information needs of people who smoke might be a more appropriate objective. Selecting an objective that is too broad or unrealistic is almost as common as tailoring the objectives to correspond to evaluation findings. Volunteer organizations and, all too often, federal legislation establish expansive objectives when the availability of funds, constraints, and the nature of these intervention programs call for a limited program with modest

Table 7-4. Objectives for a Neighborhood Health Center

Enable consumers to identify their health needs

↓

Enable consumers to meet their own health needs

↓

Meet unmet needs

↓

Provide emergent, urgent, and convenience care for at-risk populations

↓

Reduce risk factors

↓

Provide quality health care to NHC clientele

↓

Enhance continuity of care

↓

Keep people healthy

↓

Enable people to reach their greatest potential

Table 7-5. Objectives for Health Education Programs

Meeting people's information needs

↓

Changing people's attitudes

↓

Changing people's behavior

↓

Altering people's health status

objectives. When reorganization, inflation, or new leadership force an assessment, potentially good programs are discarded because they were perceived not to meet these unrealistic objectives. These programs may have made an important but less sweeping contribution.

For example, Congress established Regional Medical Programs (RMP) to reduce the incidence of heart diseases, cancer, and stroke through local action programs and physician education, without changing the patterns of medical practice. A formidable task! Time passed. The program's supporters in Congress and the administration left office. The program was attacked by the next administration, which contended that Regional Medical Programs failed to achieve their objectives. The objectives were made still broader to include renal disease and other major diseases. Program directors were issued new guidelines which dropped the reference to "preserving existing patterns of medical practice." But RMP program directors were unsure if their local constituents and funding levels would support an all out attack on practice patterns. After nearly ten years of support for 56 RMP's across the United States, the entire program was dismantled. Little was preserved.

Similarly, the ruling boards of medical societies, hospital associations, and cancer societies initiate programs and state program objectives that make failure inevitable. Medical societies have little hope of altering people's mortality and morbidity through traditional media approaches. As a result, well–run health education programs focus evaluation efforts on elements of the program under their control, measuring, for instance, the efficiency and effectiveness of their information dissemination process. Organizations sponsoring such activities (medical societies and hospital associations, for example) would be wise to band together and attempt a comprehensive study of how various modes of information alter the behavior of their intended audience.[7]

Many evaluation efforts in organizations are focused on lower–level objectives. Organizations often mistake a measurable objective for an important one. However, the value of an intervention program is associated with higher–level objectives that describe the impact of these programs on a target group. Activity (e.g., the distribution system for health education materials) cannot be substituted for the ultimate aims of the program (e.g., meeting peoples' information needs). In this case activity becomes an end unto itself and the aims of the program are lost.

If an intermediate objective is selected by the sponsor, the sequence of events that leads to the accomplishment of higher–level objectives should be clearcut. For instance, a home health care program (Table 7–3), can use "home health care visits" as an objective when visits can be clearly linked to the delivery of a specific set of services that are known to rehabilitate patients. The linkages between visits–services–rehabilitation must be reproduceable. Often linkages are taken for granted and not verified. Rehabilitation must result each time a given battery of services are provided before "visits" can serve as the program's objective. Decisions to expand or contract a program should hinge on the attainment of a high–level objective. Evaluations should focus on these objectives or on objectives with a clearcut linkage with a program's benefits.

DERIVING MEASURES FROM AN OBJECTIVE

Criteria are derived from the program's objective. The criteria are used to suggest measures, which define data that are collected in the evaluation. As shown in Table 7–6, objectives suggest criteria, which in turn suggest measures.

Table 7-6. Inferring Measures from Objectives

Objectives	Criteria	Measures
entry-level services to a community	penetration of the health center into the community	number of new enrollers vs. break-even requirements
	"one-door" medicine	strata of income enrolled vs. target
		utilization of preventive services by various age groups

For example, the guidelines and enabling legislation for Community Health Centers (previously called Neighborhood Health Centers) had "entry level health care services to a community" as their objective. The Community Health Center's "penetration into the community" may be an important criterion. High enrollment and enrollees that represent all groups in the community was an implicit desire of the program's sponsors. As a result, a criterion of "one door medicine" was implied. Enrollees should represent all income levels in the community. These criteria can be used to suggest measures. Measures could include the number of new enrollees, stratified by income and compared to targets for participation of particular income levels, and the number of patients who permit the center to break even financially. The utilization of the center's services by patients in particular age groups can be measured and compared to the number of contacts with a health delivery organization considered ideal for each age group. These norms are used to gauge the behavior of those using the community health center.

Measures for a health education program are described in Table 7-7. During the initiation phase of an educational program, the evaluation might measure the readability of the pamphlet.[8] The contact phase might consider a measure like the number of pieces of literature available for distribution. During the operational phase, the number of smokers requesting the material or the number of pieces distributed to smokers might be measured. To determine attitudinal changes, the number of smokers (or potential smokers) who read pamphlets can be measured. The number of people who learn new facts from the pamphlet could be used to measure its informational value. Behavioral changes are more difficult to determine. For example, few people who verbalize their intent to change their behavior and stop smoking, actually follow through. To complicate the evaluation, directly observing the smoker's behavior is seldom feasible. (Imagine a friend designated to report on each smoker's behavior.) Finally, an inference concerning mortality and morbidity could be drawn for a population that saw, read, and learned from that pamphlet and modified its behavior.

This process illustrates how a program evaluator deduces the measures from

Table 7-7. Measures for a Pamphlet Aimed at Smokers

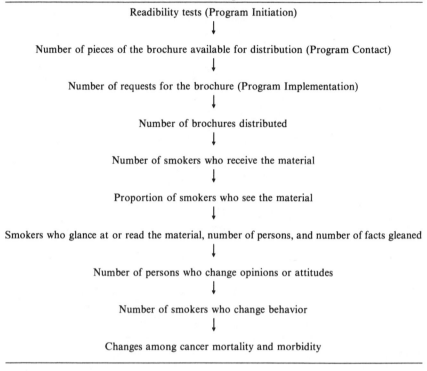

Readibility tests (Program Initiation)

↓

Number of pieces of the brochure available for distribution (Program Contact)

↓

Number of requests for the brochure (Program Implementation)

↓

Number of brochures distributed

↓

Number of smokers who receive the material

↓

Proportion of smokers who see the material

↓

Smokers who glance at or read the material, number of persons, and number of facts gleaned

↓

Number of persons who change opinions or attitudes

↓

Number of smokers who change behavior

↓

Changes among cancer mortality and morbidity

a program objective. First, objectives are carefully assessed to extract criteria which in turn are used as a means of formulating proxy measures of the program's objectives. This three–step process is required for nearly all evaluation efforts. Most evaluation projects must rely on proxy measures. The evaluator must select measures carefully so the objectives of the program being evaluated can be accurately represented.

Components of Program Objectives

Objectives may be defined so proxy measures are stated as an integral part of the objective. Objectives are defined by their components. The management by objectives literature recommends defining an objective in terms of its time frame, desired results, and performance standards.[9] Smalley contends that an objective should state yardsticks and expected values for each.[10] Gottman and Clasen describe an educational objective as specifying who will do what, under what conditions, and to what extent.[11]

These requirements suggest that intervention program objectives should specify the program's target group, the effects sought, its desired performance level and constraints. The *target group* identifies the intended recipients of the service or intervention. For example, a renal disease program should have a clear understanding of the number of people with end–stage renal disease in the region they seek to serve. The same applies to burn care centers. When planning a burn care center as a referral service, a clear understanding of the incidence of severe burns within the service region is needed to specify the scope of the program. The target group indicates those that will be served and/or those that the program seeks to influence. For instance, a multihospital system implementing a new management appraisal program must determine which executives in their operating units will be subject to the appraisal program.

The *effects* sought for the target group must be identified. In the case of services, an objective should specify what parameters in the target group should change. A service program may attempt to reduce mortality, change disability, deinstitutionalize, or provide psychological support. Renal disease programs could be focused on either mortality and/or disability: attempting to eliminate deaths due to renal disease or to return those with renal disease to an active life. The objectives for managerial interventions must also specify desired effects. For example, a multihospital system may have developed a bonus system for its laboratory supervisors. The effects sought by the bonus might include reduction in complaints from physicians, fewer errors, lower costs in the laboratory, or fewer employee grievances.

Objectives must also specify an *expected performance* level. For example, end–stage renal disease survival from a transplantation program should be 80 to 90 percent when donor and recipient kidneys are matched by tissue typing, and above 95 percent when sibling kidneys are used. No appreciable disability should result. A 75 percent referral of all severe burns in the region might be used to describe the expected performance level of a burn center. Managerial interventions might specify the number of tolerable instances of union grievances, the expected level of cost, tolerable error rates, and the like. Expected performance levels specify norms or achievement standards for the intervention program.

Finally, the objectives should specify relevant *constraints*. The most important and pervasive constraint is time. Performance is seldom meaningful unless it is measured within a specific length of time. Gauging performance for a particular time period can be used to extrapolate into the future. Another relevant constraint is budget. Intervention programs often depend upon their intensity: the number of resources allocated to carry out the program. Budget is an important constraint when generalizing a program's effects.

Thus, an objective can be defined by specifying its target group, the effects a behavior sought, expected performance levels, and constraints such as time or budget.

Group Methods to Devise Program Objectives

Many evaluation projects have advisory groups appointed to monitor results or merely to sanction the project and give it legitimacy. The members of these groups often have considerable information and insights. To exploit this knowledge, evaluators can ask the advisory groups to identify each of the components of the program's objective. For example, a national panel of experts was appointed to consult with HEW's Bureau of Community Health Services to develop an index of medical underservice. Gustafson and his colleagues had the panel suggest, cull, select, and prioritize measures of medical underservice.[12] This provided HEW's staff with priority measures to evaluate health care resource needs in various geographic regions of the United States.

Advisory groups can be asked to

—develop a hierarchy of objectives,
—select an objective from a hierarchy of objectives,
—derive criteria for the objectives,
—suggest measures for each criterion,
—specify standards or performance expectations,
—identify target groups, and
—select constraints.

Involving the advisory group in the selection of measures, performance expectations, and the like has been found to enhance their acceptance and quality.[13] Groups bring a variety of viewpoints which cause more sources of information to be considered. Mason points out that a synthesis of this information can improve the quality of the measures.[14] But as Collins and Guetzkow note, there are many barriers to full information sharing among advisory groups.[15] These barriers become intense when the advisory group's members are drawn from several organizations.[16] Each member may push personal goals such as seeking prestige or grinding a well-worn ax, before considering information their organization would agree to share. This "double filter" creates a barrier to effective group efforts.

Groups also provide an evaluator with an opportunity to enhance acceptance of objectives selected for an intervention program. Participation in the selection of objectives enhances acceptance of the evaluation process and its results.[17] Thompson calls this cooptation: involving people one hopes to influence into a policy-making role for the project.[18]

Group methods or group management techniques have been devised to overcome barriers to full participation and to stimulate acceptance. Several group management techniques can be used to elicit information from advisory groups. For instance, Delbecq and Van de Ven's *Nominal Group Technique* (NGT) has the advisory group work silently, to encourage reflection.[19] This reflective phase is followed by a systematic consideration of results. Four steps are used: silent recording of possible evaluation measures; listing the measures and giving each advisory committee member a turn, one at a time, until measurement ideas are exhausted; discussing the measures to consolidate the list and share the information about the merits of such measures; and selecting measures to be applied in the evaluation. The NGT can be used to identify objectives or criteria or to select a target group, constraints, or to specify norms. The NGT was developed to conduct broad search for information, which has been found to stimulate new ideas.[20]

Delphi surveys systematically solicit and collate judgments from an advisory group.[21] A series of questionnaires are used. The first questionnaire solicits ideas that define measures, norms, target groups, and other evaluation parameters, and asks the members to state the rationale behind their candidate measures, norms, etc. Subsequent questionnaires consolidate and feed back measures and the rationales to the advisory group. Each advisory group member can review the logic behind the arguments of others, which is thought to stimulate consensus. The final survey offers members a chance to prioritize.

Delphi is an excellent information dredge. It is also useful when confidentiality is essential, as group members can remain anonymous, and when meetings are too costly because of travel distances. But Delphi can be cumbersome, time consuming, and arbitrary. There are no rules for summarizing results.[22] Also, staff must have (or acquire) considerable knowledge of the evaluation topic to provide the necessary summaries. A large number of surveys may be needed before disagreements become apparent. Closure is often forced by the equivalent of a vote.

Hybrid group process methods have been developed to exploit the beneficial features of Delphi, NGT, and structured interaction, often called brainstorming. For instance, the *conflict-consensus* technique uses a Delphi–like survey, structured discussion, and silent recording elements of NGT.[23] Surveys are used to measure disagreement on important issues before the advisory group meeting. The survey could be used to elicit information about measures, norms, target groups, and/or other relevant parameters. For instance, members can be provided a list of objectives to prioritize by assigning an index number, using a scale like that shown below.[24]

0 = no effect in directing the program
1 = rarely dictates efforts in the program
2 = intermittently dictates efforts in the program

3 = dictates some effort in the program

4 = dictates much effort in the program

5 = dictates all efforts in the program

The average or mean value of the index number in the survey is used to identify the objective with the most support. An average of 3.00 is described as the threshold of consideration. Conflict can be defined by the variance of the index numbers assigned by the group. Coalitions in the advisory group have comparable variances.

In step two, a meeting is called. The agenda is drawn from the survey categories. First the current consensus is presented. The advisory group is encouraged to debate the appropriateness of the consensus, rather than to argue with each other. Rationale emerges via unstructured discussion. Discussion is encouraged among the group members to point out why an objective may be rated too high or too low. This discussion is directed toward the average rating, not a colleague, which encourages constructive participation from all group members. After each agenda item has been discussed, the advisory group reconsiders its original choices, using a "nominal format." The final judgments are recorded without discussion in order to encourage reflection.

This approach has been found to quickly locate the level of consensus for groups in conflict.[25] For instance, patient volume and staffing level norms for evaluating radiotherapy units based on patient values and staffing were developed and ratified in two meetings.[26]

Estimate-discuss-estimate (E-D-E) is another method synthesized from several group process techniques. Gustafson, Shukla, Delbecq, and Walster developed E-D-E to solicit parameter estimates from advisory groups.[27] A precise choice situation is necessary for E-D-E to work optimally. For instance, E-D-E can be used to estimate five-year survival rates for cancers at particular sites and given a particular stage of the disease, using various treatment modalities like radiotherapy, surgery, chemotherapy, and combinations of these (Table 7-8). First, the desired information is listed by the group without discussion. Group averages are computed and displayed to stimulate discussion. Next, the advisory group considers these initial judgments in an unstructured discussion. After this discussion the group reestimates, again following the nominal format. E-D-E has been found to be quite accurate for estimation tasks, followed by synthetic groups (surveys), committees (interacting groups), and Delphi groups.[28]

SOME BEHAVIORAL ASPECTS OF EVALUATION MEASURES

Objectives and their measures are frequently based on someone's conviction about what is desirable. It is common for objectives to be formed by an administrator without consultation from peers or the evaluator. This can lead to objectives that have deleted pertinent considerations or introduced extraneous ones. When measures are derived from a deficient objective a spurious relationship may be assessed or the intervention may stimulate responses that are inappropriate or even bizarre. For instance, some contend that inflation in health costs stemming from malpractice awards can be justified because lawsuits encourage introspection by incompetent physicians. However, the filing of a lawsuit against a competent physician creates suspicion in referring physicians, peers, hospitals, and their patients. It is bad for business, and even worse for physicians' peer associations. The pall of suspicion will continue to exist even if the case is ultimately dismissed. As a result, all physicians, competent and incompetent, have been encouraged to practice "defensive medicine" by creating the appearance that all remotely useful information has been collected by ordering batteries of diagnostic tests and consults. Physicians are also encouraged to assume that all patients are sick, which minimizes the chance that a sick person will be missed. Kerr points out that defensive medicine may even cause bad medicine.[29] Physicians are approached by patients complaining of a few stray symptoms which are classified, organized, and given a name. The patient, told what other

Table 7-8: Estimates of Survivals
For Cancer Treatment Modalities

TREATMENT MODALITIES

SITE/STAGE	Surgery	Radiotherapy	Chemotherapy	Various Combinations
Colon-Stage I				
Stage II				
Stage III				
Stage IV				
Lung-Stage I				
Stage II				
Stage III				
Stage IV				

symptoms may be expected, obligingly detects these symptoms and the physician treats the self–fulfilling prophecy as a bona fide health problem.

Deficient Measures

Deficient objectives lead to measures that may encourage behavior the intervention seeks to discourage. Orphanages, for instance, are discouraged from placing children because their budgets are based on the institution's census. As a consequence, Kerr contends that elaborate placement procedures evolved with complex placement criteria and long waiting periods so that "it is almost impossible to pry a child out of the place."[30] A health insurance company attempting to encourage accurate claim preparation, recorded the number of returned checks and letters of complaint by preparing employees. Clearly, underpayments provoke complaints, but would overpayments? When performance measures are deficient, individuals and organizations tend to ignore objectives and focus on what is being measured.

Several measures may be needed to insure that behavior will contribute to the achievement of an objective. For example, a hospital seeking to speed up the admissions process may devise an incentive scheme (the intervention) for admission clerks whereby earnings are based on the number of admission forms completed each day. This will get the admission clerks to compete for patients and, presumably, lead to faster admissions. If clerks are also responsible for support activities such as requisitioning new forms and answering phones, or for coordinational functions like relaying information on admission problems and checking out patient payment, the system will quickly break down. The clerks will respond to what is measured, which emphasizes filling out forms and ignores support and coordinational activities. The overall lack of coordination may lead to a chronic shortage of needed supplies and possibly a decline in the speed of patient admissions. Several measures are often needed to capture the full intent of an objective.

Unintended Outcomes

Table 7–9 describes how evaluations can be misinterpreted when the intervention produces extranalities or side effects. New interventions or services tend to produce unintended outcomes which may enhance or diminish the program's effectiveness. Unintended outcomes provoke consequences that the sponsor may or may not be able to anticipate.

When extranalities are positive and the consequences of the positive extranality cannot be anticipated, *post hoc objectives* are often formed by the

Table 7-9:   Interpreting Unintended Outcomes
From An Intervention Program

		CONSEQUENCES	
		Unanticipated	Anticipated
Extranalities	Positive	Post Hoc Objectives Developed	Call Attention To Program's Success
	Negative	Bizarre or Political Ramifications	Defensive Posture Established

sponsor. For example, OEO's Neighborhood Health Centers (NHC) were established to provide health care in low-income areas. OEO required each NHC to use local residents who were regular users of the centers' services to identify health needs in the area by a survey. This practice seemed desirable because it provided jobs and because the residents, through their understanding of customs in the area, seemed likely to get an accurate and comprehensive reporting of health problems. These surveys proved to be useless.[31] And training programs sponsored by OEO through each NHC failed to improve the surveys. However, the residents' knowledge of the NHC and their testimonials seemed to stimulate enrollment. These unintended benefits were used to form post hoc objectives: the objective of the surveys was changed from information gathering to marketing. Post hoc benefits are often capricious and must be verified by an independent evaluation.

Wildawsky contends that the sponsors of interventions want to see what they can get before indicating what they want.[32] As a result, objectives are often left implicit during the evaluation effort. Sponsors can then select an objective that the evaluation data appear to confirm. This process is both frustrating to the evaluator and unlikely to stimulate meaningful changes in service or intervention programs.[33]

An evaluation can be threatening, so the sponsors of intervention programs attempt to keep their objectives vague. Objectives are permitted to evolve. When inferring an objective for a retrospective evaluation (as described in a previous section), the objective can be manipulated by skillful program proponents. Those with vested interests in the program often set the objectives post hoc, after its benefits become clear. Evaluation is used merely to ratify expected outcomes. This type of evaluation has far less diagnostic value than prospective evaluations, where objectives are set before the program begins. Retrospective evaluations are encouraged because intervention programs with vague objectives may encourage innovation in the field.[34] Clever administrators encourage retrospective evaluations because they seldom contain nasty surprises.

When positive extranalities can be anticipated, they offer sponsors an opportunity to dramatize their achievements. Few sponsors miss a chance to use *windfalls* which can be used to their benefit. "Look what we have here" is followed by "...in accordance with our plans we managed to produce the following benefits for our organization." For instance, thoracic surgeons establishing an open heart surgery program in a hospital will seek "easy" cases so initial assessments of their surgery will be positive. Bitter experience has taught management engineers to implement hospital inventory control programs so early estimates of cost savings are favorable.

Bizarre outcomes occur when negative side effects are not anticipated by the sponsor. Evaluation efforts often fail to anticipate how the findings may be received by key groups. For instance, the CIA gave drugs to unsuspecting military personnel, seeking to understand how these drugs would influence the behavior of prisoners of war and CIA agents. Press coverage of these practices caused an outcry. The CIA was unable to defend the practice of using nonvoluntary military personnel to simulate how drugs might be used by foreign powers. As a consequence, the CIA agreed to a ban of *all* such evaluations.

Unanticipated negative consequences are often used by program adversaries and those seeking to discredit the program's sponsor. If an evaluation confirms the notions of the adversary, the information may be used before appropriate qualifications can be made. For example, the Nixon administration was quick to release negative findings on the Head Start program's effectiveness because Head Start was generally agreed to be one of the few Great Society programs that worked.[35] No attempt was made to discriminate between the effects of year–long programs from haphazardly operated six–week summer programs or to discuss positive features of the Head Start program. In these circumstances, the evaluator has little time to prepare program administrators for the ensuing recriminations, which may discredit any future use of evaluation by these administrators.

Finally, many negative side effects of a program can be anticipated and a *defensive posture* established. For example, neonatology programs may reduce the mortality of premature newborns, but critics contend they also result in a diminished quality of life for those that survive. The incidence of severe physical defects and retardation in children may increase as a result of neonatology programs. Advocates of neonatology programs would do well to study former patients to isolate the accuracy of these claims. A defensive posture is based on challenging the legitimacy of the claims of negative extranalities. The neonatologist can determine what is known about the survival characteristics of infants and the validity of these studies.

Similarly, public health departments often conduct screening programs which provide chest x-rays for a large population. These x-rays are often ignored by physicians, who contend that most patients referred to them with suspicious lungs stem from suspect radiographs caused by poorly trained x-ray technicians and miserable field conditions. As a result, spokesmen in medical societies state that these programs merely expose large numbers of people, in particular the x-ray technicians, to needless radiation. Public health departments should anticipate these negative side effects by dramatizing the program's benefits or by improving their process of patient referral.

Values Implicit in Objectives

The objectives of most intervention and service programs have many implicit beliefs buried in them. Suchman finds that most objectives are built on inherent, conceived, and operational values.[36] For example, several intervention programs can be envisioned which might reduce birth defects, such as cost-free prenatal care centers or genetic counseling. A genetic counseling program establishes the *inherent* value of its services by demonstrating how genetics dictates certain abnormalities. A *conceived* value for these services can be stimulated by dramatizing the impact of birth defects to the public or to legislators. Finally, an *operational* value is created in those who could benefit from genetic counseling, getting them to use the services. A failure to use the genetic counseling services suggests that people rejected the operational value of the service because it clashed with other, more important values. For instance, people's desire for freedom of choice and self-determination may outweigh all other considerations.

Similarly, the sponsor of a prenatal care center must establish the inherent values of regular monitoring during pregnancy in reducing birth defects as well as the conceived value that birth defects must be reduced. Operational values are often based on assumptions of behavior. For instance, the effectiveness of a prenatal center depends on the extent to which appointments are kept during pregnancy. Such a program assumes that pregnant women without access to prenatal care will comprehend the relationship between these services and the health of their unborn child and take advantage of the center's services. Thus, inherent and conceived values have a factual base, but often require demonstration. In contrast, an operational value must be shared by the sponsor of the program and its target group for the program to be effective. Programs often fail when the values implicit in their objectives take on special meanings for the program sponsor and for its beneficiaries.

Program objectives have validity assumptions as well as value assumptions. Value assumptions concern what the program initiators believe is "good." Suchman notes that the public health movement is based on the value assumption that government must protect people from undesirable social conditions.[37] What is good for society is often perceived to be good for the target group of the intervention. As pointed out by the birth defects example, this is not always the case. The objectives of intervention programs are often formulated by professionals and by administrators. Health education programs that attempt to get people to stop smoking assumes that if smokers can be convinced that smoking is linked to cancer and other health problems, they will give up cigarettes. The initiators of such programs, often nonsmokers, make the dubious assumption that their values can apply to cigarette users.

Validity assumptions are based on beliefs about causation. Social action programs are devised and carried out because their sponsors believed that people would benefit from the program. For instance, health planning agencies attempt to reduce the number of acute care beds, believing that excess beds have been the primary source of rising costs in the health system. The programs and services of environmental protection agencies, health and safety inspection at places of work, and compensatory education programs like Head Start were all based on this type of validity assumption.

Intervention programs are typically extensions of validity assumptions. No program is initiated unless someone has a vision and carries it out. When evaluation is built into intervention programs, these insights specify the nature of the intervention and its intended effects. Retrospective assessments must tease out these assumptions to define the intended outcomes.

MEASUREMENT SCALES

The values or numbers used by a measure can be scaled in several ways. Scaling assigns numbers to items based on one or more of their properties. Scales may be ratio, interval, ordinal, or nominal (see Figure 7–1).

A *nominal scale* provides a classification. Objects, people, or entities can be grouped to identify some characteristic of interest. The numbers or symbols that make up the classification create the nominal scale. For instance, a

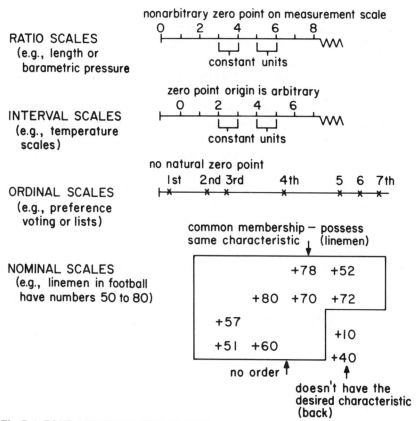

RATIO SCALES
(e.g., length or
barametric pressure

nonarbitrary zero point on measurement scale
0   2   4   6   8
constant units

INTERVAL SCALES
(e.g., temperature
scales)

zero point origin is arbitrary
0   2   4   6
constant units

ORDINAL SCALES
(e.g., preference
voting or lists)

no natural zero point
Ist 2nd 3rd   4th   5 6 7th

NOMINAL SCALES
(e.g., linemen in football
have numbers 50 to 80)

common membership — possess
same characteristic (linemen)

+78 +52
+80 +70 +72
+57
+51 +60
+10
+40
no order

doesn't have the
desired characteristic
(back)

Fig. 7-1. FOUR MEASUREMENT SCALES

mental health patient can be classified as schizophrenic, paranoid, manic–depressive, or neurotic, to create a four–item scale. To make these classifications exact, careful definitions of each category must be provided so a set of mutually exclusive classes will result. For instance, assigning numbers 50 to 80 for linemen and numbers less than 49 to backs permits an observer to classify football players by their number.

Ordinal scales provide categories and relationships among the categories. The ordinal scale can be partially or totally ordered. The ranks represent the numbers in an ordinal scale. For instance, the members of study sections often rank research grants to create a priority list. Similarly, surveys with Likert scales group responses by categories such as strongly agree, agree, disagree, and strongly disagree, to create an ordinal scale. The categorization is nominal (responses fall into distinct categories), but the categories also have some relationship to one another.

Interval scales have all the characteristics of an ordinal scale, but also specify the distance between any two categories. The mapping of categories is so precise that the size of the intervals between the categories is specified. For instance, temperature can be measured with a Centigrade or a Fahrenheit scale. The measurement unit and the zero point on the scales are arbitrary, but the scales have fixed relationships so that numbers can be transformed from one scale to the other.

Ratio scales have all the properties of interval scales with the addition of a nonarbitrary zero–point. Costs, percentages such as hospital occupancy or debt service coverage, and ratios such as nurse–patient relationships and financial indicators, are measured with ratio scales. Measures of height and length also have a ratio scale. Thus, ratio scales have four properties: equivalence, ordering, known intervals, and a defined origin.

The values from ordinal and nominal scales are called ordinal numbers, and the values from ratio and interval scales are called cardinal numbers. Cardinal numbers have the property of additivity, which is necessary to carry out the statistical tests described in the earlier chapters. The evaluator must compute parameters (e.g., means and standard deviations) to apply parametric tests demanded by t tests and ANOVA techniques.

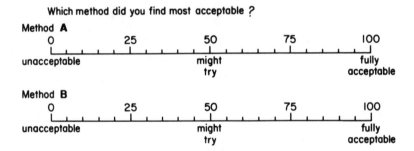

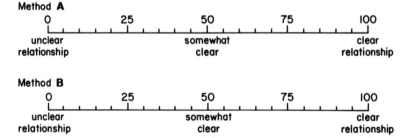

Fig. 7–2. ILLUSTRATIVE ARS SCALES

Ratio scales have advantages over ordinal and nominal scales, and evaluators try to create scales that take on their properties. For example, "anchored rating scales" (discussed in Chapter 5) attempt to define a scale interval and a zero point so responses to questions on a survey can take on ratio scale properties.[38] The anchored rating scale encourages the respondent to make fine discriminations. For instance, to detect views of the accuracy and acceptance of two methods used to construct nurse staffing models, nurse participants used the scales in Figure 7–2.[39] Each question in Figure 7–2 uses a unique set of descriptors to anchor the response scale. The descriptors are used to give meaning to the scale increments and to define the zero point on the scale.

NONPARAMETRIC METHODS OF ANALYSIS

F and t tests cannot be applied when effects are measured as ordinal numbers. Nonparametric statistical tests must be used. Segal describes several techniques that can test the similarity among ranks.[40] The *Spearman Rank Correlation* coefficient is used to compare two lists of ranks or priorities. The scores assigned to grants by agency staff and study section are shown in Table 7–10, to illustrate the computations for the Spearman coefficient.

The correlation coefficient is computed as shown below:

$$R_s = 1 - \frac{6 \sum_{i=1}^{N} d_i^2}{N^3 - N}$$

where d = the differences in ranks assigned
N = the number of objects ranked

For this example,

$$R_s = 1 - \frac{6(52)}{12^3 - 12} = .82$$

Table A–6 in the appendix is used to determine the statistical significance of this correlation. In this example the significance is .01, suggesting the staff and

Table 7-10.

Spearman Rank Correlation Coefficient*

$$R_s = 1 - \frac{6\sum_{i=1}^{N} d_i^2}{N^3 - N}$$

R_s = Spearman Correlation Coefficient
d_i = Difference in rank i
N = Number of items ranked

Grant	Scores Assigned by Staff to NCHSR Grants	Scores Computed From Study Section	di	di²
1	2	3	-1	1
2	6	4	2	4
3	5	2	3	9
4	1	1	0	0
5	10	8	2	4
6	9	11	-2	4
7	8	10	-2	4
8	3	6	-3	9
9	4	7	-3	9
10	12	12	0	0
11	7	5	2	4
12	11	9	2	4
				$\sum d_i^2 = 52$

15 point Scale
0 = Lousy
15 = Earth-shaking

*This example was adapted from Siegel, S., "Measures of Correlation and Their Tests of Significance," (p. 206) in *Nonparametric Statistics: For the Behavioral Sciences,* New York: McGraw Hill, 1956.

study section endorsed the same grants.

A *Kendall Coefficient of Concordance* compares the relationship among three or more sets of ranks. The statistic compares the degree of departure from perfect agreement among several lists of ranked items. Table 7-11 provides an illustration. To detect the amount of agreement among faculty members in the selection of graduate students, each faculty member ranked the same six applicants. The Kendall Coefficient is computed as shown below:

$$R_w = \frac{S}{1/12 k^2 (N^3 - N)}$$

where k = number of judges
N = number of objects ranked

Table 7-11: Kendall Coefficient of Concordance[a]

$$W = \frac{S}{1/12 \ k^2 \ (N^3-N)}$$

where S = sum of squares for deviations about mean rank

$$S = \sum_j (R_j - \Sigma R_j/N)^2$$

k = number of judges

N = number of objects ranked

	Applicants					
	a	b	c	d	e	f
Faculty Member #1	1	6	3	2	5	4
Faculty Member #2	1	5	6	4	2	3
Faculty Member #3	6	3	2	5	4	1
R_j	8	14	11	11	11	8

$\bar{R} = (8+14+11+11+11+8)/6 = 10.5$

Note: perfect agreement best student $1 + 1 + 1 = k$

perfect agreement least promising $6 + 6 + 6 = 18 = NK$

perfect agreement among judges would produce
3, 6, 9, 12, 15, 18 (not in this order)

no agreement, R_j will be about the same for each applicant

[a]This example was adopted from Siegel, S., "Measures of Correlation and their tests of Significance" (p. 230) in Non-Parametric Statistics for the Behavioral Sciences, New York: McGraw Hill, 1956.

S is the sum of square of observations about the mean rank, R.

$$S = \sum_{j=1}^{N} (R_j - \bar{R})^2$$

246 EVALUATION CONCEPTS AND METHODS

S is computed, from the data in Table 7–11, as

$$(8-10.5)^2 + (14-10.5)^2 + (11-10.5)^2 + (11-10.5)^2 + (11-10.5)^2 + (8-10.5)^2 = 25.5$$

R_w, the correlation coefficient, is computed as shown below:

$$R_w = \frac{25.5}{1/12(3^2)(6^3-6)} = .16$$

To test the significance of this correlation, the value S is used, and Table A–7 in the appendix must be consulted. To be significant at the .05 level, S must exceed 103.9, so the evaluation concludes that the faculty do not agree on the credentials of the applicants.

PROXY MEASURES FOR CAUSES AND EFFECTS

Measuring Effects

The objectives of intervention programs are seldom directly measurable. (Ways to identify surrogate measures for the objective were described in earlier sections of this chapter.) A good *proxy measure* ties the outcome of an intervention to the program's objectives. For example, contract hospital management is being aggressively marketed by several corporations which contend they can dramatically improve the financial performance of most hospitals. Contract management is an intervention that provides the administrative staff for the hospital, joint purchasing, labor control programs, hospital construction planning, and other special services. The hospital's board of trustees retains control of hospital policy and legal responsibilities.

The objective of contract management is to improve the hospital's financial performance while maintaining the quality of care. Several measures of performance for contract–managed hospitals are listed in Table 7–12, to illustrate how each is tied to one or more aspects of this objective.[41]

Financial indicators such as total deductions from revenue were used to suggest financial management skills in collecting reimbursements for services provided from Medicare and Medicaid. The bad–debt rate is often used to measure skills in debt collection. Days in Accounts Receivable measures the rate of collection directly. Critics of management contracts contend that the hospital's financial performance is improved at the expense of care quality. There is no accepted measure of quality, so a proxy was sought which can detect whether care levels were altered. In this case, nursing hours per patient day were tracked to demonstrate that costs were not cut by reducing the hospital's nurse–patient ratio.

Table 7-12. Proxy Measures of Contract Hospital Management
Objective: To improve Hospital performance
Intervention: Contract management

Indicators	Concept Measured
Financial Performance	
Total Deductions from Revenue	Financial management skills in reimbursement collections
Days in Accounts Receivable	Management skills in debt collection
Revenue Per Patient Day	Determine if revenue increases are due to price increases or volume changes
Operating Expenses	Exclude depreciation, rent, and interest to get a measure of partially controllable hospital costs
Total Labor Cost	Indicator of contractee's performance in labor control
Departmental Supply Cost	Indicates facility in obtaining quantity discounts through the multihospital system
Contributed Margin	Consolidated measure of financial management skills in debt collection
Other Performance Measures	
Occupancy Rate	Ability of management to stimulate demand
Nursing Hours Per Patient Day	Indicates sincerity in maintaining quality of care
Medical Specialty Fees	Reductions of costs in pathology and radiology to indicates negotiation skills

Measuring Causes

In retrospective evaluations, proxies may be needed to define measures for causal factors. Unlike prospective assessments, the intervention occurs along with several other factors. The intervention, extraneous factors, or both could have caused the measures of effectiveness to vary. For example, an evaluation of nursing home costs has a clearcut measure of effectiveness (per diem costs), but costs may be influenced by several other factors. A retrospective evaluation must define and develop measures for these factors. Proxy measures for causal factors must be derived which are mutually exclusive (measure different variables) and exhaustive (consider all possible influences). This is often a formidable task.

An evaluation framework for a retrospective evaluation of nursing home costs is shown in Table 7-13. Control status, bed size, and type of facility were called policy variables because they could be manipulated by the evaluation sponsor, a state department of health.[42] These factors were called policy variables because the policy maker (the health department) can eliminate the

Table 7-13. Proxy Measures that Influence Costs in a Nursing Home

Indicators	Concept Measured
Policy Variables	
(1) Control status Proprietary (sole, partnership, corporation) Nonproprietary	Profit motive
(2) Bed size small: 25 beds medium: 50 beds large: 100 beds	Economies of scale
(3) Type of facility Intermediate Care Facility Skilled Nursing Home	Level of care
Block Variables	
(1) Occupancy above 85% (full cost allowance) below 85% (reimbursement adjusted)	Competence of nursing home management
(2) Medicare utilization low, less than 70% high, more than 75%	Nature of patient population
(3) Staffing high nurse/patient staffing ratios low nurse/patient ratios	Quality of care

profit motive, offer incentives to increase the size of homes, and can license only intermediate care facilities. Occupancy, Medicare utilization, and staffing are called block variables because they were controlled by the management in each nursing home.

Control status was used to measure the profit motive. Nursing homes with a profit motive may have lower costs, so homes were stratified by their type of ownership (proprietary and nonproprietary) to detect the influence of this factor. Bed size (number of beds) was measured to detect the impact of economies of scale, while facility type was used to determine how level of care influenced cost. Occupancy was used as a proxy for managerial competence. When occupancy falls below 85 percent, the allowance provided by Medicare reimbursement is figured at an 85 percent rate. Hence there is considerable incentive to keep occupancy above 85 percent. The proportion of Medicaid patients in the nursing homes was selected as a proxy for patient characteristics. A high proportion of Medicaid patients suggests more care is needed, which would increase costs, compared to nursing homes with low Medicaid utilization. Finally, staffing was used as a proxy for quality of care. A low nurse–patient ratio implies that the home controls costs by using staff that cannot meet some of the needs of its patients.

Measures must be inferred for each of the policy and block variables in Table 7–11. Some measures are categorical (proprietary or nonproprietary) while others have continuous scales, but all are placed into high and low levels for each factor. The determination of levels can be difficult. Levels should be selected following a review of the literature or after consultation with experts. For instance, experts defined the home size levels as small: 25 beds, average: 50 beds, and large: over 100 beds. The data can be grouped (e.g., 0–25, 25–100, 100 and over) or placed in strata (e.g., 20–30, 40–60, 100 and up). The choice between using grouping or strata depends on the clarity of the strata and the frequency with which a stratum occurs. If nursing homes within a strata seldom occur for a particular size category, it makes a poor stratum. The most commonly occurring size ranges can be used to define the stratum. Generally, a narrow range of values for each stratum will improve the precision of statistical methods.[43]

The measures in Table 7–11 seem to meet the mutually exclusive and exhaustive tests. Other measures can be used to serve as proxies for concepts like managerial competence. Selection among these measures is often difficult. The participation of content experts through advisory groups, as described above, is always helpful in selecting measures.

MEASUREMENT TESTS

Suchman suggests two procedures to verify the merit of proxy measures in an evaluation project.[44] These procedures attempt to verify the relevance and the consistency of proxy measures of the independent and dependent variables.

Measurement Reliability

Reliability indicates a measure's consistency. A reliable measure provides similar observations when used repeatedly to measure a particular thing. When the assumed relationship between cause and effect is correct and when important causal factors have been included by the relationship, the error variance in an evaluation study becomes a measure of reliability.

Zetterberg identifies four types of measurement errors.[45] The error variance can be segregated into congruence, precision, objectivity, and consistency components. *Congruence* is the agreement among several proxy measures that measure the same thing. The variance among indicators provides a measure of congruence. For example, satisfaction and compliance (measured on the same scale) can be used as indicators of the effectiveness of a nurse–practitioner program, as described in Chapter 2. Congruence determines the amount of agreement in evaluation findings. Financial performance of a contract–managed hospital can be measured by total deductions from revenue, days in accounts receivable, contributed margin, and revenue per patient day on a daily basis (see Table 7–12). Should these measures point to distinct findings, the evaluator must account for the differences, or the findings will lack reliability.

Precision is the extent to which a particular indicator provides the same results when applied by the same observer. The variance among observers provides a measure of precision. For example, surveyors may repeat a question in a questionnaire and find that responses differ. The observer's mood may change, fatigue or boredom may set in, and other factors may influence how the surveyor gets information from a respondent. Precision measures the extent to which this has occurred. Automated observation processes such as accounting systems and unobtrusive measures typically have a high level of precision. For example, the Museum of Science and Industry in Chicago finds that the frequency of tile replacement near an exhibit is a precise and unobtrusive way to measure the popularity of their exhibits.[46]

Objectivity is the extent that an observer or process measurement obtains consistent observations when using the same measure. The variance that occurs when an indicator is repeatedly applied is the measure of its objectivity. For example, the objectivity of "days in accounts receivable" is high if several contract–managed hospitals have a comparable drop in the number of days following the initiation of contract management.

Consistency is the extent that the object being measured retains its essential characteristics. Consistency measures the change in proxy measures over time. For instance, serum cholesterol is an indicator of coronary artery disease, and blood pressure an indicator of hypertension. Unfortunately, both of these indicators have a tendency to vary independent of the status of coronary artery disease and hypertension in a patient.

To sum up, congruence is the variance among indicators, precision measures the variance between readings with the same observer, objectivity is the variance between observations, and consistency is the variance over time. The error variance in an evaluation is often made up of these factors. Block variables can be used to extract some of these measurement effects, as described in Chapters 3 and 4.

Inconsistent readings stem from several sources. Suchman identifies subject, observer, situation, instrument, and processing as causes of inconsistent observations.[47]

(1) *Subject consistency:* Transient behavior in participants (or the thing being measured) is common. For example, mood, motivation, attitude, and

the like often change during the course of the evaluation, which alters participants' attitudes and behavior. Questionnaires may fail to consider how filling out the survey may alter those being surveyed. More significantly, survey respondents may be influenced selectively by the measurement process. For instance, the survey may be more tiring to some respondents than others, producing systematic bias in these responses. In other instances transient factors may influence participants in an evaluation. For example, people who complete a questionnaire at the end of a day's work may mix their reactions to their experiences that day with the phenomonon under study. Measurement devices can also disturb physical systems. For instance, one theory of Quantum Mechanics contends that an attempt to measure properties of an electron alters these properties.

(2) *Observer reliability:* Personal factors may also influence those making observations, as well as those being observed. The behavior of the observers may influence participants and color their views.

(3) *Situational problems:* The environment in which measurements are taken may change, which can influence responses. For example, if an employee appraisal program is evaluated with some of the supervisor–subordinate meetings taking place in the boss's office and others in the cafeteria, the power symbols implicit in the boss's turf may alter the behavior, preferences, and receptivity of the appraisee.

(4) *Instruments:* Poorly worded or ambiguous survey questions may lead to random responses. Many questionnaires fail to receive a careful pretest to identify and screen out obscure questions. Standard questionnaires or survey devices are encouraged because they have known reliability. Lake, Mills, and Earle, for example, assess the reliability of many standard instruments that are useful in a wide variety of evaluation tasks.[48] Webb and his colleagues suggest physical trace measures. Bottles in trash cans can be used to measure consumption of alcoholic beverages in "dry" communities.[49] If the bottles can be redeemed nearby, the measure will systematically understate consumption because the recording process had a built-in defect.

(5) *Processing errors:* Coding and transcribing responses in large evaluation studies may introduce some random errors. Evaluators should consider how the transcription process can be simplified to reduce recording errors.

There are no absolutely consistent measures. All measures, to one degree or another, are subject to contamination. Evaluators use reliability tests to determine that portion of the residual or error variance that can be attributed to these factors. Repeated measures, repeated observations, and the like provide an important retrospective indicator of the consistency of the measurement process. In large–scale evaluations, pilot tests of the measurements process are recommended to detect the size of subject, observer, situation, instruments, and processing error variances.

Measurement Validity

Validity is the ability of a proxy measure to give meaning to the evaluation results.[50] Two informal tests of face and consensual judgments are often applied. A face valid test is based on logic. Valid proxy measures must appear to represent at least one element of an intervention program's objective. Past experience is also helpful in insuring that measures are reasonable. Advisory groups, as described earlier in this chapter, experts, and others with special insights can be asked to critique measures to determine their "consensual validity." Face and consensual validity tests are useful to screen out inappropriate evaluation measures.

Two tests of the appropriateness of evaluation results are commonly applied: correlational and predictive validity. *Correlational validity* is used when decisions must be made before feedback on accuracy can occur or such feedback cannot be obtained. Correlational (or convergent) validity relates the proxy measure of effectiveness with something else that conveys a similar meaning. Predictions can be made by experts and with a model, using the same data. If the predictions agree, higher credence can be assigned to both methods of prediction. For example, Gustafson and Halloway developed a model to measure the severity of a burn, considering the patient's percent thickness burn, percent body area affected, the age of the patient, and the patient's number of health problems.[51] To validate the severity index, the severity of a particular profile of burn patients was computed using the model and correlated with the subjective ratings of severity for these same patients made by physicians.[52] The ratings were found to agree, which gave the model some credibility.

Correlational validity is enhanced when information from different sources, derived using unique logic, is compared. For example, carbon dating is used to measure the age of artifacts. Archaeologists had difficulty verifying their predictions of age until they counted the rings of very old bristlecone pine trees and compared these age estimates with estimates based on carbon 14 traces in the same trees.[53] Carbon 14 may be underestimating by 13 percent over an age span of 6,000 years. (Tree rings provide a valid baseline if the double growth of rings in wet years occurs with about the frequency as rings that are skipped during dry years.) Bristlecone rings have been used to adjust the age of the remains of structures over a period of about 6,000 years, the age of the oldest known bristlecone pine.

Fridman reports that the depth of water penetration in obsidian can be used to measure the age of artifacts, beginning with the time when tools were first fashioned by Stone–Age men.[54] Obsidian is formed as a rock in the interior of lava flows. This rock was shaped by prehistoric man into tools and weapons. By measuring water absorption after the rock was chipped to make a utensil, the culture that made the artifact can be dated. Dating with the obsidian hydration method can be compared with carbon 14 to correlate the age estimates.

Evaluators, like archaeologists, search for base measures to verify events measured by another process. For instance, the severity index for burn patients could be correlated with days of survival, mortality, length of stay, and other outcome measures.

Predictive validity is the strongest test that can be applied. When a prediction, based on the findings on an evaluation project, can be confirmed by events, a clearcut validation can be provided. For instance, Goldberg had radiologists read x–rays to choose between a diagnosis of stomach cancer or ulcers.[55] A test of predictive validity of the diagnostic process can be made by using x–rays from postoperative patients. Similarly, pilot programs are often used to check on performance before a program is institutionalized. Tests for predictive validity are often limited by the nature of the evaluation task. For instance, evaluations based on Gustafson's index of medical underservice[56] were contentious because the index cannot be predictively validated.[57]

Sources of Bias

When a measure contains bias, it also lacks validity. Suchman identifies several causes of bias in the evaluation study, as summarized below:[58]

(1) *Propositional:* The assumptions which link the hierarchy of program objectives may prove to be invalid. Effort, for instance, may not lead to improved performance. Suchman points out that "invalid program objectives may spring from invalid theories or from invalid deductions from valid theories."[59] To illustrate, the Head Start program assumed that low–income children lacked stimulation and that organized substitutes for parental attention would improve their performance in public schools. Objectives based on this theory failed to hold up under empirical testing.[60]

(2) *Measures:* Inappropriate indices can be used. For example, survey questions may prove to be poor proxy measures for the understandability of a new program, the prospects of its implementation, or its perceived benefits. Invalid indices may result in invalid measurements. For instance, racial attitudes have been measured by clustering of blacks and whites in lecture halls.[61] These measures would lack validity when applied in many liberal universities. A recent evaluation of neighborhood health centers measured subscription rates, use of services, and the like for various income levels in the community. Unfortunately, the overriding objective in the legislation could be interpreted as "one–door medicine." Locating the NHC in low–income areas all but guaranteed that middle- and upper–income–level people would *not* use

its services. Utilization measures of the program did not indicate the reasons the neighborhood health center network failed to recruit diverse subscribers.

(3) *Sampling:* The sample drawn from an intervention program's target group may prove to be unrepresentative. The process of stratification used to select a representative target group may have overlooked an important characteristic. For example, Coleman and colleagues found that the performance of certain minorities in public schools is not influenced by the level of resources in the schools they attend.[62] These findings may be invalid because minority children seldom attend resource–intensive schools. Dropouts from experimental and control comparison groups also introduce sampling bias.

(4) *Observers:* The observer or the evaluator may introduce a bias which stems from beliefs and preconceived notions about the intended (or hoped–for) outcome of the intervention program. Investigators have become so committed to their own ideas (and administrators to their own programs) that the idea is retained in the face of contradictory evidence. Mitroff and Mason found that physical evidence from manned moon landings had no impact on those popularizing "hot" and "cold" theories of lunar evolution.[63] Several administrations (from both parties) and the U.S. Congress continue to devise programs that intensify resources in public schools in the face of evidence that school resources have little effect on a child's performance.[64]

(5) *Participants:* The views and beliefs of those representing the target group of the intervention program may cause them to deliberately misinform or distort their responses. For instance, if a study participant believes that a program is useful, he may tailor his responses to enhance the prospects the program will be adopted. And as Suchman points out, respondents often deliberately conceal information which might help scuttle the program they support for personal reasons.[65]

(6) *Setting:* The setting used to collect evaluation information may prove to be obtrusive.[66] Artificial settings may cause a program recipient to behave in an atypical manner. Similarly, field conditions often introduce biases related to the pressures of day–to–day tasks.

(7) *Analysis:* Finally, the analysis and interpretation of the data can be a source of bias. Data can be sorted so they agree with the views of important power center in the organization the evaluator seeks to impress. And data can be erroneously catalogued or manipulated.

The Relationship Between Reliability and Validity

Valid measures are usually reliable, but reliable measures may not be valid. For instance, reliable estimates of the level of effort in an intervention program may have little or nothing to do with performance. Reliability is used to detect problems in the process of measurement, and validity is built up through a series of tests and arguments.[67] Causality is the key. When the intervention program results in beneficial results, after repeated application, a strong case for its adoption is made. Pilot programs can be used to minimize investments until benefits can be confirmed in a variety of settings and for a wide range of clients or beneficiaries.

When a measure is both valid and reliable, evaluation findings have considerable credibility. Several measures with these properties provide a compelling rationale to adopt an intervention program. For instance, consider a home health care program that seeks to improve the health status of its clientele. A change in disability levels for certain diagnoses, determined by identifying each patient's degree of mobility and self sufficiency, provides valid measures of health status and strongly suggests that the home health program has merit.

SUMMARY

This chapter described several ways to identify objectives and to derive measures for the objectives of intervention programs. Objectives are often hierarchical, having causal links between adjacent levels of the hierarchy. Proxy measures are selected that consider salient elements in the program's objectives. Some behavioral aspects of using inappropriate measures and behavioral responses to extranalities, with beneficial and detrimental consequences, were discussed as an introduction to the behavior treatment of evaluation in the chapters to come. Several tests were provided to detect the reliability and validity of proxy measures applied in an evaluation. Reliability describes sources of inconsistency among distinct measures, observers, objects being measured, and over time. Validity can be determined by accumulating evidence that substantiates the evaluation conclusions. Tests of correlational validity (agreement among reliable measures) and predictive validity (anticipating a future event) can be applied.

NOTES

1. Klarman, H.E., "The Effect of Prepaid Care on Hospital Use," *Public Health Reports,* Vol. 78, November 1963; pp. 955–965. Also see Karman, H.E., "Economic Research in Group Medicine," pp. 178–193. In R.E. Beamish (ed.), *New Horizons in Health Care.* Winnipeg, Canada: First International Congress on Group Medicine, 1970.
2. "State and Local EPSDT Evaluation and Training Model," Bokanon Systems, Inc., Contract (SRS) 74–63, Social and Rehabilitation Service, U.S. Department of Health Education and Welfare, 1977.
3. Thorp, A., "The Ohio Coal Worker's Respiratory Disease Program on Evaluation," Columbus, Oh., Ohio Lung Association, 1976. The author wishes to thank Pat Findling

for bringing the Ohio Coal Miner's Program to his attention.

4. G. Nadler, *Work Design: A Systems Concept.* Georgetown, Ont.: Irwin, 1970.

5. Suchman, E.A., *Evaluation Research: Principles and Practices In Public Service 'and Social Action Programs,* Chapter 4. New York: Russell Sage Foundation, 1967.

6. Gaining approval can be difficult as higher–level objectives raise more serious questions about the value of a program. The hierarchy exposes these conflicts, making explicit what will be measured.

7. Such a study might lay to rest the contention, often advanced by health providers, that unintelligent consumption of health services is the root cause of many health system problems and that intelligent consumption, induced using media methods, can alleviate these problems.

8. Tripodi, T., P. Fellin, and I. Epstein, *Social Program Evaluation: Guidelines for Health, Education and Welfare Administration,* p. 4. Itasca, Ill.: Peacock, 1971.

9. Raia, A.P., *Managing by Objectives,* Chapter 4. Glenview, Ill.: Scott, Foresman, 1974.

10. Smalley, H., et al., "EMS System Data Requirements for Performance Evaluation," Health Systems Research Center, Georgia Institute of Technology, Grant R18HS00715–02S1, Division of Health Services Research Analysis, National Center for Health Services Research, Health Resource Administration, U.S. Dept. of Health, Education and Welfare, 1974.

11. Gottman, J.M. and R.E. Clasen, *Evaluation in Education,* Chapter 2. Itasca, Ill.: Peacock, 1972.

12. Gustafson et al., "Development of the Index of Medical Underservice," *Health Services Research,* Vol. 10, No. 2, Summer 1975.

13. Delbecq, A., "Leadership Styles in Management Conferences," *Academy of Management Journal,* Vol. 11, 1968, pp. 427–434.

14. Mason, R., "A Dialetical Approach to Strategic Planning," *Management Science,* Vol. 15, No. 4, 1969, pp. B403–B414.

15. Collins, B. and H. Guetzkow, *A Social Psychology of Group Processes for Decision Making.* New York: Wiley; 1964.

16. Nutt, P.C., "On the Quality and Acceptance of Plans Drawn by a Consortium," *The Journal of Applied Behavioral Science,* Vol. 15, No. 1, 1979; pp. 7–21.

17. Filley, A. and R. House, *Managerial Process and Oranizational Behavior.* Glenview, Ill: Scott, Foresman, 1969.

18. Thompson, J.D., *Organizations in Action,* p. 35. New York: McGraw–Hill, 1967.

19. Delbecq, A. and A. Van de Ven, "A Group Process Model for Problem Identification and Program Planning," *Journal of Applied Behavioral Science,* Vol. 7, No. 4, 1971; pp. 466–492.

20. Nutt, P.C., "An Experimental Comparison of Three Planning Methods," *Management Science,* Vol. 23, No. 5, 1977; pp. 499–511.

21. Dalky, N., *Delphi.* Santa Monica, Calif., The Rand Corporation, 1967.

22. Van de Ven, A., "An Applied Experimental Test of the Nominal, Delphi, and Interacting Decision Process," Ph.D. Dissertation, University of Wisconsin, School of Business, 1972.

23. Nutt, P.C., and P.C. Tracy, "Standards and Guidelines for a Radiotherapy Network in Wisconsin," *The Wisconsin Medical Journal,* Vol. 72, May 1973.

24. Nutt, P.C., "The Merits of Using Experts or Consumers as Members of Planning Groups," *The Academy of Management Journal,* Vol. 19, No. 3, 1976, pp. 378–394.

25. Nutt, P.C., *Quality,* p. 7–21.

26. Nutt, P.C., and P. Tracy, "Standards," p. 19–26.

27. Gustafson, D.H., R. Shukla, A. Delbecq, and G. Walster, "A Comparative Study in Subjective Likelihood Estimates Made by Individuals, Interaction Groups, Delphi

Groups, and Nominal Groups," *Organizational Behavior and Human Performance,* Vol. 9, No. 2, April 1973.
28. *Ibid.*
29. Kerr, S., "On the Folly of Rewarding A While Hoping for B," *Academy of Management Journal,* Vol. 19, No. 4, 1975, pp. 769–783.
30. *Ibid.*
31. Delbecq, A., "The Management of Decision Making Within the Firm: Three Strategies for Three Types of Decision Making," *The Academy of Management Journal,* Vol. 10, No. 4, 1967.
32. Wildawsky, A., "The Political Economy of Efficiency: Cost–Benefit, Systems–Auditing, and DPBS," *The Public Administration Review,* Vol. 26, December 1966, p. 292.
33. Manipulating objectives to match evaluation data is a common form of pseudo–evaluation, discussed in Chapter 8.
34. Rossi, P. and W. Williams (eds.), *Evaluating Social Programs: Theory, Practice, and Politics,* preface. New York; Seminar Press, 1972.
35. Williams, W. and P. Evans, "The Politics of Evaluation: The Case of Head Start," in P. Rossi and W. Williams (eds.), *Evaluating Social Programs: Theory, Practice and Politics.* New York: Seminar Press, 1972.
36. Suchman, p. 33.
37. *Ibid,* p. 42.
38. Nutt, P.C., "Comparing Methods for Weighting Decision Criteria," *OMEGA, the International Journal of Management Science,* Vol. 8, No. 2, 1980 (163–172).
39. Nutt, P.C., "The Acceptance and Accuracy of Decision Analysis Methods," The College of Administrative Science Working Paper Series. Columbus, Oh.; The Ohio State University, June 1978.
40. Segal, S., *Non Parametric Statistics For The Behavioral Sciences.* New York: McGraw–Hill, 1956.
41. Brisco, R., "An Evaluation of the Effects of Contract Management on Hospital Performance," Master's Thesis, The Graduate Program in Hospital and Health Services Administration, The Ohio State University, June 1977.
42. Hoover, S., "An Investigation of the Effects of Differences in Size, Occupancy, Medicaid Utilization, Organizational Control, and Type of Facility on Selected Costs of Nursing Homes in Ohio," Master's Thesis, The Graduate Program in Hospital and Health Services Administration, The Ohio State University, June 1978.
43. ANOVA techniques discussed in Chapter 4 are insensitive to the way strata are defined. Errors can be introduced into the analysis unless strata represent unambiguous categories or are restricted to a narrow set of values, for continuous variables.
44. Suchman, p. 115.
45. Zetterberg, H.L., *On Theory and Verification in Sociology,* pp. 50–51. Totowa N.J.: Bedminster Press, 1963.
46. Webb, E.J., D.T. Campbell, R.D. Schwartz, and L. Sechrest, *Unobtrusive Measures: Nonreactive Research in the Social Sciences,* p. 2. Chicago: Rand–McNally, 1972.
47. Suchman, p. 118.
48. Lake, D.G., M.G. Mills, and R.B. Earle, *Measuring Human Behavior.* New York: Teachers College Press, 1973.
49. Webb, et al., p. 2.
50. Suchman, p. 120.
51. Gustafson, D.H. and D. Halloway, "A Decision Theory Approach to Measuring Severity in Illness, *Health Services Research,* Vol. 10, No. 1, Spring 1975, pp. 97–106.
52. This assumes that physician ratings are the best available base line and that obtaining rating from physicians on a routine basis would be time consuming and thus costly.

53. Suess, H.E., "Bristly Cone Pine Calibration of the Radioactive Carbon Time Scale 5200 BC to Present," in I.V. Olsen (ed.), *Radiocarbon Variations and Absolute Chronology.* New York: Wiley, 1970.
54. Fridman, I., "Obsidian, the Dating Stone," *American Scientist,* Vol. 66, No. 1, January–February 1978.
55. Goldberg, L., "Simple Models or Simple Processes: Some Research on Clinical Judgements," *American Psychologist,* 1968.
56. Gustafson, D.H. et al., "An Index of Medical Underservice," *Health Services Research,* Vol. 10, No. 2, Summer 1975.
57. Wysond, G., "The Index of Medical Underservice: Problems in Meanings, Measurement, and Use," *Health Services Research,* Spring 1975.
58. Suchman, pp. 122–123.
59. Suchman, p. 122.
60. Williams and Evans, p. 256.
61. Webb, et al., p. 2.
62. Coleman, J.S., et al., "Equality of Educational Opportunity," Washington, D.C.: U.S. Government Printing Office, 1966.
63. Mitroff, I.I. and R. Mason, "On Evaluating the Scientific Contribution of the Apollo Moon Missions Via Information Theory: A Study of the Scientist–Scientist Relationship," *Management Science,* Vol. 20, No. 12, August 1974; pp. 1501–1513.
64. Coleman, et al., p. 106.
65. Suchman, p. 122.
66. Webb, et al., p. 2.
67. Suchman, p. 124.

CHAPTER 8

The Evaluation Process[1]

"But are you really the brother–in–law of a director?"
"Always. Always when the public interest requires it. I have a brother–in–law on
all the boards—everywhere. It saves me a world of trouble."

Mark Twain, *Traveling With A Reformer*

Evaluation projects stem from a need to understand the effects of planned or inadvertent interventions. After a successful unionization drive for nurses (from the administrator's perspective, an inadvertent intervention), the medical staff may request that the hospital's administration study the effects of unionization on care quality. An expansion of services in a community hospital may entice the remaining hospitals to determine the effect of these expanded services on their occupancy rates. Administrators may institute new management practices (planned interventions) and the organization's trustees may ask for an accounting of their effects. In each of these examples, one or more sponsors calls for an investigation of the merits of an intervention which is carried out by at least one evaluator. Assuming that sponsors have sufficient discretionary power and resources to commission an evaluation and that the evaluator has enough know–how to carry it out,[2] the dialogue between sponsor and evaluator dictates the success of the project.

Essential steps in an evaluation process are described in this chapter. Evaluation projects often follow a somewhat different format because the sponsor's attitudes toward evaluation and style of inquiry shape the process. Several pitfalls to these evaluation processes are identified. An improved dialogue between the sponsor and the evaluator is proposed to enhance their mutually supportive roles which may avoid some of these traps. Other traps can be predicted but not avoided. The threatening nature of evaluation causes sponsors to avoid evaluation, to carry out "pseudoevaluation" when assessment becomes unavoidable, and to attempt to rationalize the findings. Several forms of pseudoevaluation are described. In each case the evaluation process is distorted by altering essential transactions, disregarding steps in the evaluation process, or modifying information flowing from a given step in the process.

Several distorted evaluation processes are described to provide a way to predict evaluations unlikely to produce useful results. A distorted evaluation process should warn that the prospects of success for a particular project are poor.

THE EVALUATION PROCESS

An evaluation project begins when a sponsor seeks information that describes the merits of an intervention. As shown in Figure 8-1, evaluation proceeds through several stages and each stage is connected by a particular activity.[3] As a first step, the sponsor makes assumptions which define the

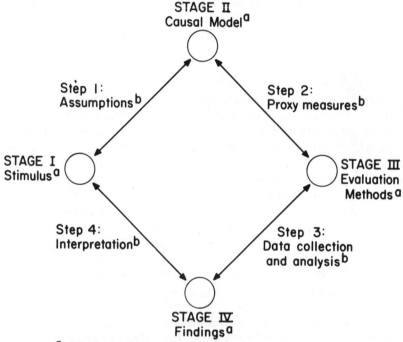

STAGE II
Causal Model[a]

Step 1:
Assumptions[b]

Step 2:
Proxy measures[b]

STAGE I
Stimulus[a]

STAGE III
Evaluation
Methods[a]

Step 4:
Interpretation[b]

Step 3:
Data collection
and analysis[b]

STAGE IV
Findings[a]

[a] Major outcomes of an evaluation project
[b] Evaluation activities that have people acting out <u>roles</u>, following cognative <u>styles</u>, and applying select <u>tools</u>.

Figure 8.1 THE EVALUATION PROCESS

[a] Major outcomes of an evaluation project
[b] Evaluation activities that have people acting out *roles,* following cognitive *styles,* and applying select *tools*

Reprinted with permission from Nutt, P.C., "Calling Out and Calling Off the Dogs: Managerial Diagnosis in Public Organizations," *Academy of Management Review,* 4:2, p. 207, (1979).

intervention (cause) and/or specify its effects. The initial model is an abstraction of the intervention and/or its effects, as seen by the sponsor. Assumptions are refined (implicitly and explicitly) by the sponsor until the abstraction confirms the sponsor's perception of reality.

The arrow linking the model and the stimulus is bidirectional. The two-way relationship suggests an interplay between the model and the stimulus. Either the emergence of new information needs or reflection may cause the sponsor to change the model. Thus causal models, which describe the merits of an intervention, are "fine tuned" by insuring that the model can provide information for decision making.

Evaluation methods are linked to the causal model by proxies selected to measure the intervention's effects. The causal model forms the basis to select an initial set of proxy measures of cause-and-effect factors. Measures are also dictated by evaluation methods. The initial set of proxy measures may restrict the range of evaluation methods that can be applied. The causal model can be changed to incorporate measures believed to be more diagnostic.

Evaluation methods (e.g., experimental or quasi-experimental designs) dictate data collection and analysis procedures which, in turn, specify the internal and external validity of the findings, as described in Chapter 6. The expected precision of the findings may suggest that a change in evaluation methods is desirable. Again the two-way arrow demonstrates that data collection and analysis are controlled by evaluation methods and by the projected level of validity in the evaluation findings.

Findings are linked to the stimulus through an interpretation. The interpretation can take several forms. The sponsor may just check to see if the findings confirm his expectations, ignoring any other interpretation. In other instances, the findings may require elaborate explanations which complicate the interpretation. The sponsor's problem may have changed during the evaluation, calling for an interpretation of the findings in the light of recent developments. These developments may involve conditions or circumstances considered only obliquely by the project. Conflict between the evaluator and the sponsor often results when evaluation findings fail to confirm the sponsor's expectations, when the findings cannot be clearly interpreted, or when the findings cannot be related to changed conditions.

The schematic representation of evaluation in Figure 8.1 will be used as a vehicle to discuss the principal stages in an evaluation project and the steps needed to carry out an evaluation.

Evaluation Stages

The Stimulus. An evaluation project begins with a directive or a need to understand the effect of a planned or inadvertent intervention. An evaluation project can be stimulated by environmental factors (externally) or within an organization (internally). External stimulants include unsatisfied claims,[4][5] new patterns of activity,[6] and conflicts.[7] Internal sources include conflicts as well as criterion checks, and problem and policy statements.[8]

Unsatisfied claims stem from the dissatisfactions expressed by the clients with the services or products of the organization. For example, demands to measure the performance of a new hospital service may come from Blue Cross in their rate review activities; from the executors of endowments and other major hospital contributors; regulatory agencies like health systems agencies; or from the hospital's clientele, its medical staff. When services are subsidized by the government, or paid indirectly through third parties like health insurance, valid dissatisfactions are more difficult to express by their consumers and harder to recognize by health organizations. Groups contending they represent consumers, like Common Cause or the Grey Panthers, may form to articulate some of these claims. When these groups garner sufficient power and visibility, organizations must make careful assessments of their demands.

New patterns of activity stem from technological advances such as full body scanners, and prompt organizations to assess their benefits. Conflict results when the medical staff, administration, and/or board members disagree on the merits of adopting new operations or services. Similarly, conflicts may occur among peers and between supervisors and subordinates. Evaluation is applied to sort out these claims and counter claims. Criterion checks are used to detect malfunctions in operations or procedures. Organizations compare revenues, costs, and other measures against standards for organizational performance. When a hospital's occupancy rates or costs per patient day drop below accepted norms, evaluation may be used to discover the causal agents. Finally, evaluation is often used to identify defensible positions for managerial policy statements. For instance, a position paper detailing union demands for higher fringe benefits may stimulate an assessment of the organization's benefit packages and its employees' productivity history. When these internal and external stimuli exceed some threshold, some form of evaluation begins.[9]

Causal Model. The causal model identifies the cause–effect relationships that merit study. The model sets out these relationships specifying a macro or micro context, the level of specificity in cause–and–effect variables, the nature of the intervention (inadvertent or planned), and the use of prospective or retrospective data. The sponsor refines the model to insure that the needed information for decision making can be provided. For instance, the U.S. Department of Defense commissioned several consulting firms to propose a "new generation of military hospitals."[10] The evaluation was devised to provide standards for military hospital construction. Several iconic models (e.g., physical shape of the facility, such as a circular design) and profiles of services common to military hospitals were used to project construction and operating costs. Causal models must be constructed with care because omissions render evaluation results—in this example, cost projections— inaccurate. Kilmann and Herden point out that the causal model will constrain all subsequent states.[11]

Evaluation Methods. Evaluation approaches include the statistical methods described in Chapter 4, and other methods such as operations research models and multiattribute utilities (MAU models).[12] The specific capabilities and requirements of evaluation methods must be fit to the causal model. For instance, an evaluation attempting to detect the effects of congressional freezes on hospital charges requires a retrospective assessment, which limits the choice of statistically based evaluation methods to time–series approaches. Generally, prospective evaluations place fewer restrictions on the selection of evaluation methods.

Findings. The results of an evaluation project are termed "findings." Findings are presented in terms of their statistical and operational significance (as described in Chapters 3 and 4), by their sensitivity to the assumptions necessary to produce them, and, as Campbell and Stanley point out, their internal and external validity.[13]

The Steps in An Evaluation Process

Assumptions. Each evaluation stage is connected by a dominant activity. To initiate an evaluation effort, assumptions are made to form a causal model. Assumptions are required because the causal model is, of necessity, an abstraction which simplifies the problem to permit detailed study. For instance, HEW evaluated a proposed "negative income tax program" to detect how direct dollar supplements would be spent by recipients. The "working poor" were included in the evaluation to determine how income supplements would influence their earnings. HEW officials dictated the premises for the study. Kershaw described these assumptions:

> [HEW] officials felt that they could predict costs for the traditional public assistance recipients under the negative income tax scheme: the aged, disabled, the very young, a family headed by a woman with small children could exercise

few labor market choices which would influence the cost of a national program. The male–headed families with an earner, however, raised substantially more serious questions: to what extent does a work–leisure trade–off operate at these income levels? Does the tax applied to a supplement have the same impact as one applied to earnings? Will a 70% tax on the (income) supplement produce a different reaction than a 50% rate? Will secondary earners leave the labor force when offered partial reimbursement through a supplement?[14]

Another set of assumptions would have dramatically altered the study. For instance, the preoccupation of economists with tax rates could have been dropped in favor of including female–headed families in the study. This would relax the rather tenuous assumption that female–headed families exercise few labor market choices.

Assumptions are rarely made conspicuous by sponsors. (Indeed, the negative income tax study may have had fewer and less–clearcut assumptions than depicted by Kershaw. In the retelling, successful, and even unsuccessful, evaluations are often reconstructed to appear as if they were rationally formulated.) The causal model must be studied to set out the assumptions implicit in the model. The motivating forces behind an evaluation seldom provide clear and internally consistent logic. Indeed, conflicting motives are common. The negative income tax evaluation was carried out to placate conservative members of Congress who demanded a careful study of program costs and participant's consumption behavior, and liberal bureaucrats, who insisted on a careful measurement of all the benefits that seemed to flow from income supplements.

Proxy Measures. Measures link the causal model and the evaluation approach. The causal model provides a list of program variables, block variables, and constraints, as well as objectives for the intervention. In the negative income tax evaluation, the program variables included the dollar amount of supplements and various tax rates on the supplement, based on income of the recipient. The range of the participant's income was a block variable. Constraints were established when the Government Accounting Office (GAO) required that participants know the purpose of the evaluation. Constraints also stemmed from the persistent threat that Congress or the GAO could subpoena records, which would prohibit assurances of anonymity to participants. Some of the causal factors in the model may resist measurement or manipulation when using an experimental or quasi–experimental design, dictating a change in the causal model and its assumptions. For example, Coleman's study of school performance and school resources was constrained by the number of high–resource schools attended by minority children.[15]

A description of how the measures of program effectiveness are derived is given in Chapter 7. Limitations in the ability to collect preferred measures may dictate changes in the causal model or dictate the choice of evaluation method. For instance, Coleman's evaluation of the status of public education could not use nonstandard academic achievement tests without being obtrusive. However, quantative test scores are generally believed more amenable to change by schools than the verbal scores used by Coleman, indicating a defect in the causal model.[16] The Head Start evaluation could have used a longitudinal design. The school performance of youngsters who had Head Start, preschool, or no preschool educational experience could have been measured in each of the first six or seven grades.[17] This evaluation approach seemed infeasible because of the lagtime and the expense involved in tracing a representative sample of youngsters.

Data Collection and Analysis. Findings stem from analysis which is dictated by the data collection device (design) that is applied. The precision of findings varies, depending on the evaluation method that is applied. Precision, and the ability to make diagnostic judgments, decline as quasi–experimental methods are substituted for experimental methods, and drop precipitously when nonevaluative methods are used. As pointed out in Chapter 3, simple stratifications of data can dramatically enhance the explanatory power of an evaluation. As described in Chapter 6, the internal and external validity of the findings should be projected considering the particulars of the evaluation project. The expected precision, scope, and other features of the findings may dictate which evaluation method should be used.

Interpretation. Evaluation findings are tied to the stimulus by an interpretation. To complete the cycle, the results of evaluation are presented to the sponsor. The findings are often generalized or extrapolated to suggest recommendations for action.

There are many very real problems in interpreting the findings of an evaluation. Polgar points out four examples of how program administrators can misunderstand evaluation information:[18]

(1) *Empty Vessel:* based on the assumption that nothing preceded the service or intervention program. The administrator ignores prior efforts, failing to build on positive features of past efforts, revealed by the evaluation.

(2) *Separate Capsule:* limits or alters evaluation findings based on the sponsor's beliefs and past practices. If evaluation confirms the sponsor's views, the likelihood of adopting evaluation information increases.

(3) *Single Pyramid:* assumes homogenity of behavior in target groups. Clients

may have different views and samples must reflect the proportion of these views in the evaluation. Multiphasic screening pilot studies attract disproportionate numbers of Jewish women, who have been found to patronize the screening program repeatedly as it moves about a city. Members of minority groups seldom seek out these services, even when they are free of charge.

(4) *Interchangeable Faces:* values which cause consumers to behave in radically different ways must not be ignored. OEO exploited cultural motifs and used local residents as employees to make their health centers conform to local values. Many contended that cultural sensitivity was a major factor in the health center's ability to get minority groups to use health care services, when many other efforts to promote health sensitivity among these groups had failed.

Interpretation is a judgmental process relying on the logical extensions of evaluation findings. For instance, Coleman found that minority youngsters were as much as 5.2 grades behind their nonminority peers in southern schools and 4.2 grades behind them in northern schools.[19] White children were 1.5 grades behind in the south as compared to northern white children. To suggest policy guides, these measures of school performance must be qualified in terms of causal factors like teacher quality and school resources, and block factors like parents' income. When the verbal achievement scores and causal and block factors were correlated, Coleman found that per–pupil school expenditures had no relationship to youngsters' school performance, and that a supportive home environment was closely related to school performance. This suggests that integration would have little effect on school achievement for minority children.

Because interpretation is judgmental, the policy guides that stem from evaluation findings are often challenged. For example, Cain and Watts took issue with Coleman's findings, contending that the evaluation had such serious methodological shortcomings that it offered little policy guidance.[20] Sponsors can seldom cope with acrimonious debates among technocrats. They tend to play it safe by disregarding controversial findings or by repeating the study. As a result, Coleman's six–month preliminary analysis of the status of the public school system provided considerable long–term support for his critics.

The reactions to evaluation findings are based on the sponsor's expectations and the way the findings are presented. As the Coleman evaluation points out, little can be done to salvage an evaluation project when its findings fail to confirm expectations in a highly contentious environment. However, most evaluations do not create this level of controversy and *mode of presentation* can have a dramatic effect on the acceptance of the findings. To be well received a presentation must stress recommendations and policy guides. Details and the methodological gyrations needed to make these recommendations and policy guides should be skipped. Sponsors have little time for details and seldom appreciate their significance. Reports and presentations that dwell on technical details are poorly received because sponsors often lack technical skills and/or because of the pressure of other tasks. Implications are stressed for administrators while extrapolations tend to be shunned in academic circles. As a result, evaluation reports stress dramatically different information from that preferred in academic circles.

A personalized presentation geared to the needs of the recipient will convey more information than traditional data–centered reports. Evaluation findings are seldom fully appreciated until they are translated from scientific into personalized terms. Mitroff, Nelson, and Mason call this type of information "mythic," and call for "myth information" systems to replace traditional reporting mechanisms.[21] Table 8-1 provides some distinctions between evaluative and mythic information.

Table 8-1. Comparing Mythic and Evaluative Information

Mythic Information	Evaluative Information
Partial, personal, interested	Impartial, impersonal, disinterested
Anecdotal, stressing cultural motifs and images	Generalizable, stressing logic or experimental inquiry
Stirs emotions in a drama	Suppresses emotions by avoiding the dramatic
Bias accepted	Bias eliminated
Repetitive and redundant	Coherent and sequential
Implicit and intuitive	Explicit and precise
Takes moral stands	Amoral

Adapted from Mitroff, I.I., J. Nelson, and R.O. Mason, "On the Management of Myth Information Systems," *Management Science,* Vol. 21, No. 4, December 1974.

Evaluation findings tend to be impersonal, amoral, and precise, and eliminate drama and emotion when most people prefer presentations that are personal and stir emotions, using repetitive arguments and taking a moralistic tone. According to Mitroff and Kilmann, a mythic presentation incorporates the evaluation findings into a story that has meaning to those who need the evaluation information.[22] For example, a multimillion–dollar statewide Neonatology Program was approved following a detailed presentation, complete with photographs, of one case: a two–pound premature infant who was currently playing Little League baseball. Documentation of case costs and profiles of the typical infant's ultimate health status were *not* presented. Ritti and Funkhouser find that successful administrators have a history of inventing themes when one is not apparent, to describe the significance of evaluation information.[23]

Closure

Ideally, information flows freely between stages of an evaluation project, as shown in Figure 8–1. As in the Coleman report, an interpretation of evaluation findings may touch off a new round of inquiry.[24] The results may suggest errors in the analysis which must be corrected, a new tack for the evaluation, or new topic which merits investigation. The sponsor's needs may have changed, or the evaluation project may become intractable. For instance, the negative income tax evaluation nearly collapsed when the prosecutor's office in Trenton, New Jersey, tried to make families in the experimental group repay "excess" welfare payments.[25] The evaluation ultimately led to Kershaw's appearance in front of a grand jury to answer charges of fraud, charged with conspiring with welfare recipients to misrepresent their welfare payments.[26] As a result, changes in the evaluation approach were required which had a profound influence on its diagnostic potential.

TRUNCATED EVALUATION PROCESSES

Figure 8.2 illustrates two ways that the evaluation process can be cut short. Sponsors and evaluators who attempt short cuts often exhibit stereotyped behavior which will be referred to as "model mania" and "data mania." Each creates problems which limit the effectiveness of an evaluation.

Model Mania

The ideal evaluation process can be shortened by following a "assumption–measures–confirmation" path. The motive behind this process is precision in the representation of the evaluation problem, provided by the causal model. It is termed model mania because the causal model and the proposed method of evaluation are repeatedly tested against perceived reality.

Model mania occurs when causal models are very difficult to construct or when the model proves to be contentious, raising many controversial questions. For example, a state mental health department with twenty or so custodial institutions sought to develop an evaluation scheme to measure the effectiveness of its institutional administrators. The task of devising a causal model for the process of mental health administration proved to be difficult. Each proposed model provided a unique conception of the administrator's role, which suggested a particular set of measures. Each of the models proved to be unacceptable to particular mental health reference groups. Cost and efficiency measures were criticized by the psychiatrists and psychologists who treat patients. Quality care measures were seen as vague and nondiagnostic,

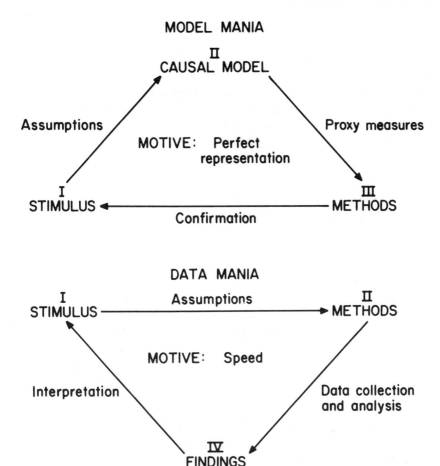

Figure 8.2 SOME TRUNCATED EVALUATION PROCESSES

Reprinted with permission from Nutt, P.C., "On Managed Evaluation Processes," *Technological Forecasting and Social Change,* Vol. 17, No. 4 (1980).

and thus unacceptable to executives in the State Department of Mental Health. The controversy led to many changes in the model in their attempts to find one that matched the implicit perceptions of the sponsor. In short, model mania led to no appreciable action in assessing the managerial competence in the institutions.

Evaluation that is focused on vague questions like measuring care quality in a hospital, or controversial issues such as the negative income tax evaluation, often results in iterative model building where model construction becomes an end in itself.[27] For instance, computer simulations for the interpretation of EKG's, refined over many years, are based on the decision process of a single cardiologist.[28] The programs are seldom compared to reconcile and merge their diagnostic queues. Similarly, operations researchers rely on standard problem representations and validate their findings by insuring that the representation fits the problem. Stimson and Stimson show how operations researchers, in their attempt to provide a perfect representation, have failed to provide timely and acceptable evaluations for the health care industry.[29]

Data Mania

The evaluation process (Figure 8–2) can also be shortened by following an "assumption–data–interpretation" path. It is termed data mania because a preference for data supersedes all other considerations. The motive fueling this process is speed.

Data mania stems from gathering data with little (if any) notion of causality and from ritualistic data accumulations. For instance, the health industry has lamented the lack of data to the point where legislation often mandates certain types of data accumulation. A recent example of data mania is the Health Planning and Resource Development Act of 1975, which requires a careful inventory of *all* health delivery resources. Apparently the resource profile is thought to have diagnostic value, helping planning agencies identify deficiencies in patterns of care delivery.

A second type of data mania is caused by sponsors who are impatient for information and impose time constraints hoping to promote a quick answer. The sponsor urges the evaluator to get some data to "size up the situation." The causal model development step is skipped, which may cause unnecessary or even misleading data to be accumulated. For example, Coleman attempted to relate school performance to school resources, teacher quality, and peer relationships.[30] Several dubious proxy measures for these causal factors and for school performance were used. Teacher quality was measured by the number of teachers in the school who had Master's degrees. Proxies for school resources included the number of laboratories and the number of books in the school library. An encyclopedia in the home served as an indicator of peer support. Verbal scores on standard achievement tests served as the performance measure.

More attention to model building (by HEW in its RFP process) could have improved these measures, reducing some of the vitriolic criticism that followed the report. For instance, a school's teacher quality could have been measured by peer recognition, salaries (compared to those in the local teacher market), or the ratings of school principals. Dollars per pupil could have been used as a measure of school resources, and time spent on home work as a measure of peer support. Why use verbal scores as proxies for achievement when quantitative scores are more amenable to change by educational instruction? This led Cain and Watts to criticize the *implicit* causal model of educational achievement used by Coleman. "...without a theoretical [causal] framework to provide order and a rationale for a large number of variables, we have no way of interpreting the statistical results..."[31]

Coleman replies, "if it were possible to know which variables have some importance in effecting [school] achievement, and to know the precise functional relationships between these variables—that is, to specify a [causal] model—then a large portion of the policy questions could be resolved."[32] Nevertheless, more attention to causal model *development* would have dramatically improved the proxies selected to measure explanatory variables, even if it did not uncover a precise functional relationship. Coleman also points out that his critics were economists and that their criticism stems from the world view of the economist:

Econometricians ordinarily deal with areas in which there are specific theoretical models. Consequently, the task becomes one of estimating values for parameters in this causal structure, and the policy results of the study lie in these parameter values. Sociologists ordinarily work in areas without such theoretical models, and the task of their empirical analysis is to gain more information about possibly relevant variables and plausible causal structures.[33]

The debate illustrates the need to carefully construct a causal model before carrying out an evaluation.

The emergence of causality from data accumulations has been advocated by well–known experimentalists like Skinner.[34] Models are expected to emerge from the data. Data accumulation has no role other than model building. This is seldom apparent to sponsors. As Coleman's study of school resources and their tie to school performance points up, sponsors did not permit the findings to serve as a preliminary to model building. Even if they had, critics were busy offering alternative explanations for the data; these must be countered. The controversy effectively prohibited a model–building phase. Administrators, pressed for evaluation results, quickly abandoned their long–range aims at the first sign of evaluation data. Thus, model building *may* emerge from the "assumption–data–interpretation" process, but such efforts are unlikely in practice. Better to build the best causal model as a study guide than to explain, as Coleman has for more than a decade, that his findings were preliminary and that HEW did not follow through on their long–range aims.

SPONSOR AND EVALUATOR PREFERENCES

Figure 8.3 provides a schematic representation of sponsor and evaluator behavior when conducting an evaluation. The sponsor dominates the left side

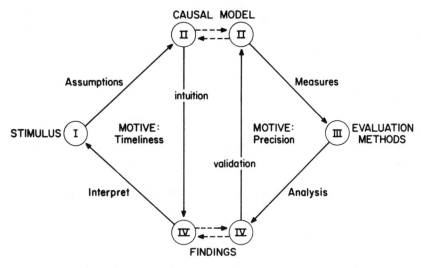

Figure 8.3 BEHAVIORALLY BASED EVALUATION PROCESSES

Reprinted with permission from Nutt, P.C., "On Managed Evaluation Processes," *Technological Forecasting and Social change,* Vol. 17, No. 4 (1980).

of the diagram. Administrators, who often become the sponsors of evaluation efforts, are constantly sifting and winnowing potential evaluation problems. When the needs for information exceed some threshold, the sponsor can allocate resources to initiate an evaluation project. The evaluator controls Stage III, methodology, in the same way the sponsor controls Stage I, the stimulus. The sponsor is unlikely to have up–to–date know–how of evaluation methods. Sponsors and evaluators share control over the development of causal models and the findings. The dialogue between evaluators and sponsors in Stage II (model formation) and Stage IV (documentation of results) leads to success or failure for the project.

Preferred Paths

The sponsor's preferred path leads to a "stimulus–model–results" evaluation process, as shown in Figure 8–3. The sponsor makes assumptions in order to build the causal model and uses the model to visualize ways to overcome problems implicit in the stimulus. Their motive is timeliness; a detailed investigation is perceived to take too long. Churchman points out that managers often believe they should be able to tease out findings without the expense and frustration of formal data collection.[35] The manager examines his causal model, may get the opinions of staff and peers, and then draws conclusions without the aid of tiresome academic fumbling. Administrators rich in experience believe they can draw on this experience to overcome the need for many evaluation projects. In Churchman's terms, the hospital administrator, nursing home operator, or public health department director knows the business and applies sound judgment to produce evaluation information. The sponsor's preferred path closes by applying intuition to link causal factors and findings (see Figure 8-3).

Most evaluators are highly skeptical of the power of intuition. All too often the experienced manager is seen selecting dubious courses of action or ignoring important problems.

When commissioned to participate in an evaluation, the evaluator treats the causal model of the sponsor as an approximation, and attempts to refine it. For instance, federal and state request for proposals, or RFP's, often list assumptions which describe an implicit causal model that the investigator is asked to study. The investigators respond with a proposal that specifies evaluation methods, describing the measures and modes of analysis believed to be appropriate. For instance, a recent federal RFP asked for proposals to study barriers that have limited the growth of health maintenance organizations.[36] To respond to the RFP, the investigator takes the implicit causal model, adds to it (suggests and refines barriers that seem to limit the growth of HMO's), and proposes a mode of study that can document these barriers. Thus the evaluator's preferred path is model–method–result. The evaluators take a statement of the causal model and refine it to derive measures, conduct needed analysis, and validate the findings against the (refined) causal model.

Improving the Evaluation Dialogue

Sponsors and evaluators adopt distinct paths because they have distinct roles and skills. Sponsors must excel in diagnostic skills. (Deciding when additional evaluation information can materially aid the organization is particularly important.) Methodological skills are the forte of the evaluator, so these skills are stressed. Neither skill can supplant the other.

Evaluators attempt to validate, using a model. The results may lack relevance because they were not exposed to the forces motivating the evaluation. Validation does not occur unless the findings are interpreted in terms of the sponsor's needs. Validation using a model leads to unread stacks of consultant and staff reports. Often, relevant and thought–provoking information fails to influence decisions in organizations because its validation lacked field testing and because the information was not carefully interpreted to the sponsor.

Sponsors can rely too often on their intuition. Churchman contends that a strict reliance on intuition leads to dogmatic managers.[37] They become professional skeptics who contend evaluation has little chance of illuminating complex issues, and relativists who believe that a mosaic of obscure contingencies dictate the success of interventions. These and other manifestations of the practical school dominate many policy–level positions in organizations. Unfortunately, many evaluation problems are counterintuitive. Recall that Coleman found that school resources did not improve school performance.[38] Being timely has little value when decisions rest on inaccurate information.

Remedies to these problems lie in the dialogue that occurs in Stage II and IV. To illustrate, the causal model may be developed *jointly* by the sponsor and evaluator, as shown in Figure 8.4. Both can educate. The evaluator learns more about the motivations behind the study and the necessity of key assumptions. The evaluator may be able to relax constraints by pointing out how evaluation methods with greater power can be used when certain assumptions are changed. This dialogue aids the evaluator and sponsor to enrich the causal model, trimming out restrictive assumptions and devising measurable program and performance factors.

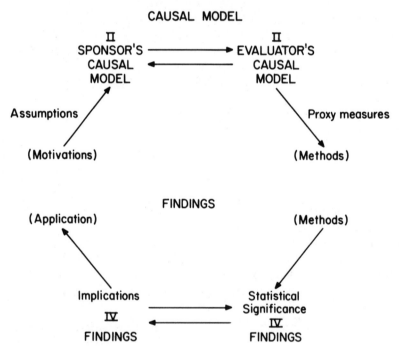

Figure 8.4 SOME DIALOGUES

Reprinted with permission from Nutt, P.C., "On Managed Evaluation Process," *Technological Forecasting and Social Change,* Vol. 17, No. 4, (1980).

Sponsor–evaluator dialogue is also essential in explaining the meaning of evaluation findings, also illustrated in Figure 8–4. Evaluators can aid sponsors by fully exploring the implications of the evaluation information. Reports or presentations should be jointly developed to describe policy guides and to provide the sponsor with an interpretation, a story, or an anecdote that can be used to illustrate key points. The evaluators must help the sponsor understand the limitations of the evaluation's conclusion–drawing power. The sponsor aids the evaluator by reemphasizing the motivation for the study and how the information will be used. Again, this dialogue permits the sponsor to make full and complete use of the evaluation information.

MANAGING THE EVALUATION PROCESS

Avoiding Evaluation

The threatening nature of evaluation sets it apart from many other collaborative staff–administrator activities. When an evaluation is conducted someone may lose, and lose badly, if the results do not support the predictions, programs, or commitments of an organization's power figures. Survival, stability, and growth are goals that often dominate the work world of administrators.[39] Evaluation focuses on past accomplishments and may turn them into deficits. For these reasons, administrators attempting to advance or maintain their power position against the intrusion of competitors often resist evaluation. In other instances, programs become highly entrenched and, as Suchman points out, are "based upon a large collection of inadequately tested assumptions and defended by staff and field personnel with strong vested interests in the continuation of the program as is."[40] Testimonials and assurances of success are periodically demanded from program administrators, forcing the administrator into a total program commitment. Such commitments entice administrators, and others with vested interests in the programs, to avoid evaluation, fearing its findings.

To avoid evaluation, administrators often engage in rationalizations, including the following:

(1) *Alleging long–range effects:* A prediction is made that the effects of a program will not show up for some time, making longitudinal studies essential.[41] For instance, a major university conducted a pilot test of a suicide prevention program, using a computer interview. The preliminary evaluation suggested that the interview was more effective than the psychiatrists. The results were put away for five years, to determine its "long–term effects."

(2) *Contending important effects resist measurement:* A contention is often made that instruments cannot detect program effects. The program is

described as having subtle, general, or small effects that will evade detection by anything but very costly evaluation and that evaluation funds could be better used to deliver program services. Programs in the War on Poverty used this rationale and often prohibited the use of any program funds for evaluation purposes. Those attempting quality–of–care studies of nursing are confronted with claims that even unobtrusive measures will (somehow) disturb the patient care process and that "tender, loving care" is not measurable anyway.

(3) *Refusing to withhold services:* Experimental and control groups may be called unreasonable because they withhold services from the needy. The Head Start and Upward Bound programs used this argument to strike evaluation funds from their appropriations.

Pseudoevaluation

Change often forces program evaluation. New patterns of activity, unsatisfied claims, conflicts, and perceived performance problems may launch an evaluation project. Suchman notes that new personnel, changes in the level of funding, and competition among programs provide difficult to reset stimuli for evaluation efforts.[42]

When evaluation can no longer be resisted, or when these rationalizations have been dismissed, those with vested interests often engage in pseudoevaluation. Pseudoevaluation is carried out to manage the evaluation process so that a thoughtful assessment of a program is impossible. Some evaluation abuses, several first identified by Suchman, are listed below:[43]

(1) *Eyewash:* An attempt to justify a weak or bad program by focusing evaluation on those aspects of the program expected to fare well. Referring to Figure 8–1, the sponsor makes assumptions and suggests causal relations that he suspects (or knows) will provide findings supportive of the program. For instance, Head Start administrators were furious because Head Start parents, known to be strongly supportive of the program, were not interviewed during an evaluation by Westinghouse Learning Corporation.[44] The evaluation of a federally supported program like comprehensive health planning agencies and OEO's neighborhood health centers were designed to provide a great many indices so program administrators could sift them and select a subset of these indices on which agencies scored well.[45]

(2) *Whitewash:* Covering up the prospect of program failure by soliciting testimonials to distract evaluation efforts. The left–hand loop in Figure 8–2, embracing the assumption–intuition–interpretation activities by sponsor, can be used to whitewash. Accreditation teams for hospitals and academic programs often act on testimonials in the form of reports and presentations which extoll their virtues, and not on formal performance measures. When

asked to assess continuing education efforts, universities solicit testimonials from past subscribers rather than engage in a careful evaluation of the benefits of the programs. The testimonial is hoped to dose the link between assumptions and interpretation. Whitewash is often successful because requests to evaluate, like the continuing education example, are pro forma: a serious attempt at assessment is not expected. In other cases, program failures are covered up by elaborate reasoning stemming from intuitive assessments, and by favorable comments in or out of context.

(3) *Submarine:* Attempt to eliminate or destroy a good program. Submarining often stems from administrative in–fighting over rights to succession or turf. Again, the left–hand side of Figure 8-2 is used, but in this case *negative* information is posited or solicited. Objective evaluation is avoided as it may reveal positive program features. The Nixon Administration selected programs that lacked a strong constituency to demonstrate they could scrap "ineffective" programs. For example, the programs, missions, and guidelines of Regional Medical Programs were altered by administrative edict so frequently and pervasively that one staffer observed that the time between the administration's changes in the program just exceeds the time necessary to understand the changes. Subsequently the Regional Medical Programs were phased out because "they failed to settle on a mission."

(4) *Posture:* Using evaluation as a gesture to create the aura of scientific objectivity. The sponsor looks good when his/her organization or unit sponsors self–assessment or appears forward–looking when new opportunities are being carefully examined. The sponsor encourages the evaluator to move through all stages (Figure 8-1), but withholds resources and personal sanction. No results are expected or even desired. Sponsors go so far as to hire and pay consultants merely to posture. It is to be hoped that the consultant will catch on, as heroic efforts to evaluate in the face of scarce resources and even scarcer legitimization will not be appreciated by the sponsor. Activities labeled "fact finding" in public agencies often signal this type of evaluation.

(5) *Substitution:* Shifting attention to less relevant, or defensible, aspects of a program to disguise failure. All stages in Figure 8-1 are covered, but the interpretation activity is selective, reporting only positive program features. These tactics are often attempted, with varying success. The Head Start administrators, once the educational benefits of their program had been discounted, tried to focus attention on its health and nutrition efforts, and its acceptance by low–income groups.[46] When sponsors also control the evaluation, substitution can be carried out with considerably more finesse. Supporters of federal water projects, under fire by environmentalists, extolled the virtues of successful projects elsewhere. In Florida, one such project would have slowed the movement of fresh water until salt water seepage would have become a serious environmental hazard. Proponents supported the project by

describing benefits of water projects in Tennessee and the Columbia river basins.

(6) *Delay:* Postponement tactics can be used to thwart evaluation. The scope of the project can be studied at length and then restudied to point out to those pushing for evaluation that a proper study takes time. After repeated failure to build a model, a case can be made that evaluation just isn't worth the effort. Or if the delays have been lengthy enough, the storm may have passed. The top loop in Figure 8-3 illustrates one delay tactic, recursive model building. Data are avoided (the lower loop in Figure 8-3) as they may contain diagnostic elements. Delay is probably the most common form of pseudoevaluation, and is often signaled by task forces, elaborate agendas, and the sudden emergence of a preference for group decision–making in otherwise autocratic administrators.

(7) *Reconstruction:* Attempts can be made to piece together programs in light of beneficial changes in performance indicators. The causal model is built to reflect the performance data. For instance, a Blue Cross organization mounted a variety of cost containment programs in response to a state's legislative mandates. First, one intervention is attempted and then another, with the last intervention often based on a spin–off of the previous program. If costs begin to show a measurable decline, a frantic search for a causal agent is mounted to reconstruct the program.

(8) *Inadvertent programs:* Data found to verify the beneficial effects of inadvertent interventions can be relabeled as planned interventions, to enhance the prestige of administrators. A causal relationship is discovered, following a routine performance audit. Serendipitous outcomes often stimulate data collection, to refine the effectiveness measures and to isolate a defensible causal agent, under the administrator's control. The sponsor verifies the veracity of the data, and then frames an evaluation question which the data can confirm. The process has but one step: intuition. For instance, a decline in hospital food service expense can be associated with a historical event of the administrator's choosing. The favorable cost picture can be attributed to recent changes in personnel, which suggests a well–run organization. Like the toothpaste ads, one in twenty studies will produce "40 percent fewer cavities" by chance alone.

(9) *Hand–picked panels:* Site visit teams are often used to evaluate programs. Outsiders often set up expectations based on experiences that are not transferable. By selecting a site visit team whose experiences, and thus biases and expectations, are similar to those operating in the program, the program can be sanctified. Or to eliminate an unwanted program, a site team may be selected whose members are likely to be hostile to the practices of the program. A clever sponsor can hand pick or prune the membership of the site team, which can dictate the outcome of the evaluation. The site team forms a causal

model consistent with their experience and searches for program practices (not performance data) that correspond to procedures or models of operation believed to be effective (typically their own). The assumption–intuition–interpretation path is followed (Figure 8.2). As Weckworth points out, site teams settle all issues, even questions of fact, with a vote.[47]

(10) *Fixed Indices:* Evaluation sponsors dictate criteria and criteria weights. Measures of the criteria are fixed to steer the evaluator toward issues the sponsor wants considered. The sponsor restricts the evaluator's scope of inquiry by dictating the measures and by restricting the evaluator's role in interpreting the results (see Figure 8.1). Interpretation is reserved for the sponsor and no dialogue is permitted (see Figure 8.2). Contract evaluation in HEW uses the fixed indices approach. Consultants are asked to determine the extent to which proposals meet certain criteria, but not to participate in criteria selection or weighting. Fixed indices are also used to create an aura of respectability for an organization. Well–endowed hospitals, for instance, publicize those indices that measure institutional solvency. Fixed indices are also used to make a point. When pupil–teacher ratios are falling, school systems compare them to other schools to justify budget increases.

Fuzzy Interpretations

As a last resort, sponsors may develop tactics to aid them in explaining away negative findings, should they occur. The results are made fuzzy to raise questions which may discredit the findings. Suchman[48] contends that even well–conducted evaluation projects can be rendered suspect when someone in a position of power makes one of several claims. These include the following:

(1) *Alleging a poorly selected target group:* The effects of the program were claimed to be understated because those who could benefit most from the services, or respond best to the intervention, did not participate in the study. In short, a biased source of the target group is alleged. Randomization makes this claim implausible, but the benefits of randomization are seldom understood, so it can be alleged anyway. A variant on this theme is to claim that those needing the services were in the control group. Again, randomization will make this claim implausible.

(2) *Claims of concentrated effects:* Some service recipients improved immensely, but the claim is made that these benefits were washed out by those who did not need the services. The selective effect argument is difficult to combat unless individual cases can be traced to isolate high benefiting participants.

(3) *Claims of faulty program mechanisms:* A more intensive program is advanced as necessary to produce positive results. This claim was advanced by

Head Start advocates, who were able to initiate "follow through," a program designed to work with low–income children after they began grade school.[49] (4) *Claim of bias:* All sorts of claims can be made which imply bias. Contending that control groups were improperly selected, measures were taken without reliability checks, and the wrong measurements were used, can discredit evaluation findings. The "Hawthorne Effect" (people responding to the evaluation situation, not the program) can always be alleged because the Hawthorne study had taken on the status of an empirical law. Cain and Watts advanced charges of bias in Coleman's evaluation of the effect of school resources on performance.[50] Controversy will tend to discredit an evaluation.

SUMMARY

This chapter described essential steps in a evaluation process. To use evaluation resources wisely dialogues, between sponsors and those who conduct evaluations, which review the causal model and the evaluation findings, were found to be essential. The threatening nature of evaluation was found to create considerable incentive for the sponsor to manage the process. Sponsors manage an evaluation by distorting the process. An evaluation process can be distorted by altering key transactions, by disregarding steps, and by modifying information that should flow between steps in the process. Several distorted process were described. Pitfalls which accompany a distorted evaluation process were discussed in the hopes that the practitioner can discriminate sincere from insincere evaluation requests and, when possible, allocate his/her time accordingly. In the final chapters we shall turn our attention to decision making and how decision makers use evaluation information.

NOTES

1. This chapter is drawn from Nutt, P.C., "On Managed Evaluation Processes," *Technological Forecasting and Social Change,* Vol. 17, No. 4, 1980.
2. In many instances, the evaluator lack essential skills and/or the sponsor lacks needed discretion to carry out an evaluation. This chapter describes the attitudes toward evaluation by competent evaluators and powerful sponsors. Some of the problems that arise when inappropriate constraints are established or accepted are described in Chapter 9.
3. This schema was proposed by Mitroff and his colleagues (Mitroff I., F. Betz, L.R. Pondy, and F. Sagasti, "On Managing Science in the Systems Age: Two Schemes For The Study of Science As A Whole Systems Phenomenon," *Interfaces,* Vol. 4, No. 3, 1974, pp. 46–58). The process has been modified to account for the similarities in procedures but differences

in the intent of evaluation and research, as identified by Suchman (Suchman, E.A., *Evaluation Research.* Washington, D.C.: Russell Sage Foundation, 1967).

4. Lindblom, C., *The Intelligence of Democracy: Decision Processes Through Adjustment.* New York: Free Press, 1965.

5. Gore, W.J., *Administrative Decision Making: A Heuristic Model,* Wiley: New York, 1964.

6. Conrath, D.W., "Organizational Decision Making Under Varying Conditions of Uncertainty," *Management Science,* Vol. 13, No. 4, 1967, pp. B487–B500.

7. March, J. and H. Simon, *Organizations.* New York: Wiley, 1958.

8. Cyert, R., and J. March, *A Behavioral Theory of the Firm.* Englewood Cliffs, N.J.: Prentice–Hall, 1963.

9. To complicate matters, this threshold may vary from one evaluation sponsor to another, dictated by personality and a myriad of other traits. Chapter 10 describes some of the ways in which decision style may influence an evaluation.

10. The studies were reported in (a) "Systems Analysis for a New Generation of Military Hospitals," Final Report Summary, Advanced Research Projects Agency of theDepartment of Defense, Contract Number DAHC 15–69–C. 035S P201. ARPA order number 1494. Arthur D. Little, Inc., April 1971; and (b) System Analysis Study towards a "new generation" of military hospitals, Vol. III: Medical Health Care Review, Advanced Research Projects Agency of the Department of Defense, Contract Number DA 1 C 15–69–C–0354, Westinghouse Electric Corporation–Health Systems Department, November, 1970.

11. Kilmann, R.H. and R.P. Herden, "Towards a Systematic Methodology for Evaluating the Impact of Interventions on Organizational Effectiveness," *Academy of Management Review,* Vol. 1, No. 3, July 1976.

12. Nutt, P.C., "The Method Variable: A Normative and Behavioral View of the Planning Process," Ohio State University, College of Administrative Science, December 1977.

13. Campbell, D.T. and J. Stanley, *Experimental and Quasi-Experimental Designs for Research.* Chicago: Rand–McNally, 1962.

14. Kershaw, D.N. "Issues in Income Maintenance Experimentation," in P. Rossi et al. (eds.) *Evaluating Social Programs,* New York: Seminar Press, 1972.

15. Coleman, J.S., E. Campbell, C. Hobson, J. McPartland, and A. Mood, "Equality of Educational Opportunity," Washington, D.C.: U.S. Government Printing Office, 1966.

16. *Ibid.*

17. Williams, W. and J.W. Evans, "The Politics of Evaluation: The Case of Head Start," in P. Rossi, et al. (eds.) *Evaluating Social Programs.* New York: Seminar Press, 1972.

18. Polgar, S., "Health Action in Cross Cultural Perspectives," in F. Howard, et al. (eds.), *Handbook of Medical Sociology,* pp. 411–414. Englewood Cliffs, N.J.: Prentice–Hall, 1963.

19. Cain, G. and H.W. Watts, "Problems in Making Policies Inferences from the Coleman Report," *American Sociological Review,* Vol. 35, pp. 228–242.

20. *Ibid.*

21. Mitroff, I., J. Nelson, and R.O. Mason, "On The Design of Management Myth Information Systems," *Management Science,* Vol. 21, No. 4, 1974, pp. 371–382.

22. Mitroff, I. and R. Kilmann, "Stories Managers Tell: A New Test for Organizational Problem Solving," *Management Review,* July 1975, pp. 18–28.

23. Ritti, R.R. and G.R. Funkhouser, *The Ropes to Know and the Ropes to Skip.* Columbus, Oh.: Grid, 1977.

24. Coleman, et al., p. 75.

25. Kershaw, p. 244.

26. *Ibid*, p. 236.
27. Kershaw, p. 224–239.
28. Computerized EKG interpretation programs were developed at the Public Health Service in HEW, the Mayo Clinic, Mt. Sinai Hospital in New York, and perhaps elsewhere.
29. Stimson, D.H. and R. Stimson, *Operations Research in Hospitals: Diagnosis and Prognosis*. Chicago: HRET, 1972, p. 414.
30. Coleman, et al., p. 97.
31. Cain and Watts, p. 74.
32. Coleman, J.S., "Reply to Cain and Watts," in P. Rossi, et al. (eds.), *Evaluating Social Programs*, New York: Seminar Press, 1972.
33. It should be pointed out that economists may disagree that their work is based on theoretical models and sociologists may not concur with the deductive role thrust on them by economists.
34. Skinner, B.F., *Contingencies of Reinforcement*, p. 81. New York: Appleton–Century–Crofts, 1969.
35. Churchman, C.W., *The Systems Approach*, p. 216. New York: Dell, 1958.
36. HMO's are prepaid prevention–oriented health care delivery organizations popularized by HEW through congressional legalization, and usually operating with federal subsidies.
37. Churchman, p. 216.
38. Coleman et al., p. 106.
39. Dill, W.R., "Business Organizations" in J.G. March, *Handbook of Organizations*. Chicago: Rand–McNally, 1965.
40. Suchman, E.A., *Evaluation Research*, Chapter 8. Washington, D.C.: Russell Sage, 1967.
41. In some cases this contention may be correct. Head Start appears to have produced effects measurable in junior high that were not apparent in the early grades.
42. Suchman, p. 143.
43. Suchman, p. 142.
44. Williams and Evans, p. 260.
45. Wholey, J.S., J. Scanlon, H. Duffy, J. Fukumoto, and L. Vogt, *Federal Evaluation Policy: Analyzing the Effects of Public Programs*. Washington, D.C.: The Urban Institute, 1971.
46. Williams and Evans, p. 256.
47. Weckworth, V., "On Evaluation: A Tool or a Tyranny," Systems Development Project, Comment Series. Minneapolis: University of Minnesota, undated.
48. Suchman, p. 144.
49. Williams and Evans, p. 261.
50. Cain and Watts, p. 74.

CHAPTER 9

Managerial Diagnosis[1]

There is a tide in the affairs of men, which, taken at the flood, leads on to fortune.

Shakespeare, *Julius Caesar*

Managers spend their professional life facing a swirling milieu of problems. Mintzberg, Raisinghani, and Theoret believe that an accumulation of stimuli must reach some threshold level before inquiry is initiated and resources are mobilized.[2] While thresholds differ, each individual manager is thought to sort acknowledged stimuli by comparing a perceived outcome (like consumer satisfaction or costs) to a norm for that outcome. This process is called "managerial diagnosis." Diagnosis is used to place problems into action and deferred categories, as well as the circular file. The diagnostic process is seldom formal, nor is it fully explicit. As a result, it may appear mysterious and, at times, even cryptic to individuals in staff positions.

Managerial diagnosis is a vitally important aspect of managerial action. Even an implicit diagnosis sets out assumptions that will direct inquiry. These assumptions stipulate both important relationships that a planning or evaluation project must consider as well as the types of results the manager will find acceptable. This chapter describes some features of the diagnostic process and provides cues to decipher the behavior and policy statements of managers who commission evaluation and planning projects.

INITIATING ACTION THROUGH MANAGERIAL DIAGNOSIS

According to Mintzberg, Raisinghani, and Theoret, managers act when opportunities, problems, or crisis situations occur.[3] Opportunities evoke voluntary actions, whereas crises create intense pressure for a response. The manager's workload is adjusted by allocating more time to crisis situations as they arise, and less time to issues that fall into other categories. No priorities are established beyond the order of crisis, problem, and opportunity.

Managers respond to time pressure by limiting the time spent on each issue. Problem and opportunity issues are not ignored, merely treated superficially. As a result, managers are thought to diagnose all issues they perceive to be important, although some will receive a very cursory examination. For instance, a hospital administrator is predicted to retain an interest in the innovations of others (opportunities) and maintain an acute concern for per diem costs (problems) while facing a large malpractice lawsuit.

The discussion in this chapter does not focus solely on strategic decisions, or on the behavior of chief executive officers in organizations. Rather, at each level of an organization, managers are seen sorting out issues into action and deferred categories. *All* problems *perceived* to be important to managers at any organizational level are considered.

Figure 9-1 provides a behavioral model of managerial diagnosis. The manager's perceived reality provides cues which are sorted into act, defer, and discard categories. These designations are frequently reconsidered, occasionally as the result of stormy encounters with important reference groups. The diagnostic process is seen as dynamic, with many false starts and misleading cues.

A decision to act is stimulated by conflict (Figure 9-1). The manager attempts to reduce this conflict through formal inquiry.[4] The stimulus is assessed to identify the assumptions which will guide inquiry. Inquiry is used to provide information that suggests a choice that reduces the manager's conflict or that points out the need for more intense information seeking. On occasion,

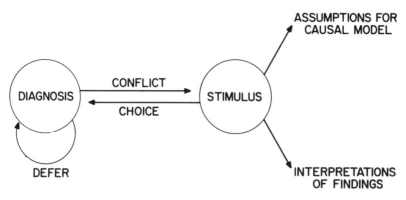

Figure 9.1 DIAGNOSIS AND THE EVALUATION PROCESS

Reprinted with permission from Nutt, P.C., "Calling out and Calling off The Dogs: Managerial Diagnosis in Public Organizations," *Academy of Management Review*, Vol. 4, No. 2, (1980).

a stimulus may contain enough information to render inquiry unnecessary. A choice is made using the available information.

CONFLICT AS A STIMULANT TO ACTION

Diagnosis begins when the manager faces a unique situation, described by an incomplete set of data. Readily available information sources, like cost–variance reports or the views of respected colleagues, are tapped to clarify the performance of current operations or planned changes.[5] This information–seeking process may be conscious or subconscious, formal or informal, and often amasses large amounts of ambiguous and contradictory data. For instance, when a hospital administrator discovers that radiation therapy equipment used in the treatment of cancer patients has been improperly calibrated for several years, the administrator may mull over the situation, discuss it with a trusted colleague, consult a lawyer, or even brush up on malpractice law, to assess the hospital's liability.

The diagnostic process pulls together *available* information and compares this information to a "norm." The norm represents a picture of the manager's expectations for efficiency, effectiveness, acceptance, innovativeness, and the like. Norms identify the manager's perception of the best attainable state of affairs.[6] They are based on past and/or projected trends, the performance of comparable organizations, expectations of key individuals or groups, or even theoretical models.[7]

Following the March and Simon typology, "norms" and "current information states" can be categorized as "good," "bland," "mixed," "poor," or "uncertain."

(1) A "good" norm anticipates several positive performance features and few negative features. For instance, a hospital financial manager may expect a bad–debt rate of 5 percent of total revenues (considered to be good) and few complaints about the hospital's collection practices. If current information finds that the bad–debt rate hovers around 5 percent, and the financial manager is unaware of complaints, the hospital's financial management can be viewed as "good."

(2) A "bland" norm has few negative features and few positive ones. For example, hospital expansions are not expected to be cost effective, but many hospital administrators believe that developing an expansion plan is necessary to deflect criticism from their medical staff. The hospital may even pay an architect to develop an expansion concept and consultants to price the plan. Even if cost estimates confirm the administrator's cost picture, the expansion plans may be submitted to regulatory bodies merely to placate the medical staff. This results in a situation with no bad features (recriminations from the

medical staff have been awarded), but no good features (the expansion cannot be justified because of its cost).

(3) A "mixed" norm has several positive and several negative features. The expectations for a new alcoholism treatment program may include plaudits of innovativeness and the inevitable problems associated with high per-case costs that occur during the initiation of a new service. High per-case costs (documented by the accounting system) and community recognition, which indicates that a program is badly needed, would suggest that the alcoholism program has mixed benefits.

(4) A "poor" norm contains few favorable expectations. Several negative features and few positive features are contained in the manager's perceptions of what is attainable. For instance, ambulatory clinics located in low-income areas anticipate high bad-debt rates and complaints about any collection attempts. Financial reports and demands by activist groups often dramatize this problem to clinic administrators.

(5) An "uncertain" norm contains little information. Uncertain norms stem from situations where the manager's experience seems not to apply. Performance data that lack a baseline or referant tend to evoke uncertainty. For instance, when Congress initiated Job Corps, Head Start, and the other Great Society programs, they had no way to judge costs, benefits, and other performance factors. Uncertainty also results when the performance associated with new programs, current operations, or the fitness of plans is unclear. Uncertainty in either norms or in current information results in evaluation to clarify norms or information states.

Comparing the five types of "norms" and five "information states," defined in the same way, identifies twenty-five unique decision situations. Table 9–1 lists all combinations of the norms and information states. For instance, when norms are uncertain, performance can be seen as good, mixed, bland, poor, or uncertain, creating five distinct diagnostic situations. Each norm can be viewed in the same way, leading to twenty-five distinct decision situations which evoke three types of responses: evaluation, planning, or deferral. Table 9–1 classifies each of these twenty-five decision situations in terms of the response the situation evokes.

The Planning Response

Planning may be carried out by a search or a formal planning process. Search is applied when a manager sorts through past experiences to suggest ideas or to get other people, like vendors, to provide ready-made solutions. Planning projects are more formal, usually involving the organization's staff or consultants. As a result, planning projects are often carried out by a

Table 9-1. Response to Conflict[a]

	Situation	Norm	Current Information State	Reponse
I. Diagnoses Calling	1.	good	uncertain	tradition evaluation
for Evaluation	2.	bland	uncertain	traditional evaluation
	3.	mixed	uncertain	traditional evaluation
	4.	poor	uncertain	traditional evaluation
	5.	poor	poor	confirmational evaluation
	6.	bland	bland	confirmational evaluation
	7.	mixed	mixed	strategy evaluation
	8.	uncertain	uncertain	norm development
	9.	uncertain	good	norm development
	10.	uncertain	bland	norm development
	11.	uncertain	mixed	norm development
	12.	uncertain	poor	norm development
II. Diagnoses Calling	13.	good	bland	planning
for Planning	14.	good	mixed	planning
	15.	good	poor	planning
	16.	bland	poor	planning
	17.	mixed	poor	planning
	18.	mixed	bland	planning
III. Diagnoses Calling for	19.	good	good	ratify current practices
Deferment (No Conflict)	20.	bland	mixed	ratify current practices
	21.	bland	good	ratify current practices
	22.	mixed	good	ratify current practices
	23.	poor	good	ratify current practices
	24.	poor	bland	ratify current practices
	25.	poor	mixed	ratify current practices

Reprinted with permission from Nutt, P.C., "Calling in and Calling out the Dogs: Managerial Diagnosis in Public Organizations," *Academy of Management Review,* 4:2, p. 206, (1979).

manager with the aid of technical personnel. The planning process may be used to seek custom-made solutions or modified solutions, which alter and adapt the practices of others.[8]

Diagnosis of situations 13 to 18 (Table 9-1) finds that performance falls below the manager's performance norms, which calls for a planning response. Planning projects stem from conflict implicit in the failure of performance to meet the manager's expectations. When the information system is believed,[9] planning is attempted in order to improve the situation by devising changes in operations or practices to improve performance.

Performance must fall below expectations before a manager will initiate a search for new ideas. This suggests that managers view planning as a last resort. This is consistent with the empirical work of Cyert and March, who found that organizations stress information gathering, not planning.[10] As a result, the manager may defer or evaluate, when planning would be a better response.

The Deferment Response

Situations 19 to 25 in Table 9–1 predict that diagnosis will result in deferral. The manager does *not* feel conflict, because his/her expectations have been surpassed. Diagnosis calls for a deferment of action and current practices are ratified.[11] The perceived difference between performance and norms may even form the basis for public statements that rationalize keeping things as they are. Neither innovation nor formal information gathering will occur in situations 19 to 25.

Deferrals may be galling to staff in situations 20, 24, and 25 (Table 9–1). In each case, current performance levels suggest that improvements can be made. Needed changes in operations and in programs may be resisted or not attempted because the manager has a pessimistic outlook, viewing the prospects of success as unlikely. According to Churchman, these managers believe that their experience is overly diagnostic, which often stands in the way of needed action.[12] For instance, a hospital administrator may reject a staff proposal to update the hospital's management information system (MIS). The current system may be perceived to have no bad features (situation 24) or good features coupled with bad (situation 20 or 25), but if the administrator's experience in getting a new MIS in operation was totally negative (late delivery, chaotic transition, and a failure to achieve the projected cost savings), anything looks good by comparison.

The Evaluation Response

Conflict in situations 1 to 12 (Table 9–1) arises out of uncertainty or because of poor performance. A diagnosis calling for evaluation is predicted when uncertainty clouds either norms *or* current information states, when expectations and performance are similar, and when current performance lacks positive features or has negative features.

March and Simon point out that a manager responds to uncertainty by seeking information.[13] In situations 1 to 4 (Table 9–1), operations or programs are perceived to have unknown performance. In these situations evaluation is initiated to clarify the unit costs, outcomes, and other features of programs, such as counseling services in a mental health center; or operations, like claim processing in an insurance agency. Assessing current performance will be called "traditional evaluation." When the manager perceives performance to be uncertain, traditional evaluation is used to clarify performance. As Leifer points out, structure is used to reduce uncertainty.[14] Traditional evaluation provides the preferred structure for managers facing situations 1 to 4. The manager reduces conflict stemming from uncertainty by commissioning an evaluation project. "Posturing" and other types of pseudoevaluation described in Chapter 8 are unlikely in situations 1 to 4 because the manager believes that performance must be clarified.[15]

In the course of an evaluation, stimulated by situations 1 to 4, it may be discovered that performance is below expectations (the norm), which provides a new situation to consider. For instance, in situation 1 the norm suggests that a "good" outcome is possible. If evaluation finds that performance is "poor," situation 1 will shift to situation 14, and planning becomes the predicted response. Also the manager may paw through the evaluation data to locate its good aspects, contending the program's effects were subtle, evaded detection, and using similar rationalizations, as described by Suchman.[16] In this case, situation 1 reverts to situation 19, and the manager ratifies the current practice. Rationalization may also change norms. Norms may be revised downward to a mixed, bland, or even poor expectation, creating situations 17, 16, and 5, respectively. Situations 16 and 17 also call for planning, while situation 5 calls for an evaluation (see Table 9-1). In short, changes in a manager's aspirations will change norms, which in turn may cause another attempt at evaluation or planning, or cause a deferment.

Evaluation is also used to clarify norms, even when current operations are seen as "good" (situation 9). In situations 8 to 12, performance is clear but expectations are not. The diagnosis calls for an evaluation to assess performance *relative* to the performance in comparable organizations or organizational units. Conflict is felt because uncertainty clouds expectations. The evaluation may appear to be pointless to the evaluator because performance is believed to be well known to those sponsoring the evaluation. The evaluation has but one purpose: to provide the manager with information that can be used to form personal norms. This type of evaluation often precedes major commitments, as when hospitals consider satellite outpatient operations. The "fitness" of plans is assessed to form norms for the manager.

Expectations become clouded with the advent of new opportunities, so changes in technology may also alter norms. For instance, benchmarks in a hospital radiology department for costs (based on the number of x-rays and the amount of personnel training) and quality (based on x-ray readability) were well understood until full body scanning was introduced. Uncertainty shrouded the performance of full body scanning, so new norms were necessary to judge quality and costs. Evaluation is used to provide information which the manager uses to form standards. In short, when the manager has uncertain expectations, evaluation is carried out to clarify the potential for change, which is used to form norms for decision making.

Past experience often influences uncertainty. When experience is thought to be relevant, uncertain information states can be explained away, which reduces conflict. To illustrate, a hospital administrator, finding that little is known about the performance of hospital–run satellite clinics, may compare the clinics to organizations he/she has managed. If the organizations seem comparable, (e.g., operated in the same manner), the manager infers norms from the previous experience. Expectations are based on the acceptance, cost, and utilization levels attainable in the setting thought to be analogous. Situations 8 to 12 shift to other situations, as dictated by the norm (e.g., good, bland, etc.) inferred by the manager.

In situations 5, 6, and 7 (Table 9–1), both norms and performance are understood. Performance is clear but either lacks positive features (situation 6), has negative features (situation 7), or both (situation 5). Evaluation is mounted because current performance has unacceptable elements in situation 5. The evaluation process is terminated at the first sign that the current information state is correct. Norms imply that little can be done. As a consequence, evaluation stops when the first trickle of data confirms the manager's views. In situation 5, evaluation provides information to confirm the necessity of retaining a program with undesirable features. A "confirmational evaluation" is also called for when current programs lack positive features (situation 6). For instance, the financial performance of hospitals is dictated by its clientele as well as its management. A poor hospital financial performance record may be unacceptable to trustees until the financial picture of comparable hospitals is drawn (norms verified) and related to the proportion of Medicaid and self–pay patients, causal factors beyond the control of the hospital. In summary, when current information suggests that norms are being met, but not exceeded, and programs or operations lack positive features, evaluation is used to confirm (defend) the manager's norms.

A confirmational evaluation often creates tension between managers and evaluators. The evaluator may believe the evaluation was unnecessary to begin with (performance was clear) and, once initiated, failed to meet rigorous standards. The manager may regard such a posture as naive; the realities of surviving in highly visible administrative positions demand defensible explanations of poor performance.

Programs with good and bad features (situation 7) are likely to receive what Wholey and his colleagues call a "strategy evaluation."[17] A strategy evaluation is used to detect whether changes in procedures can alter the negative aspects of the program's performance. For instance, a neighborhood health center may tie into a local hospital to expand its benefit package, but find that its clientele refuses to use the hospital. Concern for the cultural heritage of the client group, like using Mexican–American motifs in decorating waiting rooms and hiring bilingual triage clerks, may salvage the relationships. A strategy evaluation compares several such procedures to document their impact on utilization. To summarize: when both expectations and performance are mixed, the manager will seek information which describes how changes in procedures can ameliorate negative performance features.

In situations 5, 6, and 7, the best response, planning, is preceded by information gathering. March and Simon point out that information provided by an evaluation may alter the manager's expectations.[18] When evaluation suggests that norms are pessimistic, situations 5, 6, and 7 change to situations 15, 16, or 17; 13 or 18; and 14 (respectively), each calling for a planning response. Finally, in situations 6 and 7, a decline in expectations creates situations 20, 24, and 25. Current practices are ratified.

DECISION GROUPS AND THEIR RESPONSE TO CONFLICT

Decision groups such as United Way boards of directors or the ad hoc committees of a hospital association are postulated to seek a consensual diagnosis. As they ponder issues, "selective perception" causes each decision group member to advocate courses of action that buttress their vested interests.[19] Members of a decision group often have conflicting objectives and select information which creates a diagnosis that would benefit their constituents or themselves. Also perceptual differences may arise. Group members may have different information sources and norms which combine to suggest that evaluation (situations 1 to 12), planning (situations 13 to 18), or deferral (situations 19 to 25) is the rational response. Conflict arises because members tend to argue the merits of these different approaches without sharing the information they used to select the recommended response. As Ferrence points out, committee members present their inferences, not the information or evidence used to draw these inferences.[20] As the number of information sources increases, so does the prospect of a conflicting diagnosis.

Conflict in groups is a two–tiered process. A common diagnosis emerges when information is shared among influential group members. Effective committees are managed so members will share information.[21] Information sharing often creates a new, or synthetic, diagnosis which relaxes the group's conflict over the proper response. Once arrived at, the consensual diagnosis may also stimulate conflict, as defined by situations 1 to 25 in Table 9–1. Given a consensual diagnosis, the behavior predicted for individual decision makers will apply to groups. In short, effective groups deal with conflict by seeking a consensual diagnosis through information sharing, which leads to the same 25 situations and the responses that apply for individuals.

LINKING THE PROCESSES OF EVALUATION AND DIAGNOSIS

Evaluation projects were found to be stimulated by conflict, which stems from an unfavorable comparison of observed and expected performance and from performance uncertainties (situations 1 to 12 in Table 9–1). The decision maker feels compelled to seek information that describes or verifies performance. Figure 9–2 shows how managerial diagnosis is linked to the evaluation process described in Chapter 8.

The most common response to conflict is evaluation. Conflict goads the decision maker to suggest how, for example, costs could have escalated or to identify (or reconstruct) the objectives of an intervention program. When performance is clear, causes are sought, and when causes are clear, attempts are made to determine their effects. Assumptions are made to identify a causal relationship for exploration by the evaluation process. As assumptions are made, the process shifts from a decision to an evaluation mode. At this point, the manager's role shifts from decision maker to sponsor. The manager retains the role of sponsor until an interpretation of the findings is required. The

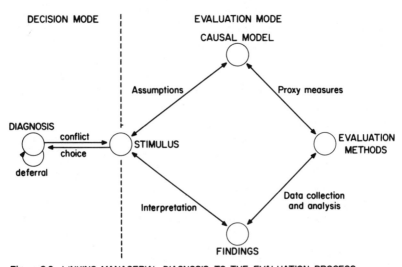

Figure 9.2 LINKING MANAGERIAL DIAGNOSIS TO THE EVALUATION PROCESS

manager shifts back into a decision mode as choices are made, as shown in Figure 9–2.

Assumptions dictate the elements of the causal model and thus play a vital role in the evaluation process. An inappropriate causal relation may be set out for study. For instance, an evaluation of factors influencing hospital malpractice awards may use the award's dollar amount as a measure of hospital risk, excluding legal fees and court costs because they are hard to determine. An evaluation of nursing home costs may assume that care quality is constant across homes, ignoring causal factors such as nurse–patient staffing ratios. When assessing the merits of contract management for hospitals, the proportion of self–insured and Medicaid patients in the hospitals, before and after the contract, may be ignored. Thus, beliefs about the measurability of objectives and the assumed tie between the intervention and the measures of its effectiveness are critical features in the assumption–building process.

Assumption Building

Thompson contends that assumptions which guide an evaluation process are drawn from the beliefs held by decision makers about the ease of measuring performance and the difficulty of relating an intervention with performance measures.[22]

Performance measure assumptions indicate the type of result the manager believes can be obtained and accurately measured. For example, the objectives of an intervention can be perceived as explicit or vague. As pointed out in Chapter 7, there is often confusion surrounding objectives. The objective can be seen as broad and vague or clear but narrow. The nature of the conflict found in the diagnosis phase may prompt a sponsor to change objectives from general to specific terms. For instance, the Job Corps program was initiated to get high school dropouts to finish high school. The success of the program in attracting those with good high school records caused a movement of its objectives from general to specific: from promoting high school to aiding the qualified to finish high school. Projects charged with measuring quality of care in a hospital ward often change objectives from specific to more general. Evaluation may attempt to measure psychological well–being, not the timeliness of medication, or infection rates. Administrators, when facing assessments, often modify their objectives to reflect their view of what seems achievable.[23] This leads the evaluation sponsor to dictate performance measures of the objective which tend to be clear or ambiguous.

The evaluation sponsor also makes assumptions about the environment (closed system or open system) and the difficulty in relating the intervention to meaningful performance measures. A sponsor may have faith in the ability of an intervention to create a given change or to produce economies. For instance, the Head Start program administrators seemed convinced that the school performance of Head Start participants would improve. This causal relation (Head Start's ability to improve school performance) seemed clear. In other instances, administrators view intervention programs with considerable skepticism. For instance, a hospital administrator may not believe that work–measurement–based labor control programs can reduce hospital costs. In this case, the causal relationship (work measurement leading to lower labor costs) would be seen as vague and ambiguous.

Environmental factors can make the causal relationship seem simple or complex. A closed system assumption would ignore outside forces, believing that these forces do not influence performance. For instance, a closed system assumption would dictate that cost savings that are realized in one hospital from improved laundry equipment should be attainable in other hospitals. An open system assumption would hold that external factors influence costs in the laundry. Costs depend on the equipment as well as the skills of available people, local labor rates, the quality of supervision, and many other exogenous factors. Thus, the sponsor's beliefs about the clarity of the link between an intervention and its effects and/or the degree of influence of the environment in which the intervention must operate frames the evaluation question. These assumptions lead the sponsor to conclude that the causal relationship tends to be clear or unclear.

Combinations of the extreme values for these dimensions define four types of assumptions which can guide an evaluation (Table 9–2). In Case I, both causal relations and performance measures seem clear. Under this assumption,

Table 9–2. Decision Rules For Evaluation Projects

| | | Beliefs About Causal Relationships | |
		known	unknown
	Clear & Measurable	Case I Optimization Decision Rule	Case II Satisficing Decision Rule
PERFORMANCE MEASURE ASSUMPTIONS			
	Uncertain & Ambiguous	Case III Feasibility Decision Rule	Case IV Social Tests As Decision Rules

Adapted from Thompson, J.D., *Organizations in Action,* McGraw-Hill, New York, p. 86, (1967).

evaluation is directed to determine the degree of "perfection" attained. Cost–benefit or cost–effectiveness measures and mathematical modeling are often recommended. The model is manipulated to reveal the optimum performance, which is compared to field observations of cost–benefit or cost–effective measures. For instance, a dietary department can use an assembly–line model to describe tray preparation and a queueing model to describe tray distribution. The quantity of trays distributed at a particular cost (a cost–effectiveness measure) permits a comparison of the model (the ideal) with actual performance for evaluation purposes.[24] The sponsor in Case I seeks to minimize the number of resources needed to achieve a desired result. The desired result is assumed to be measurable and the means to achieve the result are assumed to be known. Under this type of assumption, optimization techniques may be applied and performance may be monitored with an efficiency test.

In Case II, the sponsor believes that performance can be measured but that causal relationships are unknown. Coleman's assessment of the status of the public school system made this type of assumption.[25] A school system is made up of programs, resources, and teachers, but no one knows which of many profiles of programs and so forth is best in helping children to do well in school, as measured by standard tests. (Economists call this relationship the "educational production function.") The status of the public school system was judged by comparing the achievement of minority youngsters and the achievement of middle–class children who attended schools with various levels of resources. Hospital coronary care units monitor patients for several days following a myocardial infarction to reduce mortality. It is unclear how a different profile of resources, administrative practices, or surveillance techniques would influence mortality rates. In each example, the measures of a desirable outcome seem clear, but the means for producing the desired outcome are not. In such settings, managers tend to set targets or use standards. What March and Simon call a satisficing decision rule is used.[26] For instance, mortality rates in a coronary care unit are compared to the mortality in high–status hospitals. An optimizing rule provides a stronger test of program merit than a satisficing decision rule.

For Case III, performance measures are perceived to be either uncertain or ambiguous. No absolute and uniformly accepted standards for judging performance are believed to exist, but functioning can be observed. An empirical test is used. For example, hospitals can be observed providing care, but care is measured on one set of grounds by patients, still another by physicians, and still a third by regulators such as third–party payers and health systems agencies. Patients respond to personalized services and attention. Physicians judge hospitals in terms of the resources and facilities open to them. Blue Cross and other regulatory agencies measure the hospital's occupancy, cost per patient day, and the like. In other instances, it is convenient to contend that performance cannot be measured. For instance, health providers resist quantifying the outcomes of treatment, contending that "you can't define quality, but you know when it's missing."[27] Because a desired outcome is unclear, health organizations tend to monitor the process of care. As a result, most quality assessment activities have a reviewer, or review group, examine the process of care to determine if the process follows accepted steps. If the care process conforms to the accepted steps, care quality is labeled good, regardless of the treatment outcome. Standards applied by accreditation organizations like the Joint Commission on Hospital Accreditation, stress the availability of resources, not outcomes. Thus, accreditation is based on the capacity to act, not the actions of a hospital. The empirical test applies a feasibility decision rule, which is weaker than the satisficing test. As a result, feasibility tests are less diagnostic than satisficing tests.

In Case IV both the cause and effect relationships and the performance measures are assumed to be vague, ambiguous, or unknown. Under this assumption neither optimization, satisficing, nor workability tests can be applied. Rather, the sponsor looks for a reference group and matches performance against this group. The sponsor seeks to demonstrate that the organization's operations, services, and the like are doing at least as well as similar programs in high–status organizations. For instance, when HEW evaluated comprehensive health planning agencies (now health systems agencies), they selected a few agencies they thought were well run and compared the practices of other agencies with this reference group. This type of evaluation was predictable because the objectives of planning agencies were vague and thus difficult to measure and because few believed that the process of planning could control the unbridled growth of health services. Similarly, hospital administrators often use social tests when they attempt to demonstrate that their facilities are comparable to high–status hospitals and when they collect testimonials from well–known people. Social tests are the weakest of all decision rules and the most likely to lead to pseudoevaluation as described in Chapter 8. Evaluation using social tests often consists of little more than visiting organizations believed to be high status in order to compare practices.

A sponsor's assumptions dictate the decision rule. An inappropriate decision rule limits the value of an evaluation project. For instance, an evaluation may be required to identify an optimum level of performance. When the intervention is subject to the influence of many factors not fully understood, an optimization decision rule cannot be applied. An overly stringent decision rule may thwart the evaluation by focusing it on unobtainable goals. Sponsors that mount studies to determine "how we should be doing" in areas like hospital revenues or coronary care unit mortality assume that some absolute standard of comparison exists. On the other hand, the sponsor's assumptions may force the use of a weaker decision rule than circumstances warrant. For instance, organizations often apply a social test when a more definitive form of evaluation is possible. For example, counseling services often record the number of cases or referrals when measures of their client's behavior (a satisficing decision rule) could be used.

To insure that an appropriate decision rule is adopted, the assumptions used by the sponsor to form the causal model must be carefully inspected. The evaluator attempts to relax restrictive assumptions, following the guidelines established for the evaluation dialogue discussed in Chapter 8, so the most diagnostic evaluation can be carried out.

Interpretation—and Possibly More Evaluation

Figure 9-2 describes how the diagnostic process serves as the repository of information garnered from the evaluation process. Evaluation findings are linked to the stimulus through an "interpretation." The interpretation may consist of determining the extent to which findings confirm the decision maker's expectations. In other instances, the problem may have changed, calling for an interpretation of the findings in light of recent developments, which involve conditions or circumstances considered only obliquely by the project. If evaluation findings cannot be interpreted in terms of the changed conditions or when they fail to confirm the manager's expectations, a choice cannot be made and conflict remains. The manager (now in the role of a decision maker) may choose to discard the results or repeat the evaluation process.

NORMS AND THEIR FORMATION

Decision makers seldom disclose their norms. Barriers to disclosure include a low level of understanding or the appearance of caprice, as norms can be highly situational. To insure survival, consultation with power centers in an organization is required, and these consultations may alter the decision maker's norms.

Norms are often situational and may be changed by opportunities and by the demands of power figures. Norms stemming from opportunities are seldom revealed until all the personal benefits they offer can be extracted. For instance, a new approach for increasing reimbursement, picked up by a hospital financial manager at a continuing education seminar, may alter his "volume-adjusted revenue" expectations. These new norms are kept under wraps until the application of the reimbursement strategies can be shown to improve the hospital's revenue picture. Key members of a hospital's medical staff may successfully lobby for the latest breed of patient monitors to be placed in all the hospital's intensive care wards. The increased cost of care creates a new cost norm which an administrator must defend. Thus either opportunities or pressure can alter a manager's norms.

Disclosing norms is tantamount to losing power.[28] Managers seldom permit careful analysis of their choices, let alone analysis of the norms used to form these choices. For instance, inventory control procedures require administrators to specify how *often* they can tolerate running out of various types of hospital supplies. The hospital purchasing officer is asked to reveal his/her intuitive decision rules (norms). Managers view disclosure of this type of information as potentially damaging to their job or career, and they seldom fully comply.

Similarly, Goldberg demonstrated that the modeling can dramatically improve the reliability and validity of medical diagnosis.[29] Betaque and Gorry and Gustafson found that models which represent the process of medical diagnosis can be built by quantifying elements of the (partially) intuitive process used by physicians in diagnosing renal failure and thyroid disease.[30,31] The application of these methods has been limited by the reluctance of physicians to make their norms explicit. Physicians are threatened by the implications of "medical decision aids" and have little motivation to cooperate —to share their decision rules.

EXPLICATING NORMS

Analysts may look to a manager's behavior to infer their norms. By examining the information used to make decisions, inferences can be drawn which suggest the norms used by managers.

Recurring Decisions

When a particular decision occurs repeatedly, norms can be studied using a process called "decision analysis." Decision simulations, or actual decisions, can be analyzed to reveal norms.

Huber contends that most norms are multidimensional.[32] Several criteria must be used to judge a situation, and decision makers may attach particular weight to each criterion. For example, decisions in a surgical intensive–care unit result in interventions like closed and open chest massage, adrenaline, paddles, and the like. The occurrence of arrhythmias, augmented by EKG findings, spirometry and bloodgas readings, blood intake and urine output, and the like are routinely monitored, implying that changes in the levels of these indicators signal the need for an intervention. A decision model can be built which defines the norms used by physicians to signal the need for an intervention.

An additive decision model is constructed as shown below:[33]

$$Y_j = \sum_i b_i X_{ij}$$

where b_i = importance of criterion i
$\sum b_i = 1$

X_{ij} = criterion i (e.g., arrhythmias) for patient j
Y_j = An index for the jth patient

The norm is inferred from the levels of criteria which cause the physician to intervene. Y_j must be greater than some critical value, as shown below:

$$Y_j = b_1 X_{1j} + b_2 X_{2j} + \ldots + b_n X_{nj}$$

In some instances, some of the criteria that make up the norm have, in practice, zero weights. The decision maker behaves as though these criteria have no value in making decisions. A zero weight is implicitly assigned and the information is ignored. For instance, some physicians contend that interventions in a surgical intensive–care unit should be dictated by one criterion,[34] as shown below:

$$X_1 \text{ (arrhythmias)} > 0$$

To identify which criteria are important, regression and other correlational techniques are used to relate decisions (adrenaline, closed chest massage, etc.) to levels of each criterion. Beta weights from regression indicate the relative importance decision makers attach to each criterion when making decisions. A medical record that lists interventions and information describing patients' vital signs provides a data source for the analysis. In other instances, data archives may fail to record data with the needed precision, and behavioral simulations must be carried out. For example, Goldberg derived the norms used by radiologists in diagnosing stomach cancer by having them read x–rays from patients after surgery revealed their true condition.[35] The radiologists examined each x–ray and, using cues (criteria) they contend are contained in an x–ray, selected between a diagnosis of stomach cancer and ulcers.

Factorial designs are used to form the simulated decision tasks which permit the analyst to obtain independent estimates of weights for criteria and criteria interactions. The decision maker is confronted with several hypothetical decisions, described by levels of several criteria, and asked to make a judgment or prediction. For example, a nurse staffing model was built by considering severity indicators such as white blood count, platelets, temperature, and stage of disease (e.g., recently diagnosed, remission, relapse, terminal, or imminent death).[36] A factorial of four variables, with two levels for a linear model, is shown in Table 9–3. The decision maker (nurse supervisor) estimated the number of nursing hours needed for each patient. Decisions (hours) were correlated with the criteria levels to identify the importance of each criterion.

Similarly, physicians often balk at specifying a patient's severity, and indirect methods must be used. For example, to permit a comparison of outcomes (e.g., mortality, morbidity, length of stay) for various hospital emergency rooms, patient condition must be considered.[37] A severity index was constructed to classify the condition of patients with ischemic heart disease. Table 9–4 lists the severity criteria. A factorial of all combinations of levels for these criteria created 96 profiles ($2\times3\times2\times2\times4$), which represented two levels for primary arrhythmias, three levels for types of myocardial infarction, two levels for patient age, two for the time since the onset of symptoms, and four types of complications. Physicians skilled in the treatment of ischemic heart

Table 9-3. Patient Profiles for a Hematology Ward Using a Factorial of Severity Indicators

Patient	White blood count	Platelets	Temperature (°F)	Patient condition
1	500	0	104	imminent death
2	4,000	0	104	"
3	500	15,000	104	"
4	4,000	15,000	104	"
5	500	0	100	"
6	4,000	0	100	"
7	500	15,000	100	"
8	4,000	15,000	100	"
9	500	0	104	recently diagnosed
10	4,000	0	104	"
11	500	15,000	104	"
12	4,000	15,000	104	"
13	500	0	100	"
14	4,000	0	100	"
15	500	15,000	100	"
16	4,000	15,000	100	"

Nurse supervisors estimate the number of nursing hours by category (RN, LPN, Aid, etc.) per shift, for each of the 16 patients.

Table 9-4. Severity Criteria for Ischemic Heart Disease

Criteria	Criteria Levels
Primary arrhythmia	The existence of primary arrhythmias. 1. Significant: Ventricular fibrillation or asystole, ventricular tachycardia, or complete heart block 2. Nonsignificant: All other categories
Myocardial infarction	A diagnosis of myocardial infarction. 1. The presence of a transmural myocardial infarction 2. A nontransmural myocardial infarction 3. Myocardial infarction not diagnosed
Age	Age of Patient 1. 60 or older 2. Under 60
Time	Time elapsed since onset of symptoms (chest pain) to management 1. Symptoms persisted more than 4 hours 2. Symptoms persisted less than 4 hours
Complications	The presence of complicating conditions 1. The presence of cardiac shock and pulmonary edema, and cardiac arrest 2. Presence of cardiac shock, or pulmonary edema 3. Mild congestive heart failure 4. No complicating conditions

disease rated the severity of each of the 96 patient profiles on a continuous scale of 0 (not life-threatening) to 100 (certain death). The ratings were correlated with criteria to specify how each criterion was weighted by the panel. The weights attached to the main effects and interactions was used to form a severity index (norm).

Unique Decisions

Unique or infrequent decisions, and decisions charged with tension, must be assessed using situational information. Ritti and Funkhouser describe a way to decipher a manager's norms using what they call "informal game theory."[38] Imagine that you are an enterprising staff person in a large hospital. To enhance your prestige, you have worked tirelessly to develop an innovative plan to provide outpatient care. The outpatient care plan has been costed and tested against the perceptions of respected peers and seems tight. Naturally, having put all this effort into the plan development, you hope to retain the lion's share of the credit, and present it in this way to the administrator, who promptly rejects the idea. The payoffs for the manager are shown in Table 9-5.

In this situation, the manager may appear unenthusiastic or may block the idea. He/she has little to lose if others adopt the plan and it proves to be successful (situation III). As Cyert and March point out, decision makers are seldom penalized for a failure to innovate.[39] The manager's gains in situation I will also be modest; the staffer has seen to that. At best the manager can bask in the reflected glory of his subordinate, a small gain. But adopting a bad program is likely to create sizable personal losses for the manager (situation II). Finally, in situation IV, the manager neither gains nor loses by rejecting the plan. (Managers seldom attempt to demonstrate that they have rejected a bad idea.) Nothing was attempted, so no gain can be realized.

The staffer, understanding these norms, can attempt to salvage his/her project by adopting a cooptative or an evaluative strategy. Evaluation would attempt to demonstrate that the prospects of failure are remote. In this case the evaluation must show that the chance of success must exceed 80 percent (see Table 9-5). A rational decision maker would reject the plan even if it had an 80 percent chance of success, as shown below:

$$\text{endorse plan} = .8 \, (+1) + .2 \, (-10) = 0.8 - 2.0 = -1.2$$
$$\text{reject plan} = .8 \, (-1) + .2 \, (0) = -.8 + 0 = -.8$$

The manager will attempt to minimize his/her losses and will always reject a plan that has these payoffs.

Table 9-5: Inferring Norms Using Informal Game Theory

PLANS SUITABILITY

		Yes (.8)	No (.2)
		Situation I	Situation II
		manager gains a little	manager loses a lot
		(+1)	(-10)
	YES		
Decision			
To		Situation III	Situation IV
Endorse		manager loses a little	no payoff
Plan	NO		
		(-1)	(0)

To coopt, the manager is asked to share credit for stimulating, nurturing, or even developing the plan. While risky, this can be done by merely announcing the "contributions" of the manager or by giving implicit assurances that these contributions will be formally recognized. Cooptation increases the decision maker's payoff if the plan turns out to be successful.[40] To represent cooptation, where credit is shared equally, a payoff of +5 for situation I, and −5 for situation II, is shown in Table 9-6. In this case, with only a 50 percent chance of success, the manager's gains and losses are balanced, as shown below:

$$\text{endorse plan} = .5(5) + .5(-10) = -2.5$$
$$\text{reject plan} = .5(-5) + .5(0) = -2.5$$

A rational decision maker would endorse the plan when its chance of success was greater than 50/50.[41]

Table 9-6: Changing Payoffs by Cooptation

		PLANS SUITABILITY	
		Yes (.5)	No (.5)
		I	II
Decision	YES	(+5)	(-10)
To			
Endorse		III	IV
The Plan	NO	(-5)	(0)

SUMMARY

This chapter described the behavior of decision makers as they recognize problems which merit action. Managerial diagnosis is prompted by conflict arising out of a comparison of expectations with performance information. The diagnostic process attempts to alleviate conflict. Twenty-five distinct decision situations were described which stimulate a decision maker to commit resources for either planning or evaluation, or to defer action. The decision maker compares observed performance to expectations (norms) to select among these responses. Thus, an understanding of the decision maker's norms and when the decision maker will seek to clarify these norms, was found to be crucial to understanding the decision maker's behavior.

Evaluation was found to be the most common response, followed by deferral, which in turn was followed by planning. Evaluation and deferral were predicted in situations where planning seems more appropriate. As a result, the costs of inquiry may be inflated because evaluation may be carried out when planning seems more appropriate. Selecting the wrong mode of inquiry may discredit both planning and evaluation. At best, planning is conducted with time constraints, and at worst, not attempted at all. Evaluation, focused on situations that are unlikely to reveal anything new about performance, also loses credibility.

Managerial diagnosis was found to dictate, in a large part, the basic assumptions which guide evaluation. These assumptions can dramatically limit the usefulness of results produced by evaluation projects. The decision maker's assumption should match the most diagnostic decision rules that can be applied. Finally, a framework was provided to understand and to make explicit a decision maker's norms.

NOTES

1. This chapter was drawn in part from Nutt, P.C. "Calling Out and Calling Off the Dogs: Managerial Diagnosis in Public Organizations," *Academy of Management Review*, Vol. 4, No. 2, April 1979, pp. 203–214.
2. Mintzberg, H., D. Raisinghani, and A. Theoret, "The Structure of Unstructured Decision Process," *Administrative Science Quarterly*, Vol. 21, No. 2, June 1976, pp. 246–275.
3. *Ibid.*
4. This model has been adapted from March, J.G. and H.A. Simon, "Conflict in Organizations," *Organizations*. New York: Wiley, 1958, to describe how Mintzberg's conception of diagnosis may operate in selecting among deferment, evaluation, and planning as responses to conflict.
5. Henderson, J.A. and P.C. Nutt, "On the Design of Planning Information Systems," *Academy of Management Review*, Vol. 4, No. 3, Oct. 1978, pp. 774–785.
6. Mintzberg, Raisinghani and Theoret, p. 248.
7. Pounds, W.F., "The Process of Problem Finding," *Industrial Management Review*, Fall 1969, pp. 1–19.
8. A full discussion of the "planning response" is beyond the scope of this chapter. Interested readers are referred to Nutt, P.C., "The Method Variable," The Ohio State University, College of Administrative Science, Sept. 1977; Ackoff, R. and F. Emery, *Purposeful Systems*, New York: Aldine–Atherton, 1972; and C.W. Churchman, *The Design of Inquiring Systems*, New York: Basic Books, 1971.
9. In many circumstances performance information may be questioned. In each of the 25 situations, it is assumed that the decision maker believes the performance information is accurate.
10. Cyert, R.M. and F.G. March, *A Behavioral Theory of the Firm*. Englewood Cliffs, N.J.: Prentice–Hall, 1964.

11. When information that describes system performance is questioned, evaluation is often used to clarify the information. Situations 11 to 17 in Table 9-1 become situations 1, 2, 3, or 4 because uncertainty now characterizes the current information state, dictating an evaluation response.
12. Churchman, C.W., *The Systems Approach*, p. 215. New York: Dell, 1968.
13. March, J.G. and H.A. Simon, "Conflict in Organization," *Organization*. New York: Wiley, 1958.
14. Liefer, R., "Organizational/Environmental Interchange: A Model of Boundary Spanning Activity," *Academy of Management Review*, Vol. 3, No. 1, Jan. 1978, pp. 40–50.
15. Suchman, E.A., *Evaluation Research: Principles and Practice in Public Service & Social Action Organizations*, Washington, D.C.: Russell Sage, 1967.
16. *Ibid.*
17. Wholey, J., J.W. Scanlon, H.G. Duffy, J.S. Fukumoto, and L.M. Vogt, *Federal Evaluation Policy*. Washington, D.C.: The Urban Institute, 1971.
18. March and Simon, p. 115.
19. Dearborn, D.C. and H.A. Simon, "Selective Perception: A Note on the Departmental Identification of Executives," in Alexis, M. and Wilson, C.F., *Organizational Decision Making*, Englewood Cliffs, N.J.: Prentice–Hall, 1967.
20. Ferrence, T.P. "Organizational Communication Systems and the Decision Process," *Management Science*, Vol. 17, No. 2, 1970, pp. B83–B96.
21. Delbecq, A. and A. Van de Ven, "A Group Process Model for Problem Identification and Program Planning," *The Journal of Applied Behavioral Science*, Vol. 7, 1971, pp. 466–492.
22. Thompson, J.D. *Organizations in Action*, p. 84. New York: McGraw–Hill, 1967.
23. Suchman, p. 39.
24. Stimson, D. and R. Stimson, *Operations Research in Hospitals: Diagnosis & Prognosis*, Chicago, Ill.: HRET, 1972, Chapter 2, "A Review of Quantitative Studies."
25. Coleman, J.S., "Equal Schools or Equal Students," *Public Interest*, Vol. 1, Summer 1966, pp. 70–75.
26. March and Simon, p. 140.
27. The evaluator, of course, should respond by indicating, "You tell me how you know it's good and we'll define it!"
28. Henderson, J.C., R.R. McDaniel Jr., and G.R. Wagner, "The Implementation Operations Management/Management Science Modeling Techniques," The Ohio State University, Working Paper Series WPS 76–2, January 1976.
29. Goldberg, L.P., "Man Vs. Model of Man: A Rationale Plus Evidence For A Method of Improving Clinical Inferences," *Psychology Bulletin*, Vol. 73, No. 6, 1970, pp. 422–432.
30. Betaque, N.E. and G.A. Gorry, "Automating Judgmental Decision Making for a Serious Medical Problem," *Management Science*, Vol. 17, No. 8, 1971, pp. 421–434.
31. Gustafson, D.H. "Evaluation of Probabilistic Information Processing in Medical Decision Making," *Organizational Behavioral and Human Performance*, Vol. 4, 1969, pp. 20–34.
32. Huber, G.P., "Multi–Attribute Utility Models: A Review of Field and Field–Like Studies," *Management Science*, Vol. 20, No. 10, 1974, pp. 1,393–1,402).
33. More complex model forms can be used to describe how decision rules or norms are constructed by decision makers. For instance, "conjunctive models" suggest that indicators have critical values which must be exceeded before an action is taken. These models have cut–off points for criteria. "Lexicographic models" order criteria, and decisions are based on examining the most important criteria, as a screen, before proceeding. Criteria are used to rule out action. (Einhorn H., "The Use of Non–Linear,

Compensatory Models in Decision Making," *Psychology Bulletin,* Vol. 73, No. 3, 1970, p. 223). Huber's 1974 Literature Review (Ref. 32) finds that linear models provide the best approximation for most applications.

34. The experts (physicians) contend that only arrhythmias signal the need for an intervention. This contention raises several interesting points. First, why are SICU patients' blood, intake, urine output, and the like recorded with such compulsive precision? Why have hospitals purchased elaborate SICU monitoring systems which display EKG tracings on line, when only heart rhythm presages the need for an intervention? Why are elaborate systems designed to record unimportant indicators and why do hospitals record and store, in perpetuity, values for these unimportant indicators? These systems cannot be cost effective if the experts are correct.

35. Goldberg, "Man," p. 422–432.

36. Nutt, P.C., The Acceptance and Accuracy of Decision Analysis Methods," *Management Science* (in press).

37. This project was carried out by the author under a grant supported by the National Center for Health Services Research, with D.H. Gustafson, D.G. Fryback and J.H. Rose as the principal investigators. For details see Gustafson, D.H., D.G. Fryback, and J.H. Rose, "Severity Index Research Project Interim Report," University of Wisconsin–Madison, Center for Health Systems Research and Analysis, June 1978.

38. Ritti, R.R. and G.R. Funkhouser, *The Ropes to Know and the Ropes To Skip.* Columbus: Grid, 1977.

39. See note 9.

40. Nutt, P.C., "On the Quality and Acceptance of Plans Drawn By Consortiums," *The Journal of Applied Behavioral Science,* Vol. 14, No. 4, Winter 1978. Bargaining and political processes are described in Chapter 10.

41. For the sake of simplicity, the planning response was not included in this discussion.

Evaluation and Decision Making[1]

> ...there is nothing more difficult to carry out, nor more doubtful of success, nor
> more dangerous to handle, than to initiate a new order of things.
>
> Machiavelli, *The Prince*

DECISION STRATEGIES

Decision making is defined as a process with evaluative and judgmental phases.[2] Evaluation clarifies the properties of the alternatives and may also provide a quantitative index to describe the value of each alternative considered.[3] Judgment is used to frame the decision–making task and to sift and weigh evaluation information in order to select among alternative courses of action.[4] A decision strategy describes how analytic and forensic principles are used to carry out the evaluative and the judgmental phases of decision making. The distinguishing feature of a decision strategy is the nature and sequence of steps which pertain to gathering evaluation information and making judgments.

An *analytic decision strategy* assumes that evaluation information is highly diagnostic. Judgment is used to qualify and bring out meaning in evaluation information, so decisions often rest on interpretations of evaluative data. Analytical decision models assume that important decision criteria can be quantified and measured.

This type of strategy can be termed "mechanistic" because it represents natural processes in machinelike terms. Analytic strategies tend to make what Thompson calls a "closed system" assumption.[5] Environmental influences are largely ignored and causal relationships are simplified to permit quantification. For instance, purchasing decisions may be based on analysis of the provisions in each vendor's purchasing agreement. The relationship between quality and delivery guarantees can be balanced against penalty clauses and quantity discounts. Information from an evaluation identifies the vendor with the most favorable contract. Similarly, hospitals can let the findings of an evaluation dictate whether their laboratories should introduce technological advances like autoanalyzers. Evaluation data can dictate choice because the autoanalyzer's cost, test accuracy, turn–around time, and the like have causal relationships which permit quantification.

A *forensic decision strategy* relies on some form of debate. The debate stems from reflection or from talking with others. When using a forensic strategy, the decision maker juxtaposes the features of various options inwardly, through reflection, by considering a debate between a member of a group, or both. During the debate, the decision maker uses his/her intuition and experience to qualify and/or discard information which forms the basis for the decision.[6] As a result, forensic strategies are often homeostatic: decisions are often set out to monitor the reaction of important reference groups.[7] The intensity and nature of their reactions suggest adjustments which can lead to acceptable, if not optimal, courses of action. Forensic strategies have a somewhat jaundiced view of evaluation information. As a result, evaluation tends to be used selectively, often to confirm the wisdom of the preferred alternative or to "posture," giving the decision process the appearance of objectivity. Judgment is used to clarify the decision task and to isolate the preferred course(s) of action.

In a forensic strategy, decisions are perceived as "organic" because they deal with causal relationships which have components that resist quantification. Most of these strategies treat decision–making as "open system" where causal relations are thought to be influenced by a myriad of environmental factors that make evaluation seem both expensive and unlikely to produce usable information.[8] For instance, hospitals judge the feasibility of adding beds by announcing their intentions to expand and monitoring the reactions of regulatory agencies, banks, and other sources of capital, as well as power centers within the hospital and the community. The decision maker judges the prospects for success by contemplating the statements of important reference groups. Similarly, decisions which judge the fitness of a mental health clinic are often based on comparisons with high–status clinics. The decision is seen as organic because patient mix, medical staff quality, and a host of other factors are difficult to measure and quantify and because the relationships between these factors and cost, care quality, and the like are obscure.

Both analytical and forensic strategies have been developed which seem particularly suited for closed–system, mid–range, and open–system applications. In Figure 10.1, six decision strategies are classified according to their forensic and analytic features and their organic and mechanistic assumptions.

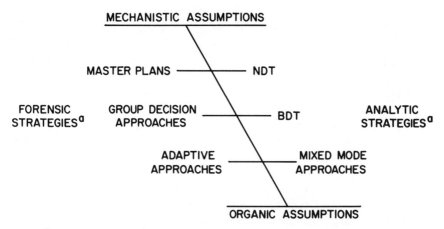

MECHANISTIC ASSUMPTIONS

MASTER PLANS ———— NDT

FORENSIC
STRATEGIES[a]

GROUP DECISION ———— BDT
APPROACHES

ANALYTIC
STRATEGIES[a]

ADAPTIVE ———— MIXED MODE
APPROACHES   APPROACHES

ORGANIC ASSUMPTIONS

[a]The role of evaluation and judgment and the extent to which factors must
be quantified are dominant assumptions of a decision strategy.

Figure IO.I SOME FEATURES OF DECISION-MAKING STRATEGIES

Reprinted with permission from Nutt, P.C., "Some Considerations In Selecting Interactive and Analytical Decision Approaches," *Medical Care,* Vol. 36, No. 2, p. 154, (Feb 1979).

MECHANISTIC STRATEGIES

Master Plans

Decisions are based on judgments which interpret a master plan.[9] The master plan provides rules governing contingencies, performance expectations, and the like, and gives procedures to interpret them for decision-making tasks. For instance, employment commission managers use a master plan which states conditions for granting unemployment, CETA, and other benefits. The manager must apply rules in the master plan to the individual circumstances of its claimants. Civil Service regulations, which govern personnel policies in many public organizations, also provide a master plan to guide decision making. The regulations must be consulted to arrive at defensible decisions concerning hiring, dismissal, transfer, and the like.

Decision groups also use master plans. For instance, an organization's "personnel committee," seeking to dismiss an employee working under a union contract, must ensure that the grounds for dismissal are supported by, or at least in harmony with, the provisions of the union contract. Federal agencies when selecting project proposals often demand that the applicant carefully describe how funds, if awarded, will be used. Funded proposals become the equivalent of master plans. For example, when federal agencies solicited emergency medical service (EMS) projects, detailed proposals were demanded. The proposals were required to identify specific objectives and a specific plan of action based on these objectives for each component of an EMS system (e.g., a 911 telephone number for reporting emergencies, vehicle dispatch, etc.) defined by those issuing the request for proposal. Funded proposals became master plans. EMS councils, composed of local EMS sponsors, were expected to derive decision premises from those in the proposal. The EMS council and others receiving federal funds, such as the Board of Directors of United Way agencies and Head Start programs, are often shocked to find that they must demonstrate how their decisions square with the premises stated in their proposal. Master plans like these allow little room for a decision group to maneuver.

Decision makers are expected to stay within their budget and display sufficient ingenuity in their judgments to avoid confrontations which lower the credibility of their organization or organizational unit. Consequently, demonstrated skill in interpreting a master plan is typically used to select decision makers. Promotion and other rewards are often based on adhering to the master plan.

Master plans are useful in decision–making environments that tend to be mechanistic and closed system. Organizations can amortize the costs of devising master plans when the environment is stable and decisions tend to recur. Careful study (or experience) should reveal decisions that occur with regularity. The mechanistic features of these decision tasks permit evaluation to associate (desirable) outcomes with particular courses of action. The decision maker(s) consults the master plan to find a situation comparable to the decision task at hand, selects a course of action, and develops a rationale for the action. Evaluation information is fit into stock situations.

For a master plan to be successful as a guide, a predictable environment is a necessity. In many organizations, master plans are pressed into service when the decision–making environment lacks the needed degree of predictability. For example, a hospital's domain (defined as the emergence or disappearance of regulating agencies, new services, public and physician support, new technology, endowments and other sources of financial support, and the like) may shift.[10] As an organization's domain shifts, decision premises shift with it and new rules (master plans) are required. Dynamic environments drive up the costs of preparing master plans and reduce their reliability. Organizations that devise master plans often fail to consider whether they will be applied in a stable environment.

Normative Decision Theory

Normative Decision Theory (NDT) is an analytic approach that demands quantative information. The decision maker, aided by an analyst, is asked to describe a set of alternatives (A_i); identify a mutually exclusive and exhaustive set of states of nature (S_j); estimate the probability (P_j) that each state will occur; indicate a preference for each alternative (A_i); implemented in an environment described by S_j; and provide a set of criteria X_k to judge the intrinsic value of A_i.[11] For example, an EMS Council may grant a franchise to provide a regional dispatching service of EMS vehicles, by considering proposals from several organizations, as shown in Table 10-1. Each proposal (A_i) is judged considering the expected levels of service volume (S_j) and the likelihood each projected level of transportation volume will occur (P_j). Evaluation information indicates the preferred course of action.

Alternatives are judged by systematically comparing their properties measured by criteria. For example, proposed EMS dispatch services can be evaluated by criteria such as their cost (C), down-time (T), and capacity (V).

Table 10-1.   Selecting Proposals for an EMS Dispatch Service
Using the NDT Decision Model

STATE VARIABLES

Dispatch Service Alternatives	State 1 EMS transports 50% less than plan estimates	State 2 EMS transports as estimated	State 3 EMS transports 50% more than plan estimates	
	$P = .15$	$P = .80$	$P = .05$	Likelihood State will occur
Proposal 1	U_{11}	U_{12}	U_{13}	
Proposal 2	U_{21}	U_{22}	U_{23}	
o o o	o o o	o o o	o o o	
Proposal n	U_{n1} Evaluation of pro-position n, if state 1 occurs	U_{n2} Evaluation of pro-posal n, assuming state 2	U_{n3} Evaluation of pro-posal n, assuming state 3	

U = Value of proposal, determined by summing the impact of several criteria to judge proposals and their importance

= $b_1 X_1$(charge to patients) + $b_2 X_2$(response time) + $b_3 X_3$(equipment provided by EMS vehicles)

(where b_1, b_2, b_3 are criteria weights that sum to 100)

Value of proposal 1 = $(.15) (U_{11}) + .80(U_{12}) + (.05)U_{13}$

Thus, a multiattribute index must be used to judge the merits of each alternative.[12] A multiplicative and an additive index are shown below:

Multiplicative Evaluation Index: $U_i = C_iV_i(1 - T_i)$
Additive Evaluation Index: $U_i = \Sigma_k b_k x_{ik}$
  where U_i = the utility of alternative i
    X_{ik} = criteria k (such as cost) for alternative i
    b_k = the weight (importance) of criteria k set by the decision maker(s)

The decision rule is called "subjective expected utility" (SEU). SEU is used because evaluation establishes a value for each alternative (A_i) by considering the probability (P_j) of each state (S_j) and the subjective weight attached to criteria (X_k) by the decision maker(s). Normative decision theory postulates that a rational decision maker seeks to maximize his subjective expected utility by selecting the A_i (alternative) with maximum $\Sigma_j P_j U_{ij}$ (utility). U_{ij} is the evaluation of alternative i in state j. The properties of each alternative A_i, measured by criteria X_k, are often influenced by S_j. For example, several levels of potential usage (S_i) for a counseling service are conceivable. The evaluation index (U_i) must consider how differential use rates influence cost, client satisfaction, and other evaluation criteria.

The decision rule is simplified when a single state exists (demand is known). The A_i with the maximum utility is determined by the criteria and the criteria weights. If the P_j and/or S_j (which indicate the likelihood of various use rates) are unknown, a "Laplace criterion" is often used ($P_1 = P_2 = P_3 = \ldots$). This merely multiplies each alternative by a constant so the values of the criteria and criteria weights again dictate the alternative with the greatest utility. (A "maximin" decision rule locates the state S_j with the highest probability P_j and picks the A_i with maximum U_i that falls in that column. Maximin, minimax, and related decision rules are suboptimal when state probabilities can be estimated.)

The NDT strategy has had many important applications. For example, the "clinical judgment" literature indicates that the NDT strategy can improve the reliability and validity of individuals or groups of decision makers facing complex decision–making tasks like medical diagnosis,[13] selecting medically underserved areas to identify priorities for HEW funding,[14] and determining the quality of care in a nursing ward.[15]

Simon and others have isolated several problems with the NDT strategy.[16] They point out that the computations for NDT are virtually impossible to complete for a broad range of complex decision–making tasks. One can seldom generate *all* relevant alternatives. And when a relevant alternative is overlooked, utility cannot be maximized. Estimating the probability for states (like use rates for a counseling service) can be a formidable task. Further, Mechanic finds that decision making is often influenced by values often not fully understood by the decision maker(s).[17] For many decision–making tasks it is not clear who should define and weight criteria. For instance, stockholders, customers, the public at large, Ralph Nader and others who contend they are surrogate citizens, funding agents, and politicians all insist that they should have a role in deciding where a public utility should locate a nuclear power plant. Consequently, computing a U_i with criteria weights specified by a decision maker(s), no matter how carefully its members are selected, can be surrounded by controversy. Huber points out that transient preferences (unstable weights b_k) make it difficult to measure preferences and that problems in gaining the confidence of the decision maker(s) to obtain preference measurements pose substantive methodological problems for the NDT.[18]

MID-RANGE STRATEGIES

Group Decision Making

Group decision making is based on what Churchman calls a "community of minds."[19] The members of a decision–making group attempt to agree on the meaning of evaluation information. When a group of experts supports a decision, it is thought to be objective.[20]

Decision making becomes a learning process in a decision group. Individuals contribute their experiences (implicit evaluations) and knowledge (implicit and explicit evaluations), which the group attempts to apply to the decision task. Groups qualify, shape, and tune the evaluation data to fit their perceptions. Inconsistent data are pruned. Forecasts of qualitative information, like the sentiments of key reference groups, are combined with quantitative information. The views of persuasive members often dictate what information is used and how it is combined to make a final judgment. Mason contends that a synthesis of this information can provide important new perspectives.[21] Participation in a decision group has been found to promote the acceptance of a decision.[22]

To establish and manage a decision–making group, its formation, cohesion development, processes, and control must be considered. *Formation* concerns the identification of members who satisfy political constraints and information needs of the decision–making task. For example, surgeons, radiotherapists, and other providers; operating agents in hospitals; and public representatives are often asked to serve on decision–making groups for a state cancer society. Consumers may be included to define service problems, administrators and elected officials to sensitize the decision group to political and resource constraints, and experts to supply technical information.[23] Collins and Guetzkow find that heterogeneous member status and expertise in a decision-making group will reduce the group's effectiveness.[24]

As the group *coalesces,* relationships are built. During this phase, influence, interpersonal relations, aspirations, and rules are determined. Delbecq points out that a leader emerges or must be identified by an appropriate power figure.[25] Collins and Guetzkow indicate that a "socio-emotional" leadership style provides social rewards such as recognition and tension release.[26] This style is best for decision-making tasks stressing acceptance. "Task leaders" contribute more information but create tension. Task leaders are best to have when the decision must be defended by logical arguments. In resource allocation tasks, veto (one person can block) and consensus (all must agree) voting rules have been found less effective than a majority rule.[27]

The methods used to manage groups are the *processes* of group decision making. When soliciting evaluation information, interacting groups are generally superior to Synthetic, Nominal, and Delphi groups.[28] Collins and Guetzkow point out that the performance of an interacting group may be improved by recognizing that[29]

(1) some information is typically excluded, and one should coax it out with social rewards;

(2) inferior group members damage results and should be screened out if possible;

(3) group members may become defensive and social rewards, through the socioemotional leader, reduce participation penalties;

(4) group members may be inhibited when status distinctions are present, as this induces competition, and when unfavorable relations among members develop;

(5) one should avoid mixing participants who want issue power with those who seek personal power; and

(6) group members who support their ideas with logical arguments and show how their ideas are consistent with past experiences of the other group members have the most influence in interacting groups.

Gustafson, *et al.,* point out that structure can be added to an interacting group by an "estimate–discuss–estimate" sequence.[30] This procedure focuses discussion and permits a systematic sharing of information by the group, which promotes agreement. Nominal groups, and other group processes that stress silent reflection, are superior in managing the activities of a decision-making group when the task is vague and must be defined by setting objectives, establishing criteria, and specifying criteria weights.[31]

Groups are aften used to bargain. In dyad (two-person) bargaining, Schilling contends that it is best to "overload" an opponent with accurate information, since these facts cannot be overlooked.[32] In contrast, the first party to compromise tends to "lose" the most in group bargaining.[33] These findings were moderated by the potential for joint rewards among bargainers.

Control of group performance is made possible by manipulating rewards and penalties. Rewarding the entire group emphasizes the task but fails to recognize important individual contributions. To cope with this, social rewards can be used to increase the contributions from nonparticipants, or the group can divide the reward according to their beliefs about each individual's contributions. Collins and Guetzkow suggest that penalties should be avoided unless the rationale of the penalty is clear and compliance can be observed.[34]

Group decision making is often carried out by stressing participation, which emphasizes the formulation and coalescing stages. Sponsors often ignore the process and control stages. For instance, Red Feather agencies and health planning under PL 89-749 and 93-641 manage their group decision making bodies by stressing participation formulas. This dramatically reduces the effectiveness of the decision group. Even when the sponsor follows each stage in the group decision model, problems may arise. Decision groups can be costly, cantankerous, hard to dismantle, unpredictable, and difficult to control. For instance, political considerations often dictate who must serve on the boards of directors of many organizations. When decisions that seem to be in the best interest of the organization threaten organizations represented by members of the board these members may engage in obstructive tactics.[35] In such situations, evaluation information is hard to introduce and is often ignored. Nonetheless, decision making groups are often the best way to get many sources of information considered and to make decisions acceptable to key administrators and their clients. For these reasons, group decision making is widely used.

Behavioral Decision Theory

Simon identifies a "decision space" (a sub-matrix of A_iS_j) to make NDT fit a wider range of decision tasks.[36] Before the search for the A_i's begins, "acceptable" states of nature are defined (levels of volume that make a service feasible). Alternatives are evaluated according to their effectiveness in these states. For example, federal agencies may require state departments of health to identify hospital emergency departments to serve as regional centers, receiving dispatched EMS vehicles. A state department of health may solicit proposals from hospitals to identify which hospitals will be designated to provide such a service. States are defined in the request for a proposal as levels of volume sufficient to operate a comprehensive emergency service in a hospital. Alternatives are sought (proposals stimulated by the health department) which fall in these states, as shown in Table 10–2. Since acceptable, not optimal, alternatives are sought, a "satisficing" decision rule is used. If acceptable alternatives are easy to find, Simon postulates that the decision maker's aspiration rises; if not, aspiration falls and an alternative with some undesirable features is adopted. Recognizing behavioral principles in decision–making is thought to interrelate the *evaluative* and *judgmental* aspects of decision making.

The satisficing and serial search aspects of the BDT strategy seems to portray the *behavior* of many decision–makers. Combining searching, learning, and decision–making is intuitively appealing. As Wildavsky points out, decision makers don't know what they want until they can see what they can get.[37] Cyert and March found that decision making in organizations was often a serial process with satisficing used as a decision rule.[38] The first acceptable alternative is typically adopted. Cravens,[39] Cyert and March,[40] Simon and Newell,[41] and others have observed that the search for new alternatives is limited to the vicinity of the current operations and practices. Decision makers move away from a familiar situation in a "progressively deepening" manner,

Table 10–2:   Judging Proposals To Provide Comprehensive Emergency Services Using the BDT Model

STATE VARIABLES (Number of Vehicle Trips Per Year)

Alternatives[a]	STATE A demand far below expectations	STATE B demand below expectations	STATE C demand at expectations	STATE D demand above expectations– convenience care visits stimulated	STATE E huge latent demand and convenience care visits stimulated
	Unknown	$P = .25$	$P = .50$	$P = .25$	Unknown
Proposal #1		U_{B_1}	U_{C_1}		
Proposal #2		U_{B_2}	U_{C_2}		
-		-	-		
-		-	-		
-		-	-		
Proposal n		U_{B_n}	U_{C_n}		

State B = .25/.75=1/3   State C = .50/.75=2/3

Value of Proposal #1 = $1/3 \ (U_{B_1}) + 2/3 \ (U_{C_1})$

Value of Proposal #2 = $1/3 \ (U_{B_2}) + 2/3 \ (U_{C_2})$

[a] Proposal from Hospitals asked to consider only states B & C.

tending to follow just a few alternatives with similar characteristics. But studies of changes in aspiration vis-à-vis a search have not found support for Simon's postulations.[42,43] Information regarding past successes (or failures) failed to influence the search. The decision–maker(s) also seems unduly influenced by uncertainty. As uncertainty increases, so does search time, care in making an evaluation, and resources allocated to the search process.[44] The BDT strategy describes what skillful decision makers *try* to do when grappling with complex decisions. Dawes contends that using BDT as a decision aid can improve decision making in many settings.[45]

ORGANIC STRATEGIES

Adaptive Decision Making

Gore and Lindblom advocate an adaptive decision–making strategy.[46,47] They believe that important decision–making tasks are organic and open system. Such decisions must consider many ill–defined variable and variable interactions, where no behavioral or normative theory exists to suggest a causal relationship among these variables, in an ambiguous and potentially threatening environment. Adaptive strategies evolved to cope with decisions that must be made under these conditions.

Judgments based on homeostatic–feedback control are the hallmark of adaptive decision making. This strategy avoids evaluation information because qualitative, not quantitative, data are believed to be diagnostic. Judgment is used to identify acceptable decisions using a "cut and try" approach.

A "tension network" identifies important decisions, as well as the partisans and/or beneficiaries of the decision.[48] A process of adjustment is used to make incremental decisions, as the views of partisans are revealed. No goals are set or even considered desirable. Explicit aims merely call for manipulation, as the organization's clients will reinterpret these aims to suit their needs.[49] The complexity of a decision–making task and its environment makes it difficult, if not impossible, for the organization to turn aside these claims. The adaptive model calls for the decision maker(s) to monitor a variety of power centers within the organization, as well as external groups. The emergence of sentiments and norms in these partisan groups are tested against current priorities. For instance, a medical school seeking to initiate a practice plan (where the clinical faculty turns over a percentage of its private practice income to the college) may suggest provisions of possible plans to monitor the reactions of the medical school faculty. The university administration can move toward the medical faculties' demands in small increments as preferences are revealed. Similarly, the American College of Surgeons may insist that an EMS council spend its grant funds to improve training for ambulance attendants. Tracking these views permits the council to move toward these "requests" in small increments as preferences are revealed. If managed with care, a partisan group may perceive the decision maker to be responsive and may moderate its requests, permitting the decision maker to shift his attention elsewhere. Good decisions find acceptance, or at least benign neglect, from affected parties. Thus decisions are not expected to correspond with any set of internally consistent logic. The decision maker merely adjusts to needs as they are expressed and *perceived* to be significant. When partisans make their wishes clear and unequivocal, the decision maker attempts to incorporate them in the final decision.

An adaptive decision strategy describes legislative decision–making and diplomacy as well as the behavior of many decision groups. Organizations must consult with the clients or beneficiaries of their services when their preferences are unknown. And to survive financially, organizations must match their priorities against those of funding agents. An equilibrium between competing interests must be maintained. Adaptive decisions result, and survival becomes the dominant decision criterion.

Some kind of rational order is required in a complex society competing for scarce resources.[50] For example, the insurance industry faces dynamic environments but has defined and quantified factors, such as probability of occurrence and the value of losses, to balance against needed investments, to form decision premises. An adaptive decision strategy seems workable only under extreme conditions, illustrated by decision tasks that are likely to resist analysis and that have a diffuse but potentially responsive reference group with a stake in the decision outcome.

The Mixed Mode Strategy

Mintzberg, *et al.*, contend that most important decisions are based on tradition and imitation.[51] In Mintzberg's studies, evaluation information was seldom sought and never applied. In contrast with the other analytic approaches, the *mixed mode* strategy recognizes that many decision makers fear unmanaged evaluation information,[52] and believe that experience is their best guide.[53] The strategy acknowledges that the manner in which decisions are made can be as important as the course of action selected. Important centers of power must be managed through their participation. Evaluation information must be carefully fitted to the decision maker's needs as they emerge. Evaluation information must also be subject to careful control: there should be no surprises. The mixed mode strategy relies on the decision maker(s) to frame causal relations for evaluation. An explicit judgmental process precedes evaluation, to define the decision's arena and goals, and follows it, to interpret the evaluation findings.

The mixed mode approach uses analysis, persuasion, bargaining, and political strategies in a particular sequence.[54] As shown in Table 10-3, the decision maker(s) considers the *arena* and *goals* of the decision task to specify an appropriate initial strategy. Goal conflict dictates that persuasion or bargaining must precede analysis carried out to provide evaluation information. The decision maker may identify a goal that has shared values through bargaining, or enlarge the goal to include the concerns of conflicting parties. If both the arena and goals are shifting, the decision maker seeks allies to build a coalition which will deal with some, if not all, issues. When an arena has been established, bargaining or persuasion may be used to set goals to guide analysis.

Goal conflicts may be managed by enlarging the goal. For example, selecting between state departments of "highway safety" and "vocational

Table 10-3:   Decision Making Strategies In The
Mixed Mode Decision Model

Decision Strategy	Arena (Scope)	Goals (Intent)	Processes
Analysis	Fixed	Fixed	Evaluation Methods
Persuasion	Fixed	Select among conflicting goals	Appeal to higher authority or search for a common goal referrent by enlarging arena
Bargaining	Fixed	Accept goal disagreement	Accept goal disagreement and define solution properties with shared values
Politics	Variable	Accept goal disagreement	Process of seeking allies, coalitions, etc., to define an arena that is acceptable to the coalition

Reprinted with permission from Nutt, P.C., "Same Considerations In Selecting Interactive and Analytical Decision Approaches," *Medical Care,* Vol. 36, No. 2, P. 154, (Feb 1979).

education" as managers of training programs for ambulance attendants can be difficult, if not impossible, if one compares the performance of each department in its educational activities. Enlarging the goals of education from meeting standards on tests to program continuity, allows an analytical strategy a chance to sort out which state department can best meet this broader goal. Alternatively, the decision maker can identify a goal that has shared values through bargaining. "Grandfather" clauses in EMS legislative bills may permit the continued operation of existing emergency transport services, forcing only new services to adopt strict requirements for the training of ambulance attendants. Analysis of the undesirable effects of grandfathering may cause controversy and result in the bill being defeated, but analysis focused on the desirable features of the bill may have a decisive effect on its passing. If both the arena and goals are shifting, the decision maker seeks allies to build a coalition which will deal with some, if not all, decisions. State departments of health may have to abandon plans which could close unstaffed emergency rooms in rural hospitals, in order to retain the support of legislators representing rural areas and county medical societies. When an arena has been established, bargaining or persuasion may be used to set goals to guide analysis, which provides evaluation information.

When decision makers ignore goal conflicts and shifting arenas, bargaining and politics will disrupt the evaluation process. Under these conditions, attempts to conduct analysis will accentuate the conflict, potentially aborting the decision. For example, Bryant's description of how General Dynamics was selected as the TFX contractor illustrates the way the decision maker, the U.S. Department of Defense, was distracted from bargaining by its preoccupation with analysis.[55] DOD policy makers and operating personnel (the Air Force and Navy) placed radically different weights on evaluation criteria used to select General Dynamics as the TFX contractor. Conflict was hidden in analytical procedures and not fully recognized until the U.S. Navy refused delivery of the F-111.

Several useful *bargaining devices* have been described in the literature. In order of increasing loss of autonomy, they include
(1) *contracting:* exchanges of resources for future performance assurances;
(2) *coopting:* absorbing representatives of unmanaged organizations or groups into existing decision–making mechanisms like directorates;
(3) *consortium:* delegating a decision task to a new decision group which represents several organizations, according to some formula;
(4) *absorption:* surrendering organizational autonomy.
Selecting an appropriate bargaining device plays a vital role in minimizing the compromises made with the decision group's members in defining goals. The arena of the decision–making task is used to identify who should serve on the

decision–making group. Goals are inferred from the mutual interest of this group. Weber showed that shared norms, norms consistent with organizational aims, can be attained when conflict is managed through inferred goals.[56]

Cooptation and consortium are mechanisms favored by many public and nonprofit organizations. For instance, EMS councils often use a consortium to allocate funds that stem from grants and contracts with third parties. The decision–making group is broadly representative of local interests and given the authority to allocate these funds among services provided by local organizations. Cooptation is often used to form a decision–making group that remains a captive of its sponsor. For example, hospital associations, health planning agencies, and community mental health centers set up such groups to garner support and legitimization from providers, politicians, and community power centers by allowing their representatives to serve on the organization's decision–making groups. The decision–making group is asked to select programs and make other decisions that balance competing interests in the group. In each case, the agendas of the members dictate the sponsor's goals, locking the sponsoring organization into activities believed to be acceptable (if not high–priority). After the goals are inferred, the decision–making group can consider and interpret evaluation information.

A political strategy considers several arenas in order to select one that provides the decision maker with a powerful set of allies. A coalition of these organizations is formed before goals are formally considered (see Table 10–3). The coalition must then bargain to infer its goals. However, a clever sponsor can skew a group's membership to include organizations known to be sympathetic to the sponsor's aims. Indeed, most successful consortia, such as kidney foundations and shared service corporations, go through this type of organizational phase. As the coalition is formed, various factions are monitored to determine their aims and how a decision group can relate to these aims. The membership of the group evolves to incorporate potentially powerful allies. After the *arena* stabilizes, bargaining is used to select program goals acceptable to the coalition. (If new allies turn up, the group may revert to the political phase.) Finally, group decision strategies are used to make judgments using analytically–derived evaluation information. To apply the mixed–mode approach, the decision maker shuttles back and forth among the decision strategies as the coalition takes shape.

Successful decision makers in public and nonprofit organizations (those that survive) are adept at applying political and/or bargaining strategies. Unfortunately, these same strategies are used to select among competing proposals and to make other important choices. Evaluation information is seldom considered or sought. Ultimately the coalition will break up under these conditions. As Filley and Grimes point out, excessive politicking, leading to repeated bargaining, strains the decision group.[57] The powerful members of a decision group must dominate each process of goal selection or see their position weaken.

STYLES OF DECISION MAKING

A "decision style" emerges from a decision maker's experience, tempered by self-selected learning episodes. McKenney and Keen point out that individuals search out occupations and tasks comparable with their perceived cognitive skills.[58] Courses in college, continuing education, and other types of learning are elected which build on these perceived strengths. This in turn reinforces a particular decision-making style.

Taxonomies of Style

Decision-making style has been conceptualized and studied in several unique ways. Beginning with Churchman[59] and Ackoff,[60] and more recently by Huysmans[61] and Doktor and Hamilton,[62] studies of style have focused on the ability of decision makers to differentiate between an object and its context. This leads to the definition of two distinct cognitive styles, called analytic and heuristic. The heuristic sees decisions as field dependent, meaning that an object cannot be separated from its context. At the other extreme, structure is used and assumptions of field independence are made. In a recent study using this taxonomy, Doktor investigated the decision-making approaches used by executives.[63] He found that (for right-handed people) the left side of the brain is used for tasks amenable to intuitive reasoning and the right is used for systematic analysis. An electroencephalogram was used to isolate brain activities of executives who worked on problems best solved by analytic and heuristic approaches. Most executives were found to rely exclusively on their preferred approach, applying it to either problem. However, in these studies the method of testing has analytic features which confound testing and the behavior the test is attempting to capture.

Style has been articulated in behavioral-environmental terms. For instance, Vroom identifies authoritarian, consultative, and group styles.[64] A decision maker with an authoritarian style makes decisions unilaterally, or as a variation, obtains information from a subordinate before making a decision. Consultative styles seek out data from several people, getting ideas and suggestions; or the decision is explored in a group setting. A group style delegates the decision to the group.

Weckworth cites studies of sibling rivalry and proposes that style may be dictated by birth order.[65] In this model, the first-born is found to be analytic and direct as well as overt. Second children are covert and make decisions by jumping between the problem and possible solutions. Third-born siblings are negotiators, and see decisions principally in terms of what is acceptable. Fourth children are like the first-born, but more pliable. Fifth-born are similar to seconds, sixth-born like thirds, etc., repeating the four-position cycle.

Driver and Mock conceptualize style in terms of the number of solutions and the amount of information used.[66] Table 10-4 summarizes their structure.

Table 10-4:   Drive and Mock's Definition of Decision Making Style

| | | AMOUNT OF INFORMATION | |
		Minimal	Maximum
	Single	Decisive Style	Hieratic Style
Number of Solutions			
	Multiple	Flexible Style	Integrative Sytle

Reprinted with permission from Drive M.J., and J.J. Mock, "Human Information Processing, Decision Style Theory, and Accounting Information Systems," The Accounting Review, July 1975.

A preference for minimal data and a single solution leads to a *decisive style*. This type of style is rigid but consistent. A *flexible style* stems from a preference for multiple solutions with minimal data. Adaptability and variety are preferred, as compared to the decisive style, which emphasizes efficiency and consistency. Those seeking a maximum amount of data and single solutions are called *hieratic*. This type of individual is very thorough—a perfectionist who emphasizes quality and rigor. Preferences for multiple solutions and maximum data lead to an *integrative style*. Integrators are experimental and very often creative.

In each of these taxonomies, the means of categorizing people by style is either subjective or tends to be unreliable. The style framework discussed in this chapter was selected because its dimensions are closely tied to both data acquisition and analysis (key elements of the decision–making models discussed in this chapter) and because instruments have been devised which can classify decision makers using this definition of style.

The Jungian Framework

The psychologist Jung proposed a typology which Mitroff and Kilman have used to identify four distinct decision styles.[67] The typology sets out distinct ways that a manager selects and analyzes data when making decisions. Data can be gathered by sensing or by intuition. *Sensation* data stress facts and details. Sensing decision makers break the decision stimulus into discrete elements. Information–gathering for a sensing individual is based on using a coding device which searches for relationships among items or looks for deviations from accepted standards.[68] For instance, a sales manager may search through reports to compare this month's sales to those in the same month a year ago, adjusted by his/her expectations for the individual salesperson. Information is coded so that significant details can be extracted from the copious information that the sales manager must process.

Intuitive data present a comprehensive picture, or a gestalt, of a decision situation which describes the decision task in its habitat. Hypothetical possibilities are drawn from the decision maker's imagination. The decision maker draws a picture which is used to create a context for the decision problem. McKenney and Keen call this a perceptive approach to information gathering. The decision maker focuses on the data to isolate their inherent patterns, rather than applying a preconceived coding strategy. For instance, an auditor examines large quantities of data to construct a picture of a hospital financial performance. Similarly, open–ended survey questions like Hackman items provide data for the decision maker to ponder.

Each type of datum has inherent strengths and limitation. Sensation data use a preconceived pattern to summarize data that may miss relevant details. For instance, cost–variance reports that discuss the performance of laundry departments in a multihospital system may not document the turnover of department heads, which may have led to poor performance described in the report. On the other hand, intuitive data may never coalesce into a coherent whole. Decision makers become overloaded with information, making them unable to build relationships in the data to devise premises upon which to base an action. For instance, content analysis, which seeks patterns in response to open–ended survey questions, may be complex, influenced by setting, mood, individual differences, and the like. Patterns remain obscure even after extensive study.

Thinking or feeling strategies may be used to analyze the data. *Thinking* relies on logic. A step–by–step process like a mathematical model is used to process data. The decision is carefully-structured so steps in processing data can be laid out in advance and followed in a sequential fashion. Thinking modes of reasoning focus on generalization. Decision makers who use them often believe they must be amoral and impersonal. The analysis, not personal considerations, should dictate choices.

Feeling personalizes the decision. When a decision maker relies on feeling, the personal circumstances of all concerned, as well as the unique nature of the decision, forms the basis for decision making. These decision makers tend to be heuristic, jumping back and forth among solution ideas and testing each one. An incubation phase follows, which leads to a flash of insight; a new idea emerges which may provide a unique or innovative response.[69]

Each mode has inherent risks. Thinking is efficient and reliable. Premises are set out and assumptions checked, permitting the rationales behind a decision to be made explicit. Unfortunately, many ill–structured decisions do not lend themselves to logic. Mintzberg, *et al.,* found that many decisions made by top management were not amenable to solution paradigms.[70] In other instances, a step–by–step analysis was often abandoned by top management because it was perceived to be time–consuming and hard to comprehend. Feeling promotes acceptance and, on occasion, innovation. But personalizing a decision may smack of favoritism or moralizing, and may cause one to miss opportunities to select a better course of action. These two ways of gathering and analyzing data can be used to identify four styles, as shown in Table 10-5.

The Systematic Decision Maker

A decision maker using a systematic decision style consciously structures the decision–making process by developing a plan to look for cues in evaluation

Table 10-5: Decision Styles

		PREFERRED DATA	
		Sensation	Intuition
PREFERRED MODE OF DATA PROCESSING	Thinking	Systematic Decision Makers	Speculative Decision Makers
	Feeling	Judicial Decision Makers	Intuitive Decision Makers

SOURCE: Adapted from Mitroff I. and R. Kilman "On Evaluating Scientific Research: The Contributions of the Philosophy of Science", Technological Forecasting and Social Change, Vol. 8, 1975 (163-174).

data.[71] The specifics of the plan may vary from one systematic decision maker to another, but each stresses hard data and logical analysis, and attempts to devise rules which can govern the decision process. The method or plan evolves. Variations and adaptations of the plan occur as it is applied to new and varied decision–making tasks.

Table 10-6 provides a comparison of the four styles using two examples. A systematic decision maker would prefer to assess performance by using objective measures for each cost center in the organization. For example, staying within prescribed budget, as measured by cost–variance reports, can be used to determine the need for managerial intervention. Evaluation measures like unit costs of services and utilization of services, compared to standards and quotas, are stressed. Capital improvement projects are compared using return on investment (ROI) criteria. The systematic decision maker validates by checking the accuracy of the accounting and financial data used to calculate return on investment.

The systematic decision maker would be most at home in an organization like a multihospital system which is centralized with a well–defined authority in its executive positions and which stresses financial viability.[72] Defining roles, assigning work, and pushing for results is the preferred leadership style of systematic administrators.

The Speculative Decision Maker

The "speculative" decision maker subjects data depicting hypothetical possibilities to logical analysis. Like the systematic decision maker, a formal

Table 10-6.   Contrasting Decision Styles

Decision Style	Systematic	Speculative
decision (1) performance appraisal	objective measures of the performance of each cost center	compare departmental performance against decision maker's view of potential
(2) capital projects	return on investment (ROI) projections, based accounting and financial data for each project.	the sensitivuty of ROI, based on cost and revenue data, to changes in demand in each project
verification	check detains of calculations and data acquisition process	examine decision in light of external factors

Decision Style	Judicial	Intuitive
decision (1) performance appraisal	objective measures of administrators	compare administrator's performance to the decision maker's view of their potential
(2) capital projects	estimates of ROI are based on the projections of experts and colleagues who jointly consider accounting and financial data for each project	estimates of ROI are sought from trusted colleagues who consider the unique features of each project
verification	acceptance by key groups	enhances organizations prestige, influence or visibility

Reprinted with permission from Nutt, P.C. "Influence of Decision Styles on the Use of Decision Models", *Technological Forecasting and Social Change,* 14:1, p. 85, (1979).

plan is often followed in the analysis, but the speculative decision maker is vitally concerned with contextual factors. Evaluation methods like sensitivity analysis, where assumptions are progressively relaxed, are preferred. The speculative decision maker devises several premises and tests them via analysis. A variety of propositions are entertained which take a broad view of the decision–making task.

A speculative decision maker prefers to assess performance by comparing work units (departments) against *his/her* view of their potential (Table 10–6). The assessment remains impersonal but uses theoretically attainable performance as a benchmark. Preferred performance measures for evaluation include the hospital's market share, service leadership or new service development, and the like. A speculative decision maker often seeks out information which describes the sensitivity of ROI calculations to dramatic drops or sharp increases in demand, before selecting among capital improvement projects. To validate, the speculative decision maker considers possible choices in the light of contextual factors such as regulation and reimbursement formulas.

The speculative decision maker prefers a hospital organization that stresses a liasion with power centers (e.g., health planning agencies and executors of hospital endowments) that regulate or influence their services, revenues, or clients. A speculative decision maker in a hospital will measure the success of the hospital against other hospitals with the same catchment area and services, seeking a competitive edge with this peer group. The ability to define problems and leadership through example are valued traits of speculative decision makers.

The Judicial Decision Maker

A judicial decision maker relies on the consensus that emerges from a decision–making group to dictate a course of action. This style often disregards general issues and focuses on human issues that appear to influence choice, describing these relationships by facts and details. Reality is a concrete proposal that a key group like a board of directors can agree on. The judicial decision maker seeks quantitative information and screens the information with a decision–making group.

A judicial decision maker assesses the performance of departments by measuring the performance of the department's administrators (Table 10–6). One preferred strategy would be management by objectives, whereby each department head is enticed to set his/her own objectives, which he/she will be measured against. Concrete evaluation measures like employee turnover, absenteeism, number of grievances, and the like, are used to form the objectives for each department. Judicial decision makers are less concerned with organizational climate, employee commitment, and interpersonal relationships because these concepts lack clearcut measures.

Decisions on capital projects are based on the judgments of experts who interpret accounting and financial data. The judicial decision maker likes to set up a meeting where experts and staff debate the merits of each project. If the group cannot be coaxed into a consensus, the judicial decision maker listens for arguments which are respected by peers and adopts the course of action that stems from an extension of these arguments. Validation occurs only when the course of action has been endorsed by centers of power important to the organization.

Judicial administrators prefer decentralized organizations with clearcut roles and work rules for all positions, stressing participative decision making. A judicial chief executive officer would judge the success of his/her organization in terms of meeting the needs and goals of its clientele, its controlling agents, and its employees. Judicial decision makers in hospitals see success in terms of keeping the medical staff happy and adherence to traditions such as being "patient oriented." Leadership stems from paying careful attention to individual needs and developing a rapport with coworkers.

The Intuitive Decision Maker

The intuitive decision maker often relies on unverbalized hunches or cues and defends his choices by relating them to previous experience. They have disdain for data, relying only on "the big picture" to extract decision–making information. Social responsibility and quality of life often form the basis for decisions. Such decision makers believe that a decision cannot be made without considering its context. Analysis is viewed as unable to capture the complexity of most important decisions. The intuitive decision maker always considers the human element in his/her decisions.

Intuitive decision makers believe that departmental performance is best measured by comparing the achievement of each administrator against the decision maker's view of the administrator's potential (Table 10–6). Satisfaction of those using the services of each department in the organization is demanded. Intuitive decision makers are also vitally concerned with consumer satisfaction and community leadership. They rely heavily on the advice of trusted peers when embarking on risky projects such as one involving a large capital investment. The advice of trusted colleagues is sought to consider the unique characteristics of each project alternative. A "good" return on investment is based on the peer's experience with similar projects. Validation of the decision hinges on the prospect that a preferred alternative will enhance the decision maker's prestige, influence, or visibility. Successful executives are believed to be the sine qua non of a successful organization.

An intuitive administrator prefers a decentralized organization with considerable delegation of authority to leaders of the decentralized units. The success of the organization would be judged in terms of its service to its community and to its clientele. Leadership is thought to stem from charismatic traits.

DECISION STYLES AND BEHAVIOR

Several investigators have shown that one of the four decision styles discussed in this chapter describes the behavior of most decision makers. Others have demonstrated that decision style influences the results of decision making. In most of these studies a "Myers–Briggs–type indicator" was used to identify an individual's decision style.[73]

A discussion of decision–making traits can be found in most organization behavior texts under the heading "leadership." For example, Hall described a consultative leader (the judicial style) and authoritarian leader (systematic system).[74] Churchman describes leaders as "devil's advocates" or charismatic (intuitive styles) and as "systems oriented" (speculative style).[75]

Several investigators have described the behavior of decision makers. The traits of systematic and intuitive styles often emerge from descriptions of how decisions were made. Systematic decision makers, trained to use a repertoire of models, can excel when one of these models, such as a quality control chart, can be used to "represent" the decision problem.[76] The model is used to specify data that should be collected and provides a format to permit a logical step–by–step analysis.

Intuitive decision makers often exhibit superior performance in poorly structured decision tasks like deciphering codes.[77] Rather than using a model, the intuitive decision maker attempts several dissimilar attacks on the problem to see where each approach will lead. Several false starts, followed by incubation, lead to a flash of insight which often breaks the code. For instance, McKenney and Keen report that production control operators in paper mills controlled the paper–making process by "tasting the broth."[78] An extensive investment of both time and resources was required before management scientists were able to devise a control process, with quantative decision rules, that worked as well as broth testing.[79] Erwing cites the skill of Estee Lauder in selecting a fragrance that has mass market appeal but points out that the internal operations of the firm during its growth and expansion were guided by systematic decision makers.[80] Mintzberg suggests some dangers in intuitive styles.

...[intuitive] managers may take these findings as a license to shroud [their] activities in darkness. The mystification of conscious behavior is a favorite ploy of those seeking to protect a power base (or to hide their intentions of creating one); this behavior helps no organization, and neither does forcing to the realm of intuitive activities that can be handled effectively by analysis.[81]

McKenney and Keen found no relationship between decision style (defined by the Myers–Briggs indicator) and performance: *no* decision style was inherently superior for all decision tasks.[82] Each had distinctive strengths.

Their studies concentrated on decision makers with systematic and intuitive styles. Seventy–five percent of their subjects used their dominant style exclusively. Mitroff and Kilmann report similar results.[83] These findings suggest that most people have a preferred style and apply it to all decision tasks they face.

Other studies provide striking confirmation of the unique decision approach adopted by each style. Mitroff and Kilman had bank officers describe how they believed loans should be made, and Nutt had health planners write an essay on the planner's view of an ideal planning approach.[84] The content of these essays was classified using the Myers–Briggs indicator. The preferred approach seems related to decision style, as shown below:

Systematic Styles: Systematic planners stressed a step–by–step planning process that isolated need, coupled need with financing, and outlined a procedure to identify ways to provide a service program within budget constraints. Systematic loan officers believed that loans should be based on a careful review of each applicant's assets and liabilities, granting loans when the rates of indebtedness to income was below a certain value.

Speculative Styles: Speculative planners preferred a planning process that was guided by generic concepts such as a formal statement of goals and objectives. The goals were described as guiding a process which develops a general model, specifying macro components of the plan. Budget constraints were seldom considered. Speculative loan officers sought a short statement of the applicant's financial position and determined why the loan was needed. The decision rules tend to be contextual: indebtedness–income ratios vary depending on the loan's intended use.

Judicial Styles: Judicial planners contended that people's needs should direct planning. Consumer surveys and small–group rap sessions were often cited as ways to judge needs. Judicial loan officers wanted to call the loan applicant's employer and others who could "vouch for" the applicant. They advocated a group session where all loan officers would share information gleaned from their applicants, with the group selecting loans to be approved from this pool of applicants.

Intuitive Styles: The intuitive planner evaluated people's needs philosophically. The plan was often described as springing from the minds of skilled planners as a consequence of carefully considering people's needs. An intuitive loan officer would want to hold an open–ended interview with each applicant and, if undecided after the interview, would prefer calling a trusted fellow loan officer to discuss the results of the interview. The applicant's personal situation was considered before granting the loan.

Most management information systems (MIS) provide information and information formats that seem best suited to systematic decision styles. A decision task was devised to test how decision style may influence the amount of information that is gleaned from such a report. Cases were constructed which depicted the clinical status of patients, using indicators of status that the nurse–supervisors contended they used when making staffing decisions.[85] Infants in a neonatology ward were described by their body weight, diagnosis, gestational age, and days since birth. Nurse–supervisors were asked to staff several units, described by various profiles of patient characteristics. A Myers–Briggs form was used to determine each nurse–supervisor's decision style.

Systematic nurse–supervisors used all available information in a highly reliable manner. (The multiple regression coefficient, which measures percent variance explained, exceeded 90 percent). The speculative and judicial supervisors were nearly as reliable information processors ($R^2 = .80$), but used fewer criteria and thus less information in their decision making. Intuitive supervisors relied on one criterion and used it in an unreliable manner ($R^2 = .40$). They also expressed dissatisfaction with the task, calling it unrealistic. These findings suggest that reports that stress partially aggregated information (e.g., cost–variance reports) will not be used to their full advantage by intuitive decision makers.

LINKING DECISION STYLES AND DECISION STRATEGIES

In practice, decision makers seem to gravitate toward a decision approach that is consistent with their personal style.[86] In the discussion to follow, the relationship between style and the decision strategies will be explored.

Systematic Styles

Decision makers with a systematic style prefer analytical decision approaches, particularly approaches that compare options using quantitative criteria.[87] A careful analysis which develops cost–benefit or cost–effectiveness information is thought to be necessary to consistently make good decisions. Unwarranted theorizing and moralizing are believed to result when qualitative information and/or personalitites clutter up decisions. In each instance, evaluation approaches are used to attach values to alternative courses of action. The evaluation arrangements of NDT, using a Laplace rule (equal criteria weights) to aggregate information is preferred. The systematic decision maker will even evaluate the premises for recurring decisions stated in master plans. The systematic decision maker sees all decisions as closed system, and becomes uncomfortable when alternatives resist quantification because they have open–system characteristics. As a result, systematic decision makers advocate that evaluation data should dictate choice. Their decisions rely heavily on the findings of an evaluation.

Speculative Styles

A decision maker with a speculative style also stresses analysis, but seeks out broader criteria with subjective elements. Decisions often follow a what–if analysis of the evaluation data in order to isolate the impact of important contingencies. As Mitroff and Kilmann point out, discovery is viewed as an important outcome.[88] Available alternatives are scored using NDT or BDT. BDT is used when the states are unclear or resist quantification. The speculative decision maker prefers a structure similar to decision theory to model the decision task, and regards those without such a structure as fuzzy thinkers.[89] Open–system decisions are made by accepting subjective information which seems to describe the decision environment. This leads speculative decision makers to prefer approaches that combine objective and subjective evaluation data like the NDT and BDT strategies.

Judicial Styles

Judicial styles are decision–task–oriented. Techniques and models are seen as useful principally for tactical decisions. Strategic decisions are viewed as unique: each should be considered on its merits. This leads judicial decision makers to advocate interactive decision processes, because they avoid the "straightjacket" of formal models and consider information from a variety of sources. Only a group decision process can cater to judicial decision makers' preference for hard data and their need to understand the views of their peers when making choices. The "community of minds" sorts through evaluation data to isolate preferred courses of action. Cost–benefit and cost–effectiveness criteria are considered, but the importance of this information hinges on its presentation and its source. A synthesis of cost–effectiveness and cost–benefit data results, based on the prejudices and synergistic insights of the group. A synthesis of this information creates understanding which is believed to lead to improved decisions. Judicial decision makers prefer group decision approaches and will attempt to use them exclusively.

Intuitive Styles

The intuitive decision maker stresses acceptance and sees decision making as a practical exercise that must cater to the whims of key reference groups. The intuitive decision maker attempts to find a way to balance conflicting claims and counter claims, which accompany most choices. The political and moral consequences of each alternative course of action is stressed. Intuitive decision makers view analytic decision strategies (e.g., NDT and BDT) with scorn because they ignore or fail to capture criteria that describe political and moral issues when assessing alternatives.[90] In their view, decisions cannot be made that are detached from the personal considerations of those affected. Group approaches are seldom used because interaction may force the decision maker to disclose information before the consequences of disclosure can be assessed. Most decision groups are seen as "pooled ignorance," and pooled ignorance, in the mind of the intuitive decision maker, seldom leads to wisdom. These views lead an intuitive decision maker to use an adaptive strategy like Model 3.[91] Intuitive decision makers prefer adaptive decision approaches, and attempt to use them exclusively.

THE IDEAL DECISION STYLE

The link between decision styles and decision strategies suggests that a strategy is seldom *used* unless it is consistent with the decision maker's style. This leads to poor decisions because each decision model has specific strengths and weaknesses. Vague and ill–structured (open-system) decision tasks may be treated to rigorous analysis. This analysis is futile because the models cannot capture or represent critical criteria which must be understood in choosing among alternatives for open–system decisions. Clear–cut (closed–system) decision tasks may receive homeostatic tinkering, when analysis can efficiently isolate a preferred (or desirable) course of action. Ideally the demands of the decision task should dictate which strategy is used.

Mitroff and his colleagues contend that the "ideal" style is that found at the center of Table 10–5 in this chapter.[92] The decision maker should be able to adopt a speculative, judicial, systematic, or intuitive style, depending on the demands of the decision–making task. It seems particularly important that strategic decisions, as defined by Mintzberg, *et al.,* should avoid endless political maneuvering when analysis can shed light on a superior course of action.[93] The mixed–mode strategy seems particularly suited to this task because it draws on elements of each decision–making style. For instance, the mixed–mode strategy allows the nature of the decision task to dictate the sequence of steps in decision making; specifying when analysis, decision groups, and politics should be applied. The mixed–mode strategy provides guides which stage decision making. The necessity and the sequence of steps is determined by the arena and goals of the decision task. To appreciate the mixed–mode strategy, a decision maker must see the value of both analytical and forensic decision approaches. This suggests that the most effective decision makers should be able to apply (personally or with the aid of staff) and understand conclusions drawn from each of the decision strategies. Effective decision makers may use an implicit form of the mixed–mode strategy to guide their decision making.

GUIDES IN SELECTING A DECISION STRATEGY

Organizational level, the nature of the task, and uncertainty identify a setting and a set of circumstances which may influence the merits of a decision–making strategy.[94] Organizations have technological, managerial, and institutional layers where decisions are made. Each layer defines a setting where a particular decision–making strategy may be best applied. The circumstances surrounding the decision–making task provide additional insights into strategy selection. In particular, uncertainty and the type of decision will be used to suggest guides.[95] Uncertainty stems from the task's uniqueness and procedural simplicity, the clarity of criteria and causal relationships, and the complexity of the decision–making environment. Information and techniques to manipulate the information can be known or unknown, identifying four types of tasks. A highly uncertain decision–making task of a particular type may demand a particular strategy when the decision occurs in a particular organizational layer. The impact of setting and circumstance is discussed in the sections that follow. Propositions are developed to suggest which decision strategy seems best, given a setting or a set of circumstances.[96]

ORGANIZATIONAL LEVEL:
ITS INFLUENCE ON THE DECISION STRATEGIES

Thompson finds that organizations have technological, managerial, and institutional layers.[97] Each layer performs unique functions for an organization. The *technological* layer carries out the core tasks of an organization. Behavioral modification treatment systems, hospital laboratories, and renal dialysis treatment programs are examples. Organizations have multiple technologies which include staff units such as accounting and personnel, as well as those units associated with their primary services.

The *managerial* layer is devoted to coordination: allocating resources among technical units, serving as a conduit of information, and mediating disputes. The managerial layer is used to deal with the dependencies among the technical units. For example, disputes between nursing and the medical staff and between the medical staff and hospital laboratory regarding quality, standing orders, the timeliness of actions, and the like, are mediated by the managerial layer.

The *institutional* layer of an organization develops policy, garners resources, and seeks public support. In short, the institutional layer spans the boundary between the organization and its environment. A key task is to predict and develop contingency plans which cope with anticipated environmental changes. When the environment becomes unstable, liaison arrangements are initiated which funnel information to the institutional layer. Institutional decision makers accept many appointments with related organizations to keep tabs on the flow of events. Also, the organization may surrender some autonomy to have outsiders serve on their board of directors, as well as to maintain open information channels.

The Technological Layer

A closed–system assumption is often reasonable for the technological layer, making master plans and NDT potentially useful strategies. This layer is sealed off from environmental influences, and thus analytical methods and master plans may be used more often than in the coordinational and institutional layers.[98] However, decision–making tasks seem far too variable to recommend the exclusive use of analytical methods merely because the decision arises in the technological layer. Task factors will be required to guide the selection of a strategy in this layer.

The Managerial Layer

The management of dependencies is the primary role for the managerial layer. Thompson defines dependencies as pooled, serial, or reciprocal.[99] Admitting clerks in a hospital have pooled dependencies: each job tends to be self–contained. Serial dependencies occur when one unit (or individual) performs a service that becomes the starting point for another unit. Laboratory, x-ray, and hospital admitting all perform functions which must precede surgery, so these functions have serial dependencies. Reciprocal dependencies describe relationships among people or work units which are highly interdependent. Surgical teams and boards of trustees are examples.

The complexity of the decision environment for the decision maker in the managerial layer of an organization is dictated by the number and types of dependencies he must manage. Several reciprocal dependencies represent a complex environment. The complexity surrounding the decision–making task helps to identify an appropriate decision strategy.[100]

Thompson contends that pooled dependencies should be coordinated by standardization through rules, procedure, and precedent; serial dependencies by plans, schedules, or targets; and reciprocal dependencies by mutual adjustment of the dependent units.[101] Forensic strategies, which stress interaction or reflection, seem best suited to these tasks. Master plans are recommended to make decisions dealing with the coordination of pooled units, group methods for serial coordination, and adaptive approaches for reciprocal coordination.

Self–contained units in an organization find that master plans are valuable when decisions are routine. The master plan provides an efficient and a just mechanism to resolve minor disputes. Decisions that adhere to precedent and accepted rules are likely to be accepted, and require comparatively little time. However, the master plan has few prescriptions for the nonroutine decisions. When self–contained units disagree over policy, budget, and similar issues, other decision–making approaches are needed.

Decision makers managing serially coordinated units should use group decision–making approaches. Serially coordinated units can often resolve disputes when the affected parties share information and establish mutually acceptable performance targets. The group provides a hearing for those affected to share information and settle on a solution. However, serially coordinated units may have dramatically different status and power within the organization, in addition to other characteristics which render group approaches ineffective. For instance, to resolve problems of patient flow between admitting and surgery, serially dependent departments' group approaches dictate that both departments be represented in a decision group. Clearly, admitting clerks will find it difficult to effectively confront surgeons in such a setting. Similarly, group methods may be helpful in resolving disputes between radiology and cardiology over poor x-ray quality, but less so in resource allocation decisions.

Adaptive approaches seem necessary when a decision involves reciprocally dependent units. These units have highly complex relationships which must be understood before action can be taken. A decision maker applying an adaptive approach publicizes a tentative action and collects information by monitoring the reactions from reciprocally dependent units. For instance, new personnel policies for surgical teams with a high turnover in their surgical nursing staff could be tested in this way. However, when those affected by a decision tend to react in a hypersensitive manner, the adaptive strategy may provoke problems as well as solve them. Some decisions involving reciprocally coordinated units will be routine (suggesting master plans), and others may benefit from analysis to sort out the complexity which surrounds the decision. Again, the nature of the decision task is an important factor in selecting a decision approach.

To delegate decision making to the technological level, managers should require units with pooled dependencies to develop rules and procedures. Those with serial dependencies should be required to prepare decision plans which test criteria and weights, to apply when decisions arise. Units with reciprocal dependencies are asked to specify adjustment patterns or the group processes they will use when the need for decision making arises.

The Institutional Layer

The institutional layer establishes the organization's structure, and structure creates many of the coordinational problems that the managerial layer must resolve. The ideal structure minimizes coordination effort and thus costs. Units are grouped according to their dependencies. Reciprocally dependent units are grouped first, then serially dependent units are assembled, followed by macro groups constructed along functional lines. Because they select the organization's structure, decision makers in the institutional layer are largely responsible for the complexity of decision making at the managerial level of the organization. To simplify decision making, the organization's structure can be realigned to minimize coordination. Administrators at the institutional level, preoccupied with coordinational problems referred up the hierarchy, should consider realigning their organization to reduce unnecessary coordinational complexity.

Devising arrangements to reduce the uncertainty is a key role of executives at the institutional level of an organization. The environment is analyzed to isolate its effect on the organization's services. While on the surface, adaptive strategies seem well suited for decision making at the institutional layer, they leave considerable residual uncertainty in their wake. Again the nature of the task seems a dominant factor in selecting among decision strategies.

Summary

Organizational level provides some guidance in the selection of a decision-making approach. Applying analytical approaches in the technical layer, a forensic strategy in the managerial layer, as dictated by the complexity of coordination, and an adaptive approach in the institutional layer, was recommended. However, these guides can be far more definitive when the influence of the decision-making task is considered.

JUDGING THE EFFECTIVENESS
OF A DECISION-MAKING STRATEGY

Indicators that will be used to suggest the merits of a decision strategy are listed below:

Cost: Cost is incurred in both the development and maintenance of a decision-making strategy. Decision makers may adopt low-cost decision-making aids because they have few resources to underwrite their activities, beyond their own time.

Timeliness: The delay between the occurrence of a decision-making task and choice is a measure of timeliness. The time required to apply a decision-making strategy may create a delay. In decision making, speed may be a practical virtue because those with power in an organization may have a history of demanding "short-fuse" decisions.

Validity: A strategy's accuracy can be measured when a choice suggested by the strategy can be verified by events. Decision makers should seek decision-making aids with a successful track record.

Reliability: A consistent decision-making strategy will produce the same choice in repeated applications when conditions and evaluation information remain constant. To defend their actions, decision makers may have to demonstrate how they have responded in a consistent manner.

Flexibility: Flexibility refers to the ability of a decision-making strategy to incorporate *judgmental* and *qualitative* data. Decision makers faced with open-system conditions may prefer a strategy that enables them to fold in the experiences and intuitions of peers.

Omission: Omission refers to a judgment stemming from a particular approach, which does not deal with one or more of the evaluation criteria. For instance, decisions by health planning agencies that omit community need when considering hospital expansions may be overturned or lead to a decline in the planning agencies' credibility.

Acceptance: Acceptance describes how elements of a particular strategy can pave the way for the implementation of a decision. For example, group methods promote acceptance through participation of affected groups in the decision-making process.

Decision–making strategies are suggested which seem best for various levels of uncertainty and for particular types of decision–making tasks by considering how cost, timeliness, validity, reliability, flexibility, the risk of omission, and acceptance are influenced when a particular strategy is used.

SELECTING A DECISION–MAKING STRATEGY TO COPE WITH UNCERTAINTY

The level of uncertainty provides several guides which aid in the selection of a strategy.[102] Uncertainty is defined by the stability and homogeneity of the decision–making environment, in temporal and procedural terms, and by the quantifiability of the decision task.[103] In Table 10–7, low, moderate, and high uncertainty are defined using these factors. In the discussion that follows, propositions are presented which show how cost, timeliness, validity, consistency, flexibility, omission, and acceptance are influenced when a decision–making strategy is applied when there are varying levels of uncertainty.

Uncertainty Stemming From Procedures and Frequency of Occurrence

Van de Ven and Delbecq define uncertainty in terms of "analyzability," the extent decision procedures exist, and "variability," the frequency with which similar decisions occur.[104] Analyzability describes the difficulty of an information search and the amount of thinking time necessary to make a decision.[105] The existence of a procedural base for decision making, no matter how complex, defines the high end of the continuum. Experience and intuition must be used when analyzability is low. Variability refers to the number of times that a particular kind of decision task is faced. Table 10–8 illustrates some decision–making tasks classified using the Van de Ven and Delbecq typology.

When analyzability is low and the task is unique, the decision makers have little to guide them in selecting among alternatives. High uncertainty results. For example, a hospital administrator attempting to strip privileges from a medical staff member, uses a one–time heuristic search for information. Uncertainty is low when tasks are recurring and have clearcut decision procedures, even if sophisticated techniques are used. A recurring task may permit the sponsor to systematize the decision through programming. Inventory control procedures in hospitals are examples. In other instances, management by exception principles can be followed. Moderate uncertainty results when decisions are either unique (but amenable to analysis) or when the task is repeatable, but decision–making procedures must be established.

Table 10-7. Attributes Which Describe The Uncertainty of Decision Tasks

TASK ATTRIBUTES	LEVEL OF UNCERTAINTY		
	LOW	MODERATE	HIGH
Temporal and Procedural	frequent with known procedures	infrequent, with known procedures or frequent with unknown procedures	unique with unknown procedures
Quantifiability	criteria & cause-effect known	criteria partially given and/or cause-effect relations unknown	criteria & cause effect relations unknown
Task Envorinment	stable and homogeneous projects	moderate number of projects some with stable demand or use rates	shifting and heterogenous projects

Reprinted with permission from Nutt, P.C., "Some Condsiderations in Selecting Interactive and Analytical Decision Approaches," *Medical Care*, 17:2, p. 162, (1979).

Table 10-8: Using Analyzability and Variability Factors To Classify Decision Making Tasks

		Variability of Decision Task		
		Low	Moderate	High
Analyzability of Decision Tasks	Low	Behavioral Modification Procedures	Psychological Counseling	Research
		Coronary Care Units	Burn Care	Neonatology
			Legal Services	Legislation
	Moderate	Computerized EKG Interpretation	Paramedics	Hospital Architecture
		Medical Histories Taken By Computer	Nurse-Practitioners	Trauma Units
	High	Inventory Control Models for Hospital Supplies	Pharmacy	Hospital Admitting
		Distillation of Hospital Chemicals	Hospital Dietary Department	

Preferred decision-making strategies may be suggested by the amount of uncertainty in the task, described by its variability and analyzability:[106]

Proposition 1: Uncertainty is low when a logical base for decision making has been derived and decisions are recurring. Mechanistic strategies should be used. Decisions based on master plans and NDT are consistent, valid, and can be timely, with a low cost, but have only moderate flexibility. Both rely on a statement of rationale to enhance acceptance. *Master plans* are preferred because costs can be amortized. The open system strategies in Figure 10–1 are undesirable. Adaptive models have low reliability and validity, critically important decision attributes. Mixed-mode models are unnecessarily costly and take too long to carry out.

Proposition 2: Uncertainty is moderate when *decision tasks are unique.* The costs of applying a master plan are often prohibitive. The information needed is both hard to obtain and probabilistic in nature. *Analytic models* like NDT are preferred because they can achieve consistency and validity, when their high cost and low timeliness can be justified. Flexibility and acceptance are moderate. Group decision approaches are efficient, timely, flexible, and promote acceptance, but lack reliability and validity.

Proposition 3: Uncertainty is also moderate when *decision procedures are unknown,* which calls for a mid-range strategy. *Group decision approaches* are preferred over analytical models (BDT). Neither strategy has high reliability or validity, but the group is often flexible, promotes acceptance, and may be timely with low cost.

Proposition 4: Highly *uncertain* decision tasks result when the tasks are unique and procedures unknown, which calls for an organic strategy. A open system strategy is required. The adaptive decision approach is timely and has low cost. A *mixed-mode strategy* is preferred because it has less risk of omission, more reliability and flexibility, and promotes acceptance, with modest sacrifices of cost and timeliness. Validity is seldom achievable when the decision is unique and procedures are unknown. Analytical decision strategies cannot be applied until the decision task is simplified.

Quantifiability and Uncertainty

Thompson suggests that decisions can be classified by the clarity of both the "criteria" and "cause–and–effect relationships" in the decision task.[107] For example, inventory control procedures for supply items in hospitals have exploited the clarity of criteria (ordering and holding costs) and knowledge of how usage rates of supplies vary with census and other factors to apply analytic decision strategies and optimizing decision rules. When criteria are known, but cause–effect relations are not, only satisficing decisions can be made. For example, a hospital administrator defending the continued use of vein grafts by the hospital's thoracic surgeons, can only compare his hospital's case-adjusted mortality rates with hospitals whose surgeons use myocardial revascularization. The open heart program is judged satisfactory if mortality is comparable to that in other hospitals. Instrumentality tests are used when criteria are unknown, but cause–effect relationships are thought to be clear. Quality assessment programs in hospitals often use check lists to insure that accepted procedures were followed, because desirable outcomes are undefined. Social tests are applied when neither criteria nor cause–effect relations are known. Hospitals mimic organizations perceived to have prestige and add open heart surgery, radiotherapy, dialysis, and other esoteric services for these reasons.

Uncertainty can be defined in terms of the precision of decision criteria and the clarity of cause–effect relationships imbedded in the decision task. Uncertainty is high when *both* criteria and cause–effect relationships surrounding decision tasks are unknown, and uncertainty is "low" when both are clear. Moderate uncertainty occurs when cause–effect relations are unknown, because satisficing criteria can be used. Uncertainty increases when criteria are unknown.

Proposition 5: Uncertainty is low when cause–and–effect relationships are known and evaluation criteria are clear; optimization can be sought and *mechanistic strategies* are preferred. NDT can be reliable and valid, have low to moderate cost, and can be timely with little risk of omission. Master plans are used when decisions can be based on historical performance trends, using exception checks. When uncertainty is low, flexibility is unimportant. A master plan can be inexpensive, valid, and timely. Consistency and acceptance can be high and risk of omission low, but depend on the skill of the decision maker(s).

In a relatively certain environment, data systems based on master plans *can* be constructed to monitor important performance indicators. For example, standard EMS reporting forms can be used to track utilization or cost performance of a vehicle dispatch service, 911 telephone systems, training programs for ambulance attendants, and the like.

Proposition 6: Moderate uncertainty, stemming from unknown cause–effect relations, suggests a *satisficing* decision rule and a mid–range strategy. When acceptance is important, group methods can be used to process evaluation data. In all other circumstances, *analytical* strategies (e.g., BDT) are preferred because they have a low risk of omission and provide reliable decisions. Group approaches are somewhat more flexible. Both the forensic (group) and the analytic BDT strategy can be timely and inexpensive in this environment. Validity cannot be measured because of the uncertainty associated with the cause–effect relationships.

In Proposition 6, the inability to define an optimal or ideal outcome forces the use of relative standards. For example, behavioral modifications experts in mental retardation centers set reading, dressing, and other behavioral performance goals according to what they believe is attainable for each patient. The desired behavior (criteria) for patients such as autistic children, are clear, and various treatment procedures are attempted until this behavior is observed.

Proposition 7: Moderate uncertainty, due to unknown criteria, requires *instrumentality* tests. Checklists (adherence to accepted procedures) and quotas, using proxy measures, serve as evaluation criteria. A forensic decision approach is required. A group approach is preferred because of its acceptance, flexibility, and low risk of omission, which in this environment is more important than the low reliability associated with *group decision making.* Both the group and the BDT approaches can be inexpensive and timely, but neither is likely to be valid.

In Proposition 7, validity is undefined. Instrumentality tests are *not* related to outcomes, so no checks of decision accuracy can be made. For instance, utilization review committees in hospitals do not measure, or even consider, care quality factors. As a result, acute–care hospitals which provide tertiary care services often base their assessments on utilization quotas and adherence to accepted medical practice because quality–of–life factors have not been defined. Generally a forensic decision strategy is preferred when uncertainty is moderate because of unknown decision criteria.

Proposition 8: Uncertainty is high when criteria are ambiguous and cause–and–effect relations unknown. Performance is measured by comparisons with *reference groups,* mimicking the activities of organizations that have been labeled successful. An organic strategy must be used and adaptive strategies are preferred. Adaptive approaches can be timely and flexible, with modest cost, but lack consistency and acceptance because of their inherent capriciousness, and have a high risk of omission. Both adaptive and mixed mode strategies lack validity because of the ambiguity surrounding the decision task.

Proposition 8 depicts decision making in organizations when both the means and their desired ends are unclear. Decisions are often made by imitating the behavior of similar high–status organizations. For instance, health planning agencies mimic the practices and organizational arrangements of agencies labeled "highly successful" by HEW. The Bureau of Health Planning and Resource Development in HEW used an idealized model of a health planning agency to judge the fitness of a given agency.

Uncertainty Produced By The Task Environment

Thompson argues that "environment" is an important aspect of uncertainty.[108] Environmental uncertainty may be related to the number of services and the stability of the demands for each service in an organization. Uncertainty is defined by the "homogeneity" and "stability" of the organization's services. For example, a hospital with a heterogeneous service profile would have a heavy commitment to ambulatory care through a network of outpatient clinics; would maintain several tertiary care services, such as renal dialysis and open heart surgery; and would provide long–term, rehabilitative, and restorative care. Environment also considers the laws or regulations that influence the organization and the organization's key benefactors. When demand, type of services, benefactors, and regulations are heterogeneous and subject to many changes, an uncertain environment results. For example, health planning agencies have both shifting budgets and shifting mandates or objectives, making decisions in this environment highly uncertain. Decision making may be mechanistic when environmental attributes are known and can be understood. For example, well–endowed community hospitals without competitors in their service area, and located in states that permit cost–based reimbursement and limit the planning agency's control over expansion plans, have a comparatively certain decision environment. Uncertainty is low in stable, homogeneous environments and high in shifting, heterogeneous ones.

Proposition 9: Decision making in *stable and homogeneous environments* (low uncertainty) can be made using a mechanistic strategy. *Master plans* are preferred because they can be timely, inexpensive, flexible, and reliable, depending on the skills of the decision makers. When validity is critical, analytical approaches may be needed to demonstrate the wisdom in the master plan's conclusions. A demonstration makes the rationale behind the decision clear, which promotes acceptance.

For example, if the demands for a service are growing at predictable rates, decision rules like maximum utility can be used to make decisions. Recurring decisions justify the construction of master plans to guide the decision–making process.

Proposition 10: Decision premises for *stable* but *heterogeneous* environments (moderate uncertainty) should be derived for each homogeneous sector. Optimization is attempted for each sector, and satisficing criteria are applied for multisector decisions. *Analytic* decision approaches (NDT and BDT) are preferred because they can be reliable and valid for each sector. A forensic approach is used to compare multisector alternatives. A group strategy will suboptimize, which lowers the validity of allocation decisions but enhances their acceptance. Modest timeliness, cost, risk of omission, and flexibility result.

By deriving decision premises for each service sector, Proposition 10 contends that the decision maker must suboptimize. For example, in resource allocation decisions, public health departments often allocate available funds to each service area or department with a satisficing criterion. A project for immunization that scores lower than projects for sanitation or children's services, using various effectiveness and demand criteria, may be approved to equate expenditures across these service areas. An equity standard is used. For instance, for–profit hospital systems often equate research and development and training expenditures with those of their prime competitors.

Proposition 11: Decision making in a *shifting but homogeneous* environment (moderate to high uncertainty) requires *adaptation*. Plans are prepared to associate decision premises with anticipated shifts in service characteristics. Organic strategies provide useful decision frameworks. *Mixed–mode approach* is preferred because it is more flexible, timely, promote acceptance, and have less risk of omission than other strategies. Neither the adaptive nor the mixed-mode strategy is likely to achieve valid or consistent decisions in shifting environments.

Proposition 11 suggests that the environment requires decision makers to place a high premium on adjustment. Flexible arrangements are needed to move into new areas of opportunity. For instance, EMS decision groups must constantly monitor changes in attitudes toward projects by foundations and legislatures and others to permit rapid environmental adjustment.

Proposition 12: Decision making in *heterogeneous* environments which are also *shifting* (highly uncertain) requires inspirational and highly adaptive decision makers and decision aids. Organic strategies are required. The adaptive approach can be timely with low cost, but has low acceptance; and risk of omission is high and undetected, as little accurate feedback can be observed. Flexibility occurs only through highly competent decision makers. *The mixed-mode approach* is preferred because it improves acceptance and reliability, and lowers risk of omission.

Organizations with many shifting constituencies, each with a fluctuating commitment, face heterogeneous and shifting environments. Charities like Red Feather or United Way agencies face an uncertain environment because they must serve several users with volatile annual revenues. Regional Medical Programs also faced a highly uncertain environment because their legislative and bureaucratic mandates and budgets were constantly shifting. Proposition 12 suggests that coordinating decisions for many shifting services requires a highly adaptive and skillful manager. In these settings, a mixed-mode strategy can help structure the decision tasks, which improves their manageability.

Summing Up The Influence Of Uncertainty

The mixed-mode decision strategy should be used when decision-making tasks are *highly uncertain*. Adaptive approaches were found to be capricious, potentially lowering acceptance, with considerable risk of omission and low reliability, because they rely exclusively on judgment. The timeliness and low cost of adaptive decision approaches are outweighed by the acceptance, flexibility, and lowered risk of omission associated with the mixed-mode strategy. In uncertain environments, none of the strategies can provide high consistency or a basis for judging the prospects of valid decisions.

Group decision making is preferred for most *moderately uncertain* decision tasks when the group reconciles available evaluation information. A group approach and BDT can be used sequentially to provide evaluation information for a decision group to interpret. Reliability, while hard to achieve in group decisions, can be enhanced by using a group processes to systematically consider evaluation data. Group methods, if properly managed, can be timely, inexpensive, flexible, promote acceptance, and make few omissions. Moderate uncertainty makes it hard to make valid decisions or to judge the prospects of validity in decisions, using any of the six decision strategies.

Recurring decision tasks with low uncertainty can use master plans. (Decision Theory and similar approaches provide a basis for constructing the master plan.) Unique decisions associated with little uncertainty should be made using an analytical approach (NDT). This strategy can be valid, reliable, with low risk of omission, and favorable cost and timeliness. The flexibility to include qualitative data is seldom essential in relatively certain environments. Acceptance depends on how the rationale used to make decisions is presented to affected parties. These conclusions are summed up in Table 10–9.

SELECTING A DECISION STRATEGY CONSIDERING THE DECISION PROBLEM

Guides which aid in the selection of a decision strategy are also based on the nature of the decision–making problem. Table 10–10 summarizes four

Table 10-9. Preferred Criterion and Decision Approaches for Various Levels of Uncertainty

| | | DOMINANT DECISION APPROACH | |
		FORENSIC	ANALYTIC
	LOW	Judgements based on Master Plans (preferred, recurring decisions)	Optimize using NDT (preferred, unique decisions)
UNCERTAINTY	MODERATE	Agreement by the decision group (preferred to promote acceptance)	Satisficing using BDT (preferred to promote reliability)
	HIGH	Acceptance to reference group using adaptive approaches	Synthesis of information from a coalition using a mixed mode approach (generally preferred)

Table 10-10. Types of Decision Problems

		INFORMATION REQUIRED	
		Known	Unknown
		Type I	Type II
METHODS TO	Known	Representational Decision Problem	Empirical Decision Problem
MANIPULATE		Type III	Type IV
INFORMATION	Unknown	Informational Decision Problems	Search Decision Problem

Adapted from McKenney, J.L. and P. Keen, "How Managers' Minds Work", *Harvard Business Review,* p. 816, (July–Aug 1973).

distinct types of decision problems, adapted from the McKenney and Keen typology.[109] In this typology, the decision maker's information needs and methods which are useful in manipulating the information may be known or unknown. When both seem clear, a Type I or a *representational decision problem* results. This type of problem has a clearcut definition of the needed data and has a method to process the data. The decision maker merely arranges the data according to the dictates of the method. For example, decisions which involve expanding the service capacity of an airport or a hospital outpatient clinic can be modeled by Queuing Theory. The Queuing Theory model dictates the needed information (arrival and service times) and the analytic methods which frame cost–service time trade–offs. Similarly, an inventory control model specifies both the needed data (e.g., the costs of orders, stock–outs, and holding inventory), and how to arrange the data in a format that permits analysis. The former example illustrates nonrecurring decisions, while the latter offers the opportunity to establish an automatic or a semiautomatic decision system. For instance, inventory control systems can be programmed to initiate an order when an information system indicates that stock has fallen below a specific level. The quality of the decision depends on the fit of the model to the decision problem. A poor fit leads to decisions that ignore important issues.

Proposition 13: Representational decision problems should use mechanistic decision strategies. A master plan is preferred for recurring decisions and formal analytical models in all other instances. This leads to decisions that are consistent, valid, and timely, with only modest cost. Risk of omission increases if the model's representation of the problem is incomplete. Flexibility is poor but seldom essential. Acceptance is often low but may been enhanced by a demonstration of validity.

NDT provides a less than ideal decision strategy for this type of decision task. A special purpose model is preferred over the general purpose NDT. When models are fit to the decision task to derive principles and rules for a master plan, validity can be enhanced and risk of omission reduced without adversely affecting cost, timeliness, or reliability.

A Type II or an *Empirical decision problem* uses known methods of analysis to generate data. Deductive methods are used to frame the decision task. A causal model is proposed to suggest relationships, so data can be collected to weight the importance of factors in the model. Methods such as experimental designs and regression, which can be used to weight the importance of model factors, are used.[110] After parameters in the model have been empirically derived and validated, the decision maker can relax key assumptions to determine the sensitivity of options to changes in use rates and the like. For example, when policy makers became concerned about nursing–home costs, an evaluation was initiated to identify nursing–home factors that may influence cost, such as ownership status (profit or nonprofit), size, nurse–patient ratios, and occupancy.[111] Policy options, such as altering the size of the nursing home, may be considered in light of possible changes in the environment, such as various growth rates for an elderly population. Policy options may also be studied in light of contextual factors. For example, an evaluation to detect the risk associated with malpractice lawsuits, naming hospitals as defendants, related the size of the award to the severity of the injury, the hospital's service intensity and size, time until settlement, type of alleged error, incident location, claimant factors (age and sex), and mode of disposition (trial, out–of–court, arbitration).[112] Mode of disposition offers several policy options which can be assessed by relating each option (before trial, arbitration, etc.) with contextual factors (severity, time until settlement, claimant factors).

Proposition 14: Empirical decision problems must consider the context of the decision task. Mid–range strategies are preferred, and analytic approaches are essential. For Type II decision problems, the BDT strategy is preferred because BDT can be consistent, timely, and potentially valid, although validity is strictly inferential. Cost and flexibility are moderate. Risk of omission is high. Acceptance depends on a demonstration that consistency is enhanced compared to forensic approaches such as group approaches.

Group methods are frequently used to deal with empirical decision tasks. For instance, public organizations often appoint task forces to settle questions of fact. Disputes over the productivity in local and state governmental agencies or the economic impact of a convention center in a community get side–tracked by committee rhetoric. The "fact–finding" committee seldom finds much new information, but does create the aura of action. Decision consistency, timeliness, and validity (when obtainable) are adversely affected when group decision making is substituted for the BDT strategy for this type of decision task.

Unknown methods with known data results in a Type III or an *informational decision problem*. Type III problems stress induction. Facts and circumstances that surround the decision task are assembled in various ways to isolate a preferred course of action or to serve as a basis from which to draw conclusions. Decision groups are preferred for sifting the data. A synthesis is sought which can reconcile the data into a new pattern that suggests a preferred course of action. For instance, collective bargaining decision groups are used to bring out information on safety, wages, productivity, grievances, profitability, and the like. The decision group reconciles conflicting facts by writing a contract that can be endorsed by both the union and management.

Proposition 15: Informational decision problems must rely on mid-range strategy; a forensic strategy is preferred. For this type of decision problem, none of the six strategies can be consistent, and each has considerable risk of omission when applied to Type III decision problems. Validity is undefined. Group methods are preferred because they are flexible, promote acceptance, and can be timely with low cost, given proper management.

Evaluation can be used in an informational decision problem if the decision group can pose an evaluation question and has the resources and patience to wait for an answer. Evaluation, when used to support a group process, can greatly improve decision consistency. Poor decisions may still result because evaluation questions may be framed obscurely, either intentionally or through ignorance.

A Type IV or *search decision problem* describes decision tasks that have unknown methods and unknown data requirements. The decision maker must search for cues and explanatory concepts which can be used to judge the merits of alternatives. Search problems often follow open–system assumptions and deal with strategic decisions. For example, consider a community mental health center having a tax–support windfall and choosing between adding new services, expanding current services, or maintaining the status quo. Little is known about demand, revenues, and potential benefits (remission rates) for these options, so the decision maker must search for methods which can provide the needed information.

Proposition 16: Organic strategies seem best for *search decision problems.* The mixed–mode model (compared to the other models) is flexible, can be timely and consistent with a low risk of omission, and promotes acceptance. No model can be valid or have low cost when dealing with search decision problems.

The adaptive decision strategy is often viewed as capricious, which lowers acceptance.[113] The adaptive strategy also has considerable risk of omission and low consistency because the strategy relies exclusively on judgment. Mintzberg and his colleagues suggest that an adaptive decision strategy may prematurely terminate search, which increases risk of omission.[114] The advantages of the adaptive strategy (timeliness and low cost) seem to be outweighed by the advantages of the mixed–mode strategy: increased acceptance, consistency, and lowered risk of omissions.

Summing Up The Influence Of Task Factors

The mixed–mode decision strategy was found to be best for "search" types of decision problems. But adaptive decision strategies seem to be preferred by decision makers when they face search problems.[115] Applying a mixed–mode type of decision strategy may improve both the acceptance and consistency of search–type decisions in public organizations.

Group methods were recommended for "informational" decision problems because groups, when properly managed, can be timely, inexpensive, flexible, and promote acceptance. Reliability, while difficult to achieve in a group setting, may be enhanced when the decision group sponsors an evaluation process. The performance of task forces and other types of decision groups often set up by public agencies may be dramatically improved when the decision group reconciles evaluation information generated by an evaluation process the group initiated.

The recommended decision strategy for "empirical" decision strategies is deductive, using the evaluative framework of the BDT model to isolate causal relationships. Group strategies are often applied by public organizations to this type of decision problem, which was found to lower the decision's consistency and timeliness.

Automatic decision systems which can be incorporated into a master plan were recommended for "representational" decision problems. When applied to a representational decision problem, the NDT model was found to lower validity and increase the risk of omission because its general–purpose approach creates, at best, an approximate fit to the decision task.

CONCLUSIONS

In this chapter, six decision strategies, recommended to guide decision making in organizations, have been described and critiqued. Advocates of these strategies often contend or imply that a particular strategy should be used exclusively.

A structure was provided to classify the decision strategies according to how they consider environmental influences and the dominance of analytic or forensic procedures. Evaluation and judgment were found to have distinct roles in each strategy. Evaluation principles were used to provide information in analytic decision strategies. Information stems from debate in a forensic decision approach. The decision strategies were placed along a continuum so strategies that assumed away most environmental influence would fall at one extreme and strategies that considered such influences as having overriding importance at the other. Because decision strategies can be categorized in this way, it seems likely that their benefits are selective.

To test the notion of selective benefits, each decision strategy was assessed considering aspects of the decision task. Most organizations face each of the decision tasks and experience various levels of uncertainty, as discussed in this chapter. Decision makers in these organizations should have a repertoire of decision strategies and skills to apply them. With such skills, decision strategies can be fit to tasks amenable to their procedures. Fitting decision–making strategies to the nature of the decision task was found to have a favorable effect on cost, timeliness, risk of omission, flexibility, acceptance, consistency, and validity of decisions.

NOTES

1. The material in this chapter was drawn from Nutt, P.C., "Some Considerations in Selecting Interactive and Analytical Decision Approaches," *Medical Care,* Vol. 36, No. 2, 1979, pp. 58–73; "Fitting Decision Strategies to Decision Problems in Public Organizations," College of Administrative Science, Working Paper Series, Columbus, July 1979; "Models for Decision Making in Organizations: Some Contextual Variables That Stipulate Optimum Use," *Academy of Management Review,* Vol. 1, No. 2, 1976, pp. 84–98; and "The Influence of Decision Styles on the Use of Decision Models," *Technological Forecasting and Social Change* Vol. 14, No 1, June 1979, pp. 77–93.

2. Simon contends decision making involves search, intelligence, and choice. In this chapter, *evaluation* provides information based on a systematic search and rules to interpret this information (intelligence). *Choice* describes how the decision maker uses intuition and experience to qualify evaluation information (another type of intelligence) when selecting among alternative courses of action. The evaluation–judgment dichotomy is also consistent with Mintzberg and his colleagues, who describe decision making in terms of evaluation and choice routines. (Simon, H.A., *Administrative Behavior.* New York: Macmillan, 1947; Mintzberg, H.A., D. Raisinghani, and A. Theoret, "The Structure of Unstructured Decision Processes," *Administrative Science Quarterly,* Vol. 21, No. 2, 1976.)

3. Huber, G.P., "General Models—Decision Making," in G. Nadler, *Work Design: A Systems Concept.* Georgetown, Ont.: Irwin, 1970.

4. Mintzberg, H., D. Raisinghani, and A. Theoret, "The Structure of 'Unstructured' Decision Processes," *Administrative Science Quarterly,* Vol. 21, No. 2, 1976, pp. 246–275.

5. Thompson, J.D., *Organizations In Action: Social Science Bases Of Administrative Theory.* New York: McGraw-Hill, 1967.
6. Churchman, C.W., *The Systems Approach.* New York: Dell, 1968.
7. Lindblom, C.E., *The Intelligence Of Democracy: Decision Process Through Adjustment.* New York: Free Press, 1965.
8. Mintzberg, Raisinghani, and Theoret, "Decision Processes."
9. Weber, Max, "The Essentials of Bureaucratic Organization: An Ideal-Type Construction," in Translated by A.M. Henderson and T. Parsons (eds.), *The Theory of Social and Economic Organization.* Oxford: Oxford University Press, 1947.
10. Thompson, *Organizations.*
11. Huber, "General Models."
12. Huber, G.P., "Multi-Attribute Utility Models: A Review of Field and Fieldlike Studies," *Management Science,* Vol. 20, No. 10, 1974, pp. 1,393–1,402.
13. Goldberg, L.P., "Man vs. Model of Man: A Rationale Plus Some Evidence for a Method of Improving on Clinical Inferences," *Psychology Bulletin,* Vol. 73, No. 6, 1970, pp. 422–432.
14. Gustafson, D.H., R. Shukla, A. Delbecq, and G. Walster, "A Comparative Study in Subjective Likelihood Estimates Made by Individuals, Interaction Groups, Delphi Groups, and Nominal Groups," *Organizational Behavior and Human Performance,* Vol. 9, No. 2, April 1973.
15. Huber, G., V. Sahney, and D. Ford, "A Study of Subjective Evaluation Models," *Behavioral Science,* Vol. 14, No. 6, 1969, pp. 483–489.
16. Simon, H.A., "A Behavioral Model of Rational Choice," in Alexis, M. and Wilson, C. (eds.), *Organizational Decision Making.* Englewood Cliffs, N.J.: Prentice-Hall, 1967.
17. Shull, F.A., "Matrix Structure and Project Authority for Optimizing Organizational Capacity," *Business Science Monograph #1,* Southern Illinois University Business Research Bureau, Carbondale, Ill., October 1968.
18. Huber, "Utility Models."
19. Churchman, C.W., *The Design of Inquiring Systems.* New York: Basic Books, 1971.
20. Mason, R.W. and I.I. Mitroff, "A Program for Research on Management Information Systems," *Management Science,* Vol. 19, No. 5, 1973, pp. 475–487.
21. Mason, R.O., "A Dialectical Approach to Strategic Planning," *Management Science,* Vol. 14, No. 8, 1969, pp. B403–B444.
22. Hall, R.H. *Organizations: Structure and Process,* Englewood Cliffs, N.J.: Prentice-Hall, 1972.
23. Delbecq, A., A. Van de Ven, and D.H. Gustafson, *Group Techniques for Program Planning,* Glenview, Ill: Scott, Foresman, 1975.
24. Collins, B. and H. Guetzkow, *A Social Psychology of Group Processes for Decision Making,* New York: Wiley, 1964.
25. Delbecq, A., "The Management of Decision Making in the Firm: Three Strategies for Three Types of Decision Making," *Academy of Management Journal,* Vol. 10, No. 4, 1967, pp. 329–339.
26. Collins and Guetzkow, *Social Psychology.*
27. Burnberg, J.G., L.P. Pondy, and C.L. Davis, "Effect of Three Voting Rules on Resource Allocation Decisions," *Management Science,* Vol. 16, No. 6, 1970, pp. B356–B371.
28. Delbecq, Van de Ven, and Gustafson, *Group Techniques.*
29. Collins and Guetzkow, *Social Psychology.*
30. Gustafson, D.H., et al., "The Development of an Index of Medical Underservice," *Health Services Research,* Summer 1975, pp. 168–180.
31. Nutt, P.C., "User Preference as a Basis to Select a Planning Method," *AIDS Proceedings,* Vol. 8, Nov. 1976.

32. Schilling, T.C., *The Strategy of Conflict*, Cambridge, Mass.: Harvard University Press, 1963.
33. Cummings, C.C. and D.C. Harnett, "Bargaining Behavior in a Symmetric Bargaining Triad: The Impact of Risk Taking Propensity, Information, and Terminal Bid," *The Review of Economic Studies*, Vol. 36, No. 4, 1969, pp. 485–501.
34. Collins and Guetzkow, *Social Psychology*.
35. Nutt, P.C., "On the Acceptance and Quality of Plans Drawn By Consortiums," *The Journal of Applied Behavioral Science*, Vol. 15, No. 1, 1979, pp. 7–21.
36. Simon, *Behavioral Model*.
37. Wildavsky, A., "The Political Economy of Efficiency: Cost/Benefit Systems Analysis, and PPBS," *The Public Administration Review*, Vol. 26, No. 4, December 1966, pp. 292–310.
38. Cyert, R.M. and J.G. March, "Organizational Expectations," in *A Behavioral Theory of the Firm*. Englewood Cliffs, N.J.: Prentice–Hall, 1963.
39. Cravens, D.B., "An Exploratory Analysis of Individual Information Processing," *Management Science*, Vol. 16, No. 10, 1970, pp. B656–B670.
40. Cyert and March, *Behavioral Theory of the Firm*.
41. Simon, H.A. and A. Newell, "Human Problem Solving: The State of the Art in 1970," *American Psychologist*, Vol. 26, No. 2, 1971, pp. 145–159.
42. Lanzetta, J.T. and V.T. Kanaroff, "Information Cost, Amount of Payoff, and Level of Aspiration as Determinants of Information Seeking in Decision Making," *Behavioral Science*, Vol. 7, No. 4, 1962, pp. 459–473.
43. Streuffert, S. and S.C. Streuffert, "Effects of Increasing Failure and Success on Military and Economic Risk Taking," *Journal of Applied Psychology*, Vol. 54, No. 5, 1970, pp. 393–400.
44. Conrath, D.W., "Organizational Decision Making Under Varying Conditions of Uncertainty," *Management Science*, Vol. 13, No. 8, 1967, pp. B487–B500.
45. Dawes, R.M., "A Case Study of Graduate Admissions: Applications of Three Principles of Human Decision Making," *American Psychologist*, Vol. 26, 1976, pp. 180–187.
46. Gore, W.J., *Administrative Decision Making: A Heuristic Model*, New York: Wiley, 1964.
47. Lindblom, *The Intelligence of Democracy*.
48. Gore, *Administrative Decision Making*.
49. Dearborn, D.C. and H.A. Simon, "Selective Perception: A Note On the Departmental Identification of Executives," in Alexis, M. and C.Z. Wilson, *Organizational Decision Making*. Englewood Cliffs, N.J.: Prentice–Hall, 1967.
50. Shull, *Matrix Structure*.
51. Mintzberg, et al., *Decision Processes*.
52. Suchman, E.A., *Evaluative Research*. Washington, D.C.: Russell Sage Foundation, 1967.
53. Churchman, *The Systems Approach*.
54. March, J.G. and H.A. Simon, *Organizations*. New York: Wiley, 1958.
55. Bryant, S.E., "TFX–A Case in Policy Level Decision Making," *Academy of Management*, Vol. 8, No. 1, 1964, pp. 54–70.
56. Weber, C.E., "Inter–Organizational Decision Processes Influencing the EOP Budget," *Management Science*, Vol. 12, No. 4, 1965, pp. B69–B93.
57. Filley, A.C. and A.J. Grimes, "The Basis for Power in Decision Processes," *Academy of Management Proceedings*, Vol. 10, December 1967.
58. McKenney, J.L. and P. Keen, "How Managers' Minds Work," *Harvard Business Review*, May–June 1974, pp. 79–90.
59. Churchman, C.W., *Prediction and Optimal Decision*, Englewood Cliffs, N.J.: Prentice–Hall, 1961.

60. Ackoff, R.L., *Scientific Method: Optimizing Applied Research Decisions*. New York: Wiley, 1962.
61. Huysmans, J., *The Implementation of Operation Research*. New York: Wiley–Interscience, 1970.
62. Doktor, R.H. and W.F. Hamilton, "Cognitive Style and the Acceptance of Management Science Recommendations," *Management Science,* Vol. 19, No. 8, 1973, pp. 884–894.
63. Doktor, R.H., "EEG Research on MS Implementation Barriers," The XXII TIMS International Meeting, Kyoto, Japan, July 1975.
64. Vroom, V.H., "A New Look at Managerial Decision Making," *Organizational Dynamics,* Spring 1973, pp. 66–80.
65. Weckworth, V.E., "Birth Order: Does It Determine Management Style?" *Hospital Financial Management,* May 1978, pp. 8–13.
66. Driver, M.J. and T.J. Mock, "Human Information Processing, Decision Style Theory, and Accounting Information Systems," *The Accounting Review,* July 1975, pp. 490–508.
67. Mitroff, I.I. and R. Kilmann, "On Evaluating Scientific Research: The Contributions of the Philosophy of Science," *Technological Forecasting and Social Change,* Vol. 8, 1975, pp. 163–174.
68. McKenney and Keen, *Managers' Minds.*
69. Maier, N.F.R., *Problem Solving and Creativity In Individuals and Groups*. Brooks/Cole, 1970. Maier found that successful decision makers faced with poorly structured tasks, followed a search–incubation–insight process. When confronted with ill-defined tasks, success was often linked to following this sequence of steps. McKenney and Keen, Doktor and Hamilton, and Mintzberg find that success in solving tasks like those used by Maier is closely associated with an "intuitive style." This style can be misleading and inefficient when applied to tasks that *have* definition and structure.
70. Mintzberg, et al., *Decision Processes.*
71. McKenney and Keen, *Managers' Minds.*
72. Mitroff, I.I. and R. Kilmann, "Stories Managers Tell: A New Tool for Organizational Problem Solving," *Management Review,* July 1975, pp. 18–27.
73. Myers, I.B., and K.C. Briggs, "Manual for the Meyers–Briggs Type Indicator," Princeton, N.J.: Educational Testing Service, 1963. Lake, Miles, and Earle critique several such instruments. (Lake, D., M. Miles, and R. Earle, Jr., *Measuring Human Behavior,* New York: Teachers College Press, 1973.)
74. Hall, *Organizations.*
75. Churchman, *The Systems Approach.*
76. Henderson, J.L. and P.C. Nutt, "On the Design of Planning Information Systems," *Academy of Management Review,* Vol. 3, No. 4, 1978, pp. 774–785.
77. McKenney and Keen, *Managers' Minds.*
78. McKenney and Keen, *Managers' Minds.*
79. This does not imply that "broth testing" is a superior control device. The skill must be passed on in a reliable manner by selecting people amenable to training in broth testing to advocate intuitive styles in this type of application.
80. Erwing, D.W., "Discovering Your Problem Solving Style," *Psychology Today,* December 1977, pp. 69–74.
81. Mintzberg, H. "Planning on the Left Side, Managing on the Right," *Harvard Business Review,* July–August 1976, pp. 50–58.
82. McKenney and Keen, *Managers' Minds.*
83. Mitroff and Kilman, *Stories Managers Tell.*
84. Mitroff I. and R. Kilmann, "On the Importance of Qualitative Analysis in Management Science: The Influence of Personality Variables on Organizational Decision Making,"

University of Pittsburg mimeo, 1973; describes the loan office example. The relationship between preferred planning approach and decision style appeared in Nutt, P.C., "User Preference As A Basis to Select A Planning Method," *American Institute of Decision Science Proceeding*, Vol. 8, Nov. 1976.

85. Nutt, P.C., "Decision Style and the Design of a MIS," Ohio State University Mimeo, 1979.

86. When decision makers are presented with an unfamiliar model congruent with their style, they quickly endorse it.

87. These decision styles are described in Nutt, P.C., "The Influence of Decision Style on The Use Of Decision Models," *Technological Forecasting and Social Change*, Vol. 14, No 1, June 1979, pp. 77–93.

88. Mitroff and Kilmann, *Stories Managers Tell.*

89. Churchman, *The Systems Approach.*

90. Mitroff and Kilmann, *Stories Managers Tell.*

91. Doktor and Hamilton, *Cognitive Sytle.*

92. Mitroff and Kilmann, *On Evaluating Scientific Research.*

93. Mintzberg, et al., *Decision Processes.*

94. Nutt, P.C., "Models for Decision Making In Organizations: Some Contextual Factors That Stipulate Optimal Use," *Academy of Management Review*, Vol. 1, No. 2, 1976, pp. 84–98.

95. Nutt, P.C., "Some Considerations in Selecting Interactive and Analytical Decision Approaches," *Medical Care*, Vol. 36, No. 2, 1979, pp. 152–167.

96. A proposition states the relationship between two or more causal factors which summarizes current knowledge about a particular causal system.

97. Thompson, *Organizations in Action.*

98. Nutt, *Models for Decision Making.*

99. Thompson, *Organizations in Action.*

100. Nutt, *Models For Decision Making.*

101. Thompson, *Organizations in Action.*

102. Nutt, *Selecting Interactive and Analytical Decision Approaches.*

103. Traditionally, uncertainty is defined in terms of a decision's state of nature, following the structure of NDT or BDT. This definition, and others like it, lack sufficient generality to define low, moderate, and high levels of uncertainty and how levels of uncertainty influence each of the six decision models. See Conrath, D. "Organizational Decision Making Under Varying Levels of Uncertainty," *Management Science*, Vol. 13, No. 8, 1967, for a critique of the state of nature as a definition of uncertainty.

104. Van de Ven, A.H. and A.L. Delbecq, "A Task–Contingent Model of Work Unit Structure," *Administrative Science Quarterly*, Vol. 19, No. 2, 1974, pp. 183–197.

105. Perrow, C., "A Framework for the Comparative Analysis of Organizations," *American Sociological Review*, Vol. 32, No. 2, 1967, pp. 194–208.

106. These propositions considering uncertainty were taken from Nutt, P.C., "Some Considerations in Soliciting Interactive and Analytical Decision Models," *Medical Care*, Vol. 36, No. 2, 1979.

107. Thompson, *Organizations in Action.*

108. *Ibid.*

109. McKenney and Keen, *Managers' Minds.*

110. Operations research techniques, forecasting, experimentation, and the like can also be used to represent the decision problem.

111. Caswell, R.J. and W.O. Cleverley, "Cost Analysis of Ohio Nursing Homes," National Health Planning Center (HRR–0029393) Washington, D.C.

112. Nutt, P.C. and S.M. Emswiler, Factors Influencing the Size of Malpractice Awards in Hospitals, *Academy of Management Proceedings,* Vol. 22, April 1979, pp. 88–101.
113. Mintzberg, Raisinghani, and Theoret, "Decision Processes."
114. *Ibid.*
115. *Ibid.*

Index